Current Controversies in Foot and Ankle Trauma

Editor

MICHAEL P. SWORDS

FOOT AND ANKLE CLINICS

www.foot.theclinics.com

Consulting Editor
MARK S. MYERSON

March 2017 • Volume 22 • Number 1

ELSEVIER

1600 John F. Kennedy Boulevard • Suite 1800 • Philadelphia, Pennsylvania, 19103-2899

http://www.theclinics.com

FOOT AND ANKLE CLINICS Volume 22, Number 1
March 2017 ISSN 1083-7515, ISBN-13: 978-0-323-50977-0

Editor: Lauren Boyle
Developmental Editor: Meredith Clinton

Foot and Ankle Clinics (ISSN 1083-7515) is published quarterly by Elsevier, Inc., 360 Park Avenue South, New York, NY 10010-1710. Months of issue are March, June, September, and December. Periodicals postage paid at New York, NY, and additional mailing offices. Subscription price per year is $320.00 (US individuals), $489.00 (US institutions), $100.00 (US students), $360.00 (Canadian individuals), $588.00 (Canadian institutions), $215.00 (Canadian students), $460.00 (international individuals), $588.00 (international institutions), and $215.00 (international students). To receive student/resident rate, orders must be accompanied by name of affiliated institution, date of term, and the *signature* of program/residency coordinator on institution letterhead. Orders will be billed at individual rate until proof of status is received. Foreign air speed delivery is included in all *Clinics* subscription prices. All prices are subject to change without notice. **POSTMASTER:** Send address changes to *Foot and Ankle Clinics*, Elsevier Health Sciences Division, Subscription Customer Service, 3251 Riverport Lane, Maryland Heights, MO 63043. **Customer Service: 1-800-654-2452 (US and Canada). From outside of the United States and Canada, call 314-447-8871. Fax: 314-447-8029. E-mail: JournalsCustomerService-usa@ elsevier.com (for print support); JournalsOnlineSupport-usa@elsevier.com (for online support).**

Reprints. For copies of 100 or more, of articles in this publication, please contact the Commercial Reprints Department, Elsevier Inc., 360 Park Avenue South, New York, NY 10010-1710. Tel.: 212-633-3874; Fax: 212-633-3820; E-mail: reprints@elsevier.com.

Contributors

CONSULTING EDITOR

MARK S. MYERSON, MD
Medical Director, The Foot and Ankle Association, Inc; Institute for Foot and Ankle Recon at Mercy, Baltimore, Maryland

EDITOR

MICHAEL P. SWORDS, DO
Michigan Orthopedic Center, Chief, Orthopedic Surgery, Director of Orthopedic Trauma, Sparrow Hospital, Lansing, Michigan

AUTHORS

JOHN G. ANDERSON, MD
Orthopaedic Associates of Michigan, Foot and Ankle Division, Grand Rapids, Michigan

JAN BARTONÍČEK, MD
Department of Orthopaedics, First Faculty of Medicine, Central Military Hospital Prague, Charles University, Prague; Department of Anatomy, First Faculty of Medicine, Charles University Prague, Prague, Czech Republic

STEPHEN K. BENIRSCHKE, MD
Department of Orthopaedics and Sports Medicine, Harborview Medical Center, University of Washington, Seattle, Washington

DONALD R. BOHAY, MD, FACS
Orthopaedic Associates of Michigan, Foot and Ankle Division, Grand Rapids, Michigan

MICHAEL P. CLARE, MD
Director, Foot and Ankle Fellowship, Florida Orthopaedic Institute, Tampa, Florida

WILLIAM S. CRAWFORD, MD
Texas Foot and Ankle Orthopaedics, Fort Worth, Texas

MARK S. DAVIES, FRCS(Tr&Orth)
London Foot and Ankle Centre, Hospital of St John and St Elizabeth, London, United Kingdom

BRYANT HO, MD
Hinsdale Orthopaedics, Hinsdale, Illinois

JOHN KETZ, MD
Department of Orthopaedics, University of Rochester Medical Center, Rochester, New York

NATHAN J. KIEWIET, MD
Drisko, Fee, and Parkins Orthopedic Surgery, Independence, Missouri

PATRICIA ANN KRAMER, PhD
Departments of Anthropology and Orthopaedics and Sports Medicine, University of Washington, Seattle, Washington

PHILLIP PENNY, DO, MA
Department of Orthopedic Surgery, Mclaren Greater Lansing, Lansing, Michigan

RUPESH A. PUNA, MBChB, FRACS (Orth)
Clinical Orthopaedic Foot and Ankle Fellow, University of Toronto, Toronto, Ontario, Canada

STEFAN RAMMELT, MD, PhD
Professor, Head of the Foot & Ankle Section, University Center for Orthopaedics and Traumatology, University Hospital Carl-Gustav Carus, Dresden, Germany

ANTHONY SAKELLARIOU, FRCS(Tr&Orth)
Surrey Foot and Ankle Clinic, Mount Alvernia Hospital, Guildford, Surrey, United Kingdom

ANDREW SANDS, MD
Chief, Foot and Ankle Surgery, Downtown Orthopaedic Associates; Chairman, AO-ASIF Foot and Ankle Expert Group; Clinical Associate Professor of Orthopedic Surgery, Weill Cornell Medical College, New York, New York

BRUCE J. SANGEORZAN, MD
Professor, Department of Orthopedics and Sports Medicine, Harborview Medical Center, University of Washington, Seattle, Washington

TIM SCHEPERS, MD, PhD
Trauma Surgeon, Trauma Unit, Academic Medical Center, University of Amsterdam, Amsterdam, The Netherlands

JOHN R. SHANK, MD
Department of Orthopedic Surgery, Colorado Center of Orthopaedic Excellence, Colorado Springs, Colorado

MATTHEW C. SOLAN, FRCS(Tr&Orth)
London Foot and Ankle Centre, Hospital of St John and St Elizabeth, London, United Kingdom; Surrey Foot and Ankle Clinic, Mount Alvernia Hospital, Guildford, Surrey, United Kingdom

MICHAEL P. SWORDS, DO
Michigan Orthopedic Center, Chief, Orthopedic Surgery, Director of Orthopedic Trauma, Sparrow Hospital, Lansing, Michigan

MATTHEW P.W. TOMLINSON, MBChB, FRACS (Orth)
Clinical Head of Orthopaedics, Middlemore Hospital, Auckland, New Zealand

MICHAL TUČEK, MD
Department of Orthopaedics, First Faculty of Medicine, Central Military Hospital Prague, Charles University, Prague, Czech Republic

BRIAN M. WEATHERFORD, MD
Illinois Bone and Joint Institute, Glenview, Illinois

Contents

Preface: Current Controversies in Foot and Ankle Trauma   xi

Michael P. Swords

Open Reduction and Internal Fixation Versus Primary Arthrodesis for Lisfranc Injuries   1

Brian M. Weatherford, Donald R. Bohay, and John G. Anderson

Management of injuries to the tarsometatarsal (Lisfranc) joint complex continues to generate heated debate. Arthrodesis of the Lisfranc joint complex has historically been reserved as a salvage procedure for failed treatment. Recently, primary arthrodesis has emerged as a viable treatment alternative to open reduction and internal fixation for these injuries. The objective of this article was to examine the current literature regarding open reduction and internal fixation versus primary arthrodesis of Lisfranc injuries.

The Role of Percutaneous Reduction and Fixation of Lisfranc Injuries   15

Rupesh A. Puna and Matthew P.W. Tomlinson

To be able to perform percutaneous fixation of Lisfranc injuries, this article emphasizes that an anatomic reduction must be mandatory. When uncertainty remains as to whether closed reduction is anatomic, formal open reduction is recommended because accuracy of reduction is correlated with long-term outcome. Closed injuries with minimal displacement, bony avulsions, and skeletally immature individuals seem the most appropriate indications for percutaneous fixation. Not all injuries are ideal for this method of treatment, and this is an area that needs to be more clearly defined in the future.

Syndesmosis Stabilisation: Screws Versus Flexible Fixation   35

Matthew C. Solan, Mark S. Davies, and Anthony Sakellariou

Orthopedic surgery is not short of situations where there is controversy regarding optimum management. Treating ankle syndesmosis injuries is an example where practice varies widely and there are many questions that remain unsatisfactorily answered. When addressing the type of syndesmosis stabilization that is required it is essential to ascertain the extent of instability. Only then can a logical approach to restoring the ankle mortise be achieved. Fixation of fibula shaft fractures and posterior malleolus fractures can restore sufficient stability to render syndesmosis stabilization unnecessary. The indications and techniques for stabilizing the distal tibiofibular joint are reviewed with clinical examples.

Late Treatment of Syndesmotic Injuries   65

Michael P. Swords, Andrew Sands, and John R. Shank

Normal syndesmosis anatomy and alignment are essential to ankle function. Although injuries to the syndesmosis are common with ankle injuries, accurate diagnosis and reduction continue to be a challenge. Late reconstruction for syndesmosis is reviewed. A surgical technique for late reconstruction is outlined in detail.

Calcaneal Fracture Management: Extensile Lateral Approach Versus Small Incision Technique   **77**

Nathan J. Kiewiet and Bruce J. Sangeorzan

Calcaneal fracture management has historically been a controversial topic and represents an area of sustained interest over the past several decades. The authors review current methods for calcaneal fracture fixation with an extensile lateral approach and small incision techniques. Early reports of small incision techniques have reported promising outcomes and reduced risks for complications. These techniques may be beneficial to reduce the risk of soft tissue complications and improve the rate of recovery.

Early Fixation of Calcaneus Fractures   **93**

Michael P. Swords and Phillip Penny

The treatment of calcaneus fractures is controversial. Historically, most operatively treated fractures have been approached with a lateral extensile incision requiring delay in operative treatment until swelling has improved. There is a current trend and interest in small incision approaches allowing, and in some cases requiring, earlier operative fixation. Clinical scenarios amenable to consideration for early fixation are reviewed. The sinus tarsi surgical approach and reduction techniques are outlined in detail.

Managing Complications of Calcaneus Fractures   **105**

Michael P. Clare and William S. Crawford

Calcaneus fractures remain among the most complicated fractures for orthopedic surgeons to manage because of the complexity of various fracture patterns, the limited surrounding soft tissue envelope, and the prolonged rehabilitation issues impacting function after successful treatment. Despite this, appropriate management of complications associated with calcaneus fractures is critical for the complete care of this injury, whether treated operatively or nonoperatively. The authors present the common complications encountered with fractures of the calcaneus and management thereof.

Gastrocnemius or Achilles Lengthening at Time of Trauma Fixation   **117**

Stephen K. Benirschke and Patricia Ann Kramer

Gastrocnemius equinus is a frequent comorbidity with traumatic injuries of the foot and ankle. Gastrocnemius lengthening at the time of definitive treatment facilitates obtaining and maintaining an anatomic reduction of the injury. The lengthening procedure is accomplished in 5 steps and results in fewer long-term, problematic sequelae.

Posterior Malleolar Fractures: Changing Concepts and Recent Developments   **125**

Jan Bartoníček, Stefan Rammelt, and Michal Tuček

Injuries to the posterior malleolus are of prognostic relevance in ankle fracture-dislocations. The three-dimensional outline of the fragments as reflected by computed tomography classification, involvement of the fibular notch, and the presence of intercalary fragments seem to be of greater therapeutic relevance than the size of the fragment and amount of the articular surface involved. Operative treatment aims at reconstruction of the posterior tibial plafond, the fibular notch, and the integrity of the posterior inferior tibiofibular syndesmosis. Direct open reduction and fixation of posterior malleolus fragments via posterior approaches is biomechanically more stable than indirect reduction and anteroposterior screw fixation.

Primary Arthrodesis for Tibial Pilon Fractures **147**

Bryant Ho and John Ketz

Staged primary ankle arthrodesis is a viable option for high-energy pilon fractures that are nonreconstructible, in patients with delay in treatment or multiple medical comorbidities, or in patients with peripheral neuropathy. Small retrospective series demonstrate high union and low wound complication rates, although further studies are needed to determine the long-term results. Ankle arthrodesis offers decreased complication rates while eliminating the potential of posttraumatic ankle arthritis pain.

Chopart Injuries: When to Fix and When to Fuse? **163**

Stefan Rammelt and Tim Schepers

Chopart joint injuries have a profound effect on global foot function. Surgical treatment aims at joint reconstruction and axial alignment with restoration of the normal relationship of the lateral and medial foot columns. Internal fixation is tailored to the individual fracture pattern and achieved with resorbable pins, Kirschner wires, screws, and/or anatomically shaped minifragment plates. If instability persists, temporary joint transfixation may be achieved with Kirschner wires or bridge plating. Primary fusion sacrifices essential joints and should be reserved for severe initial cartilage damage. Corrective fusion becomes necessary for malunited Chopart joint injuries with rapidly evolving posttraumatic arthritis.

Treatment of Peripheral Talus Fractures **181**

John R. Shank, Stephen K. Benirschke, and Michael P. Swords

Peripheral talus fractures include injuries to the lateral process, posteromedial talar body, and talar head. These injuries are rare and are often missed. Nonunion with conservative treatment is high and excision can lead to joint instability, rapid arthrosis, and earlier need for arthrodesis. Open reduction internal fixation of most peripheral talus fractures is critical to achieving a good outcome. Open reduction leads to more rapid union and ability to mobilize the ankle and subtalar joints, quicker revascularization of the talus, and lower rates of arthrosis. Surgical treatment can lead to substantial functional improvement and a slowing of the degenerative process.

Complex Foot Injury: Early and Definite Management **193**

Tim Schepers and Stefan Rammelt

Complex foot injuries occur infrequently, but are life-changing events. They often present with other injuries as the result of a high-energy trauma.

After initial stabilization, early assessment should be regarding salvagability. All treatment strategies are intensive. The initial treatment includes prevention of progression ischemia/necrosis, prevention of infection, and considering salvage or amputation. Definitive treatment for salvage includes anatomic reconstruction with stable internal fixation and early soft tissue coverage followed by aggressive rehabilitation. Prognosis after complex injuries is hard to predict. The various stages of the treatment are reviewed and recommendations are made.

Index   **215**

FOOT AND ANKLE CLINICS

FORTHCOMING ISSUES

June 2017
Current Updates in Total Ankle Arthroplasty
J. Chris Coetzee, *Editor*

September 2017
The Flatfoot: What Goes Wrong with
Treatment
Kent Ellington, *Editor*

December 2017
Treatment of Acute and Chronic Tendon
Rupture and Tendinopathy
Selene Parekh, *Editor*

RECENT ISSUES

December 2016
Bone Grafts, Bone Graft Substitutes, and
Biologics in Foot and Ankle Surgery
Sheldon Lin, *Editor*

September 2016
Minimally Invasive Surgery in the Foot
and Ankle
Anthony Perera, *Editor*

June 2016
New Ideas and Techniques in Foot and
Ankle Surgery: A Global Perspective
John G. Anderson and Donald R. Bohay,
Editors

March 2016
Joint-Preserving Osteotomies for Malunited
Foot & Ankle Fractures
Stefan Rammelt, *Editor*

RELATED INTEREST

Orthopedic Clinics of North America, April 2016 (Vol. 47, No. 2)
Common Complications in Orthopedics
James H. Calandruccio, Benjamin J. Grear, Benjamin M. Mauck, Jeffrey R. Sawyer,
Patrick C. Toy, John C. Weinlein, *Editors*
Available at: http://www.orthopedic.theclinics.com/

THE CLINICS ARE NOW AVAILABLE ONLINE!
Access your subscription at:
www.theclinics.com

FOOT AND ANKLE CLINICS

FORTHCOMING ISSUES

June 2017
Current Update on Foot and Ankle Surgery
J. Chris Coetzee, Editor

September 2017
The Flatfoot: What Goes Wrong in Treatment and Rehabilitation
Kent Ellington, Editor

December 2017
Treatment of Acute and Chronic Tendon Rupture and Tendinopathy
Selene Parekh, Editor

RECENT ISSUES

December 2016
Bone Grafts, Bone Graft Substitutes and Bone Stimulators in Foot and Ankle Surgery
Stephen A. Brigido

September 2016
Minimally Invasive Surgery in the Foot and Ankle
Anthony Perera, Editor

June 2016
New Ideas and Techniques in Foot and Ankle Surgery
John G. Anderson and Donald R. Bohay, Editors

March 2016
Bone Tumors and Other Tumor-Like Formation
Hideji Kawanabe, Editor

RELATED INTEREST

Orthopedic Clinics of North America, April 2016 (Vol. 47, no. 2)
THA: Complications and Outcomes
Michael J. Taunton and John J. Callaghan, Editors
Available at: http://www.orthopedic.theclinics.com

Preface

Current Controversies in Foot and Ankle Trauma

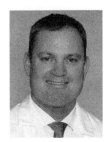

Michael P. Swords, DO
Editor

This issue of *Foot and Ankle Clinics of North America* covers a variety of controversial topics in foot and ankle trauma. At times, clinical decisions are straightforward, black or white, yes or no decisions. It is hoped that this issue provides some discussion of topics that fall into the gray. Controversy is defined as a prolonged public dispute or debate concerning a matter of opinion. Some of the work presented you may agree with—some you may not. It is intended to make you think and stimulate discussion. The authors collectively bring a vast amount of knowledge and experience to this issue. I have had many conversations with them on how to best treat complex foot and ankle trauma and the myriad complications we deal with while treating these injuries. I hope you find their insights as valuable as I do.

I would like to dedicate this issue to my wife, Christy, and children, Grace, Mike, Mary Kate, and Caroline. My involvement in foot and ankle trauma is not a solo endeavor. They have been with me on the journey from the beginning. I thank them for their love, support, and understanding.

Michael P. Swords, DO
Michigan Orthopedic Center
Sparrow Hospital
2815 South Pennsylvania Avenue
Suite 204
Lansing, MI 48910, USA

E-mail address:
foot.trauma@gmail.com

Foot Ankle Clin N Am 22 (2017) xi
http://dx.doi.org/10.1016/j.fcl.2016.10.001
1083-7515/17/© 2016 Published by Elsevier Inc.

foot.theclinics.com

Open Reduction and Internal Fixation Versus Primary Arthrodesis for Lisfranc Injuries

CrossMark

Brian M. Weatherford, MD[a],*, Donald R. Bohay, MD[b], John G. Anderson, MD[b]

KEYWORDS

- Tarsometatarsal joint • Midfoot • Lisfranc • Open reduction and internal fixation
- Arthrodesis

KEY POINTS

- Lisfranc injuries represent a broad spectrum of pathology and therefore one treatment may not adequately address all injury patterns.
- Anatomic reduction is required to restore the function of the midfoot regardless of the treatment chosen.
- Primary arthrodesis has shown improved outcomes for certain injury patterns.

INTRODUCTION

The unique anatomy of the tarsometatarsal (Lisfranc) joint complex allows for effective force transfer and propulsion during gait. Injuries to the Lisfranc joint complex are rare and frequently missed on initial presentation.[1,2] If missed or treated inappropriately, Lisfranc injuries may result in chronic pain and disability.

Operative treatment of these injuries continues to generate significant controversy. Undoubtedly this is because, at least in part, Lisfranc injuries represent a broad spectrum of pathology, from the subtle sprain to the high-energy crush injury. Modern surgical treatment of tarsometatarsal injuries has emphasized achieving and maintaining anatomic reduction with open reduction and internal fixation.[3,4] Prompt diagnosis, anatomic reduction, and stable fixation has demonstrated improved outcomes over historical treatments, yet modern series still demonstrate rates of posttraumatic arthritis ranging from 25% to 94%.[5]

The authors have nothing to disclose.
[a] Illinois Bone and Joint Institute, 2401 Ravine Way, Glenview, IL 60025, USA; [b] Orthopaedic Associates of Michigan, Foot and Ankle Division, 1111 Leffingwell Avenue Northeast, Grand Rapids, MI 60025, USA
* Corresponding author.
E-mail address: bweatherford@ibji.com

Foot Ankle Clin N Am 22 (2017) 1–14
http://dx.doi.org/10.1016/j.fcl.2016.09.002

Historically arthrodesis of the tarsometatarsal joints has been considered a salvage procedure[6]; however, primary arthrodesis (PA) of Lisfranc injuries has recently emerged as a viable alternative to open reduction and internal fixation (ORIF).[7] Despite promising early results, the role of primary arthrodesis in the management of Lisfranc injuries has yet to be defined.

ANATOMY
Osseous Anatomy

The osseous structure of the Lisfranc joint complex is composed of the articulations of the wedge-shaped metatarsal bases with their corresponding tarsal bones. Critical features of the osseous anatomy include the following:

- The cuneiforms and metatarsal bases have a trapezoidal configuration, with the second metatarsal base and middle cuneiform serving as the "keystone" of the transverse arch[8] (**Fig. 1**)

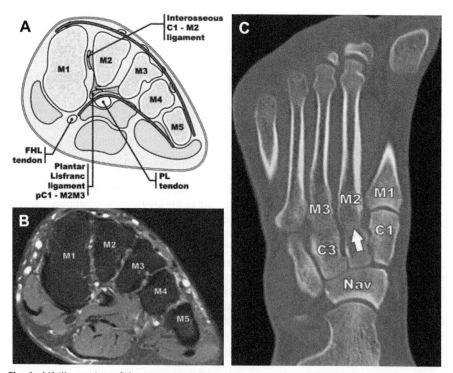

Fig. 1. (A) Illustration of the "Roman arch" architecture of the metatarsal bases with second metatarsal as the keystone. The interosseous or Lisfranc ligament(C1–M2) and plantar oblique ligament (pC1–M2M3) are seen. (B) Coronal T2 MRI sequence demonstrating the Roman arch configuration of the metatarsal bases with the second metatarsal base serving as the keystone. (C) Axial long-axis CT cut. The white arrow highlights the recessed position of the second metatarsal in the mortise. Note the flat joint surfaces. C1, medial cuneiform; C3, lateral cuneiform; M1, first metatarsal; M2, second metatarsal; M3, third metatarsal; Nav, navicular. (*From* Siddiqui NA, Galizia MS, Almusa E, et al. Evaluation of the tarsometatarsal joint using conventional radiography, CT, and MR imaging. Radiographics 2014;34(2):515; with permission.)

- The middle cuneiform is recessed, allowing the second metatarsal base to lock in to a mortise configuration (see **Fig. 1**)
- The individual articulations of the tarsometatarsal and naviculocuneiform joints are "flat on flat" with little inherent stability (see **Fig. 1**)

Ligamentous Anatomy

As there is little inherent stability of the tarsometatarsal articulations, the ligamentous restraints of the Lisfranc joint complex are critical. Several aspects of the ligamentous anatomy of this region confer additional stability and are crucial to understanding patterns of instability.

- The dorsal ligaments are weaker than the plantar ligaments and typically fail first under tension[9,10]
- The transverse intermetatarsal ligaments secure the bases of the second through the fifth metatarsals; however, no such ligament exists between the first and second metatarsals[11]
- A complex of dorsal, interosseous, and plantar ligaments secures the medial cuneiform to the second metatarsal to lock in the mortise configuration
- The interosseous ligament is the strongest ligamentous restraint of the Lisfranc joint complex, and is commonly referred to as the Lisfranc ligament[9] (**Fig. 2**)

Functional Anatomy

The midfoot acts as a lever or "leaf spring" to absorb impact between heel strike and foot flat so as to transition to the next phase of the gait cycle.[12] The functional anatomy of the tarsometatarsal joints is perhaps best understood by the 3-column classification of the midfoot[13] (**Fig. 3**). The medial column is composed of the medial naviculocuneiform joint and the first tarsometatarsal joint. The middle column consists of the lateral

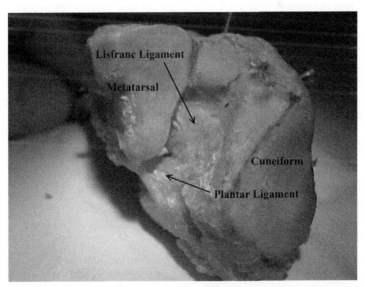

Fig. 2. Cadaveric specimen demonstrating the orientation of the Lisfranc (interosseous) ligament and the plantar oblique ligament. (*From* Panchbhavi VK, Molina D 4th, Villarreal J, et al. Three-dimensional, digital, and gross anatomy of the Lisfranc ligament. Foot Ankle Int 2013;34(6):877; with permission.)

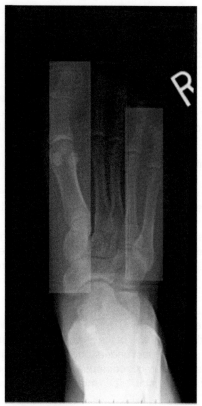

Fig. 3. AP foot radiograph with the 3 columns of the foot shaded. Yellow shading corresponds with the medial column. Red corresponds to the middle or intermediate column and green represents the lateral column.

naviculocuneiform joints and second and third tarsometatarsal joints. The lateral column is composed of the articulations of the fourth and fifth metatarsal bases with the cuboid.

- The medial and middle columns function as a unit with very little motion seen across these articulations during gait
- The lateral column is mobile and essential for shock absorption when the foot strikes an uneven surface
- The articulations of the medial and middle column are nonessential and can be sacrificed yet still maintain the function of the midfoot[12]
- Arthrodesis of the joints of the lateral column is poorly tolerated and significantly increases plantar forefoot pressure[14,15]

MECHANISM OF INJURY

Lisfranc injuries can be grouped into either direct or indirect mechanisms. Many of these injuries result from a crushing injury to the dorsal aspect of the foot. These high-energy mechanisms may result in significant soft tissue disruption, and may even require staged treatment with external fixation similar to tibial pilon fractures.[16] Compartment syndrome and open injuries are more commonly seen with crush mechanisms.[17]

Indirect mechanisms account for most injuries and are typically seen with an axial and/or rotational force applied to a plantar flexed foot.[18] The weaker dorsal ligaments typically fail under tension, leading to dorsal displacement of the metatarsals. Abduction or torsional mechanisms may lead to fracture of the base of the second metatarsal. Significant abduction moments may even lead to compression fracture of the cuboid.[19]

DIAGNOSIS
Physical Examination

Even with subtle injury patterns, patients will typically present with difficulty with weight bearing; however, in subtle athletic injuries, patients may experience pain only during explosive movements. Plantar arch ecchymosis is highly associated with Lisfranc injury[20] (**Fig. 4**). Pain may be reproduced with direct palpation of the Tarsometatarsal (TMT) joints, as well as with passive abduction stress of the midfoot while stabilizing the transverse tarsal joint.

In patients with high-energy injuries, careful attention should be directed to the soft tissue envelope. Closed injuries with fracture blisters signify a substantial soft tissue insult that would benefit from delayed management or even staged internal fixation (**Fig. 5**). The presence of tense swelling and increasing pain should alert the clinician to the possibility of compartment syndrome.[21]

IMAGING
Initial Imaging

Initial imaging of suspected Lisfranc injuries should consist of anteroposterior (AP), lateral, and 30-degree oblique views of the foot. Certain radiographic landmarks are scrutinized on each image to rule out Lisfranc injury.

- On the AP view, the medial border of the second metatarsal should align with medial border of the middle cuneiform.
- On the oblique view, the medial border of the fourth metatarsal and the medial border of the cuboid should be collinear.
- The lateral view should demonstrate alignment of the dorsal cortices of the metatarsals with their corresponding tarsal bones.
- Avulsion fracture off the base of the second metatarsal or medial cuneiform, known as the "fleck" sign, signifies disruption of the Lisfranc ligament.[18]

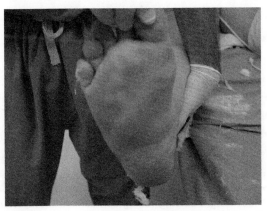

Fig. 4. Clinical photograph of a patient with Lisfranc injury demonstrating the presence of plantar arch ecchymosis.

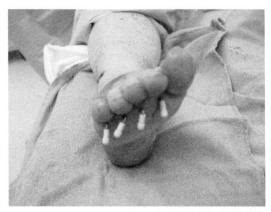

Fig. 5. Clinical photograph of a patient with a high-energy injury temporarily stabilized with percutaneous wires.

Dynamic Imaging

It is imperative to assess how the midfoot behaves under physiologic load in patients suspected of midfoot trauma. Stress radiographs are an essential imaging modality to diagnose subtle instability.

- Weight-bearing radiographs should be obtained in all patients suspected of midfoot injury (**Fig. 6**).
- A pronation-abduction stress radiograph may unmask instability in patients unable to bear weight[22] (**Fig. 7**).

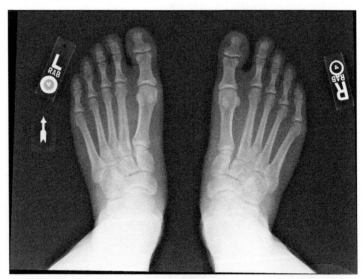

Fig. 6. Bilateral AP foot weight-bearing radiograph demonstrating lateral subluxation of the second metatarsal and intercuneiform widening in a patient with a history and examination suspicious for subtle instability.

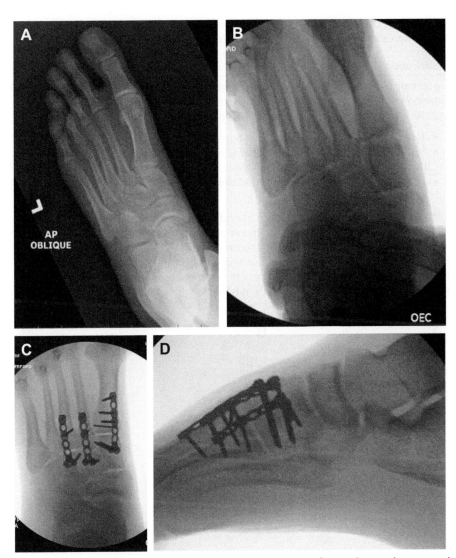

Fig. 7. (*A*) Non–weight-bearing AP radiograph demonstrating first and second metatarsal base fractures suggestive of Lisfranc injury. (*B*) Intraoperative stress view demonstrating instability across first TMT joint and second and third metatarsal base fractures. (*C*) AP intra-operative image demonstrating a joint-sparing technique with dorsal bridge plating of the first, second, and third TMT joints. (*D*) Lateral fluoroscopic image demonstrating dorsal bridge-plating technique.

Advanced Imaging

Computed tomography (CT) and MRI can be useful adjuncts in the evaluation of a pa-tient with a Lisfranc injury. Caution should be used, however, if using CT or MRI to rule out Lisfranc injury. Neither imaging modality is dynamic and therefore instability may present despite normal or equivocal findings. CT scan can be particularly useful for preoperative planning to delineate areas of articular comminution and nondisplaced fracture lines. Disruption of the plantar oblique on MRI has been highly correlated with intraoperative instability on examination under anesthesia.[23]

Classification

The classification proposed by Myerson and colleagues[18] is perhaps the most commonly used to describe Lisfranc injuries (**Fig. 8**). The classification divides injuries in terms of joint congruity, location of involvement, and direction of instability.

- Type A injuries are those with total homolateral joint incongruity.
- Type B injuries are subdivided into injuries involving the medial column in isolation (B1) and those involving the lateral rays (B2).
- Type C injuries are divergent patterns with either partial (C1) or total (C2) incongruity.

The Myerson classification provides a helpful framework for understanding patterns of injury. The system accounts for patterns of instability that may extend to the intercuneiform or naviculocuneiform joints and implies that the energy imparted may dissipate in different locations as it enters and exits the midfoot. Although previously thought to not be predictive of outcome, one recent study has found increased rates of symptomatic posttraumatic arthritis in patients with type C injury patterns.[24]

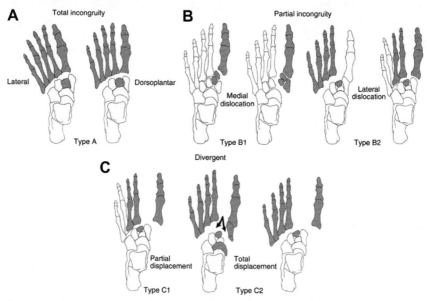

Fig. 8. Classification of tarsometatarsal joint injury. The shaded areas represent the injured or displaced portion of the foot. (*A*) Type A, total incongruity, which involves displacement of all 5 metatarsals with or without fracture at the base of the second MT. The usual displacement is lateral or dorsolateral. These injuries are "homolateral." (*B*) In type B injuries, 1 or more articulations remain intact. Type B1 represents partial incongruity with medial dislocation. Type B2 represents partial incongruity with lateral dislocation; the first TMT joint maybe involved. (*C*) Divergent injury pattern, with either partial (C1) or total (C2) displacement. The arrows in C2 represent the forces through the foot leading to a divergent pattern. (*From* Myerson MS, Fisher RT, Burgess AR, et al. Fracture-dislocations of the tarsometatarsal joints: end results correlated with pathology and treatment. Foot Ankle 1986;6:228; with permission.)

MANAGEMENT
Nonoperative

Successful nonoperative management of Lisfranc injuries is predicated on ruling out instability. Midfoot injuries suspicious for instability by history and examination merit further investigation with weight-bearing or manual stress radiographs. If a high index of suspicion remains with equivocal findings on stress imaging in the office setting or advanced imaging, an examination under anesthesia is a reasonable next step. Patients should be counseled and consented for surgical fixation should the examination under anesthesia demonstrate instability.

In patients with stable injury patterns, the treatment consists of non-weight-bearing immobilization for a period of 4 to 6 weeks. Once the immobilization is removed, patients are allowed to progress weight bearing as tolerated with a course of physical therapy focusing on gait and balance. Return to function and resolution of pain and swelling may take 4 to 6 months.

Operative

Open reduction and internal fixation

Modern treatment of Lisfranc injuries has evolved to include open approaches with anatomic reduction and rigid internal fixation of the medial and middle columns, typically with transarticular screw fixation. Kuo and colleagues[25] examined the outcomes of 48 patients following ORIF of Lisfranc injuries at a mean follow-up of 52 months The rate of posttraumatic arthritis was 25%, with both arthritis as well as patient outcomes significantly correlated with the quality of reduction. Six patients (12.5%) required conversion to arthrodesis during the study period. There was a trend toward increased arthritis in the subgroup with primarily ligamentous injuries despite anatomic reduction (40% vs 18%), leading the investigators to suggest this patient population may benefit from PA. Abbasian and colleagues,[26] in contrast, found no significant difference in functional outcomes and rates of arthritis in a matched cohort of 58 patients with either ligamentous (n = 29) or combined (n = 29) injury patterns. Radiographic arthritis was seen in 27% of ligamentous injuries compared with 31% of osseous injuries; however, only 1 patient in each treatment group required conversion to arthrodesis during the study period (3%). The investigators theorize that the standardized postoperative protocol of prolonged cast immobilization (3 months), implant removal (3 months), and use of an arch support for 4 to 6 weeks following initiation of weight bearing may contribute to the improved results in the ligamentous cohort. Dubois-Ferrière and colleagues[24] recently reported the outcomes of 61 patients at 2 to 24 years following ORIF (n = 50) or PA (n = 11) of Lisfranc injury. Radiographic arthritis was seen in 72% of patients, with 51% of patients having symptomatic posttraumatic arthritis. Symptomatic arthritis was significantly correlated with a nonanatomic reduction, Myerson type C injury pattern, and smoking status. Those patients with symptomatic arthritis had significantly worse functional outcome scores. Despite more than half of patients having some form of symptomatic arthritis, overall functional outcome measures were not significantly different from prior studies and only 4 patients required conversion to arthrodesis.

Primary arthrodesis

Despite the recent renewed interest in primary partial arthrodesis of acute Lisfranc injuries, few studies have examined the outcomes of this treatment in isolation. Reinhardt and colleagues[27] evaluated 25 patients at a mean of 42 months following PA of primarily ligamentous (n = 12) or combined osseous and ligamentous (n = 13) injuries. American Orthopaedic Foot and Ankle Society midfoot scores were not significantly different between the primarily ligamentous or combined injuries following arthrodesis and patients reported an average return to 85% of their preinjury activity level. Four patients (16%) developed a nonunion and 3 patients (12%) had signs of radiographic adjacent joint degeneration at the time of final follow-up. MacMahon and colleagues[28] evaluated the outcomes of 38 patients who underwent PA, specifically as it relates to return to sports and physical activity. Although patients expressed a high rate of satisfaction with the surgical outcome, only 64% returned to their preinjury level of athletic participation. No cases of nonunion were reported and 1 patient developed symptomatic adjacent joint arthritis.

Open reduction and internal fixation versus primary arthrodesis

Two randomized studies have directly compared the results of PA with ORIF of Lisfranc injuries. Ly and Coetzee[7] randomized 41 patients to either ORIF (n = 20) or PA (n = 21) for primarily ligamentous injury patterns with a minimum 2-year follow-up. The arthrodesis group had significantly improved functional outcomes, higher returns to preinjury activity levels, lower rates of reoperation, and less pain at final follow-up. In the group that underwent open reduction, 15 (75%) of 20 patients developed radiographic arthritis and 5 patients (25%) required conversion to arthrodesis for symptomatic posttraumatic arthritis. Routine removal of transarticular screws was not performed in the ORIF group. Henning and colleagues[29] found no significant difference in either (short form musculoskeletal function assessment) SMFA or Short Form-36 scores at 2-year follow-up in 32 patients randomized to either PA or ORIF for both ligamentous and combined injury patterns. There was a significantly higher rate of secondary surgery in the ORIF group; however, all but 1 of the reoperations were for elective implant removal as part of the study protocol.

DISCUSSION

Modern techniques of open reduction and rigid internal fixation have offered improved results compared with historical treatments, such as flexible wire fixation.[30] Achieving and maintaining an anatomic reduction has clearly been shown in multiple studies to correlate with the development of arthritis and patient outcome.[24–26,31] Despite appropriate treatment, many patients still progress on to degenerative changes. Although radiographic arthritis does not always correlate with patient outcome, up to 51% of patients will experience symptomatic arthritis at long-term follow-up[24] (**Fig. 9**). Secondary arthrodesis after failed ORIF is technically more demanding and may compromise patient outcome.[32]

The current treatment of Lisfranc injuries with transarticular screw fixation raises several interesting questions. Although this is accepted practice for the midfoot, perhaps the syndesmosis is the only other periarticular injury in which a similar technique is used. Imagine treating a tibial plateau fracture with anatomic reduction followed by temporary or permanent transarticular screw fixation. One would reasonably expect the knee joint to have significant stiffness and limited function following such treatment. Abbasian and colleagues[26] argue that, to maintain anatomic reduction following ORIF, prolonged cast immobilization is required to allow for the build of "solid and reliable scar formation."

Whether or not to remove the implants following transarticular screw fixation remains controversial. If the screws are not removed, how does this treatment function any differently from an arthrodesis? Ideally the patient forms a painless, stable pseudarthrosis. Joint-sparing techniques, such as dorsal plating, have been advocated as a way to avoid the potential pitfalls of transarticular screws.[4] Small series have shown promising results with this technique; however, the treatment is still reliant on the

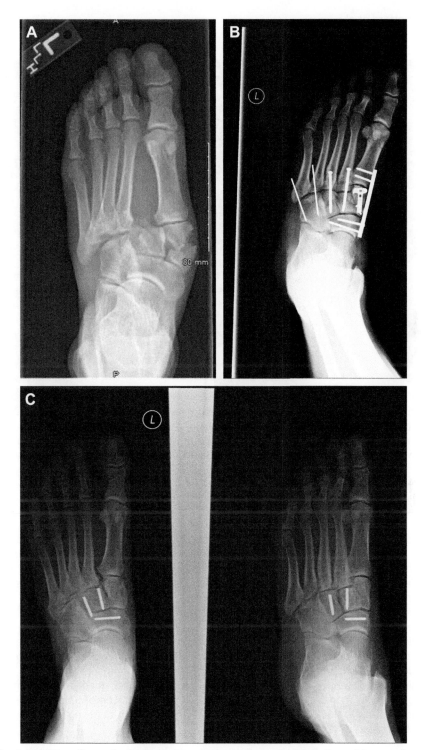

Fig. 9. (*A*) AP radiograph demonstrating divergent fracture dislocation with comminuted fracture of the medial cuneiform. (*B*) Postoperative radiograph showing anatomic reduction and stable fixation with the use of a medial bridge plate to span the comminuted medial cuneiform and maintain medial column length. (*C*) Follow-up radiograph demonstrating posttraumatic arthritis and broken implants retained in the cuneiforms and navicular.

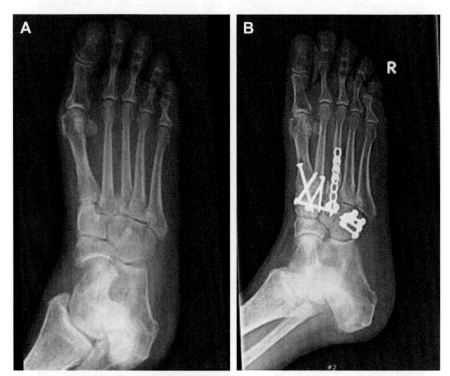

Fig. 10. (*A*) Oblique foot radiograph demonstrating Lisfranc injury including comminuted third metatarsal base fracture and displaced cuboid fracture. (*B*) Oblique foot radiograph following PA of the first, second, and third tarsometatarsal joints and ORIF of the cuboid.

formation of a physiologic amount of scar tissue across inherently unstable articulations. Again, if the implants are not removed with a second surgery, then these joints are potentially permanently immobilized.

PA is a viable alternative to ORIF with several potential advantages (**Fig. 10**). Arthrodesis can approximate the functional anatomy of the medial 3 tarsometatarsal joints with solid bone healing instead of scar tissue formation. Successful arthrodesis minimizes or eliminates the risk for later symptomatic posttraumatic arthritis of the midfoot. Additionally, arthrodesis does not necessarily obligate the patient to a secondary surgical procedure for implant removal.

Despite these advantages, PA has several current limitations. Enthusiasm for this procedure must be tempered by the fact that no long-term data exist regarding the function of patients following PA for Lisfranc injury. Perhaps, similar to ORIF, the results of PA may diminish with time. Only one study to date, that of Ly and Coetzee,[7] has demonstrated superiority of this treatment technique compared with ORIF. The remaining studies have all found equivalent, but not superior, functional outcomes compared with modern series of ORIF. PA is not without complication. Rates of nonunion of up to 33% have been reported.[14] Adjacent joint degenerative changes have been seen in 12% of patients.[27]

SUMMARY

The wide spectrum of pathology that falls under the category of "Lisfranc injury" renders it unlikely that any one treatment can fit all patterns of injury. There can be no argument that the outcome will be wildly different with a low-energy incomplete ligamentous injury versus a crushing injury with soft tissue compromise, regardless of the treatment chosen. This would be analogous to comparing the outcomes of a rotational ankle fracture with a tibial pilon fracture with the expectation that the results might be similar.

Treatment of unstable tarsometatarsal joint injuries remains a challenge. PA appears to offer improved outcomes for patients with complete primarily ligamentous injuries. The role of PA in patients with incomplete ligamentous injuries or combined osseous and ligamentous patterns has yet to be clearly defined. Some investigators have proposed algorithms that differentiate treatment based on incomplete versus complete patterns of ligamentous injury.[33] Although this approach is rational, the evidence to support differentiating treatment based on the degree of ligamentous instability is scant. Further well-designed prospective studies comparing ORIF with PA are needed to more clearly define the role of each treatment in the management of these complex injuries.

REFERENCES

1. Cassebaum WH. Lisfranc fracture-dislocations. Clin Orthop Relat Res 1963;30: 116–29.
2. Aronow MS. Treatment of the missed Lisfranc injury. Foot Ankle Clin 2006;11(1): 127–42, ix.
3. Benirschke SK, Meinberg E, Anderson SA, et al. Fractures and dislocations of the midfoot: Lisfranc and Chopart injuries. J Bone Joint Surg Am 2012;94(14): 1325–37.
4. Stern RE, Assal M. Dorsal multiple plating without routine transarticular screws for fixation of Lisfranc injury. Orthopedics 2014;37(12):815–9.
5. Sheibani-Rad S, Coetzee JC, Giveans MR, et al. Arthrodesis versus ORIF for Lisfranc fractures. Orthopedics 2012;35(6):e868–73.
6. Sangeorzan BJ, Veith RG, Hansen ST Jr. Salvage of Lisfranc's tarsometatarsal joint by arthrodesis. Foot Ankle 1990;10(4):193–200.
7. Ly TV, Coetzee JC. Treatment of primarily ligamentous Lisfranc joint injuries: primary arthrodesis compared with open reduction and internal fixation. A prospective, randomized study. J Bone Joint Surg Am 2006;88(3):514–20.
8. Kelikian AS, editor. Syndesmology, in Sarrafian's anatomy of the foot and ankle: descriptive, topographical, functional. Philadelphia: Lippincott, Williams and Wilkins; 2011. p. 208–12.
9. Solan MC, Moorman CT 3rd, Miyamoto RG, et al. Ligamentous restraints of the second tarsometatarsal joint: a biomechanical evaluation. Foot Ankle Int 2001; 22(8):637–41.
10. Kaar S, Femino J, Morag Y. Lisfranc joint displacement following sequential ligament sectioning. J Bone Joint Surg Am 2007;89(10):2225–32.
11. de Palma L, Santucci A, Sabetta SP, et al. Anatomy of the Lisfranc joint complex. Foot Ankle Int 1997;18(6):356–64.
12. Hansen ST Jr. Functional anatomy of the foot and ankle, in functional reconstruction of the foot and ankle. Lippincott Williams and Wilkins; 2000. p. 22.
13. Chiodo CP, Myerson MS. Developments and advances in the diagnosis and treatment of injuries to the tarsometatarsal joint. Orthop Clin North Am 2001;32(1): 11–20.
14. Mulier T, Reynders P, Dereymaeker G, et al. Severe Lisfrancs injuries: primary arthrodesis or ORIF? Foot Ankle Int 2002;23(10):902–5.

15. Nadaud JP, Parks BG, Schon LC. Plantar and calcaneocuboid joint pressure after isolated medial column fusion versus medial and lateral column fusion: a biomechanical study. Foot Ankle Int 2011;32(11):1069–74.
16. Kadow TR, Siska PA, Evans AR, et al. Staged treatment of high energy midfoot fracture dislocations. Foot Ankle Int 2014;35(12):1287–91.
17. Thakur NA, McDonnell M, Got CJ, et al. Injury patterns causing isolated foot compartment syndrome. J Bone Joint Surg Am 2012;94(11):1030–5.
18. Myerson MS, Fisher RT, Burgess AR, et al. Fracture dislocations of the tarsometatarsal joints: end results correlated with pathology and treatment. Foot Ankle 1986;6(5):225–42.
19. Weber M, Locher S. Reconstruction of the cuboid in compression fractures: short to midterm results in 12 patients. Foot Ankle Int 2002;23(11):1008–13.
20. Ross G, Cronin R, Hauzenblas J, et al. Plantar ecchymosis sign: a clinical aid to diagnosis of occult Lisfranc tarsometatarsal injuries. J Orthop Trauma 1996;10(2): 119–22.
21. Dodd A, Le I. Foot compartment syndrome: diagnosis and management. J Am Acad Orthop Surg 2013;21(11):657–64.
22. Coss HS, Manos RE, Buoncristiani A, et al. Abduction stress and AP weightbearing radiography of purely ligamentous injury in the tarsometatarsal joint. Foot Ankle Int 1998;19(8):537–41.
23. Raikin SM, Elias I, Dheer S, et al. Prediction of midfoot instability in the subtle Lisfranc injury. Comparison of magnetic resonance imaging with intraoperative findings. J Bone Joint Surg Am 2009;91(4):892–9.
24. Dubois-Ferrière V, Lübbeke A, Chowdhary A, et al. Clinical outcomes and development of symptomatic osteoarthritis 2 to 24 years after surgical treatment of tarsometatarsal joint complex injuries. J Bone Joint Surg Am 2016;98(9):713–20.
25. Kuo RS, Tejwani NC, Digiovanni CW, et al. Outcome after open reduction and internal fixation of Lisfranc joint injuries. J Bone Joint Surg Am 2000;82-A(11):1609–18.
26. Abbasian MR, Paradies F, Weber M, et al. Temporary internal fixation for ligamentous and osseous Lisfranc injuries: outcome and technical tip. Foot Ankle Int 2015;36(8):976–83.
27. Reinhardt KR, Oh LS, Schottel P, et al. Treatment of Lisfranc fracture-dislocations with primary partial arthrodesis. Foot Ankle Int 2012;33(1):50–6.
28. MacMahon A, Kim P, Levine DS, et al. Return to sports and physical activities after primary partial arthrodesis for Lisfranc injuries in young patients. Foot Ankle Int 2016;37(4):355–62.
29. Henning JA, Jones CB, Sietsema DL, et al. Open reduction internal fixation versus primary arthrodesis for Lisfranc injuries: a prospective randomized study. Foot Ankle Int 2009;30(10):913–22.
30. Schepers T, Oprel PP, Van Lieshout EM. Influence of approach and implant on reduction accuracy and stability in Lisfranc fracture-dislocation at the tarsometatarsal joint. Foot Ankle Int 2013;34(5):705–10.
31. Stavlas P, Roberts CS, Xypnitos FN, et al. The role of reduction and internal fixation of Lisfranc fracture-dislocations: a systematic review of the literature. Int Orthop 2010;34(8):1083–91.
32. Rammelt S, Schneiders W, Schikore H, et al. Primary open reduction and fixation compared with delayed corrective arthrodesis in the treatment of tarsometatarsal (Lisfranc) fracture dislocation. J Bone Joint Surg Br 2008;90(11):1499–506.
33. Coetzee JC. Making sense of Lisfranc injuries. Foot Ankle Clin 2008;13(4): 695–704, ix.

The Role of Percutaneous Reduction and Fixation of Lisfranc Injuries

Rupesh A. Puna, MBChB[a],*, Matthew P.W. Tomlinson, MBChB[b]

KEYWORDS

- Lisfranc injuries • Lisfranc fracture/dislocation • Percutaneous fixation
- Percutaneous fracture fixation • Role of percutaneous fixation

KEY POINTS

- To be able to perform percutaneous fixation of lisfranc injuries, the authors emphasize an anatomic reduction must be mandatory.
- When uncertainty remains as to whether closed reduction is anatomic, the authors recommend formal open reduction because accuracy of reduction is correlated with long-term outcome.
- Closed injuries with minimal displacement, bony avulsions, and skeletally immature individuals seem the most appropriate indications for percutaneous fixation.
- The authors admit not all injuries are ideal for this method of treatment, and this is an area that needs to be more clearly defined in the future.

INTRODUCTION

Since Jaques Lisfranc (1790–1847) described an amputation through the tarsometatarsal (TMT) joints during the Napoleonic Wars in 1815,[1–3] injuries to the TMT joint complex have become eponymous with his name.

These injuries usually consist of unstable fracture-dislocations or purely ligamentous injuries with subluxation through the TMT and adjacent joint complexes in the midfoot[3,4] and are regarded as serious injuries with the potential for significant morbidity and long-term sequelae resulting in permanent disability.[5,6]

Poor results with traditional treatments of these injuries, such as closed reduction and casting[7] or supervised neglect, have led to the development of techniques to reduce the Lisfranc joints anatomically and provide stable internal fixation with screws[8–13] or plates[14] or to fuse the unstable joints primarily.[9,11,15]

The authors have nothing to disclose.
[a] Division of Orthopaedic Surgery, St Michael's Hospital, University of Toronto, 30 Bond Street, Toronto, Ontario M5B 1W8, Canada; [b] Counties-Manukau Health Orthopaedics, Middlemore Hospital, 100 Hospital Road, Otahuhu, Auckland 2104, New Zealand
* Corresponding author.
E-mail address: rupeshpuna@yahoo.com

Open reduction and internal fixation has become the gold standard treatment of these injuries during the past 4 decades,[8,10,12–14] using the principles of internal fixation developed by the AO group and others[16]; however, with the advent of less invasive surgical approaches to orthopedic injuries to better preserve the soft tissue envelope, there is now more interest in techniques that allow percutaneous reduction and fixation of these injuries.[17]

Crucial to this concept is the need to be able to achieve an anatomic reduction prior to any attempt at fixation because outcomes have been shown to correlate with accuracy of reduction.[4,18] If this is unable to be accomplished using closed reduction techniques, then the surgeon should consider proceeding to open reduction and internal fixation if the soft tissues allow it or waiting for the swelling to subside and returning for open reduction and internal fixation at a later date.

For this aforementioned reason, the authors tend to use percutaneous methods only in cases of an anatomic reduction likely to be easily achieved; this is elaborated on further.

INCIDENCE AND PREVALENCE

The incidence of Lisfranc injuries is reported as 1 per 55,000 persons yearly in the United States, which makes up approximately 0.2% of all fractures.[14,19,20] This may be underestimated, however, because studies have shown that up to one-third of Lisfranc injuries can be missed on initial presentation.[13,19,21] Given that the long-term natural history of untreated or missed lisfranc injuries is for persistent instability, deformity, and arthritis,[5,6] it is imperative that a timely diagnosis is made and appropriate management undertaken during the acute phase, because delayed treatment is associated with inferior outcomes.[6,22,23]

MECHANISM OF INJURY

Both direct and indirect mechanisms are responsible for injuries to the TMT joint complex.

The most common mechanisms are indirect injuries.[19] These can be either high-energy injuries, such as those associated with motor vehicle accidents or falls from a height, or low-energy injuries, such as those sustained during athletic activity.[20] Most often, these involve a combination of longitudinal force applied to the forefoot, which is then subject to rotation and compression.[24] Excessive plantarflexion and abduction forces are the most common indirect mechanisms leading to TMT joint complex injury.[25]

Direct injures are less common and are usually sustained from crush injuries in which the metatarsal bases undergo either dorsal or plantar displacement.[22] These injuries can be associated with significant soft tissue trauma, vascular compromise, skin compromise, and/or compartment syndrome.[7,26]

ANATOMY

The TMT articulations consist of both osseous and ligamentous components. The osseous component is divided into 3 columns. The medial column consists of the medial cuneiform and the first metatarsal. The middle column consists of the middle and lateral cuneiforms and their respective articulations with the second and third metatarsals. The lateral column contains the cuboid and fourth and fifth metatarsals.[27] The trapezoidal shape of the medial 3 metatarsal bases and their associated cuneiforms produce a transverse or Roman arch configuration.[28,29] The keystone to the transverse arch is the second TMT joint, which results from the recessed middle cuneiform lying 8 mm proximal to the medial cuneiform and 4 mm proximal to the lateral cuneiform.[30]

The ligamentous component consists of groups of ligaments defined by their course and location.[31] Transverse ligaments attach the second through fifth metatarsal bases. There are no such ligaments between the first and second metatarsal base.[26,31] Between the medial cuneiform and second metatarsal, however, lie 3 groups of ligaments (dorsal, interosseous, and plantar). The oblique interosseous ligament represents what is referred to as the Lisfranc ligament, which is the strongest component of this complex (8–10 mm wide and 5–6 mm thick).[14,32] The Lisfranc ligament has also been noted to be variably arranged with either a single or double bundle configuration. This is supported by dorsal and plantar ligaments. The plantar ligament divides into 2 bands – a deep band that inserts into the base of the second metatarsal and the superficial band that inserts into the base of the third metatarsal.[33] On average, the interosseous ligament is 4.5 times larger than the dorsal ligament and twice as large as the plantar ligament.[34]

CLINICAL FINDINGS

A history suggestive of either a direct or indirect Lisfranc injury mandates a thorough examination directed at looking for signs associated with the injury. Other than midfoot pain and swelling, important clinical signs that may aid in the diagnosis of an occult Lisfranc injury include the plantar ecchymosis sign, which consists of an ecchymotic area over the plantar aspect of the midfoot[35]; a positive gap sign, where diastasis is noted between the hallux and second toe[36]; and the toe-up sign, which represents an irreducible Lisfranc injury due to interposition of a slip of the tibialis anterior tendon preventing reduction.[37,38]

Other clinical signs and tests that may be of benefit in the diagnosis include the passive pronation-abduction test described by Curtis and colleagues[39] performed by manipulating the forefoot into pronation and abduction with the hindfoot fixed and detecting instability, an inability to bear weight on tiptoes,[20] and the piano key test stressing the first and second TMT joints in a dorsoplantar direction, in abduction-adduction, and also divergently.[14]

As part of the authors' routine assessment, evidence of significant ankle equinus is also looked for. It is the authors' belief that equinus contractures can contribute to treatment failure in this group and consideration should be given to gastrocnemius recession or Achilles lengthening where appropriate.

Compartment syndrome, especially in the context of a high-energy injury, should be looked for and treated if necessary. Significant pain and tense swelling are the most common findings and, if indicated, decompressive fasciotomies may be required in an emergent fashion to prevent long-term sequelae.[40] Patients requiring decompressive fasciotomies through dorsal incisions are not usually suitable for consideration of percutaneous reduction and fixation and are normally fixed open, but a medial approach does not preclude the possibility.

RADIOLOGIC FINDINGS

As many as one-third of Lisfranc injuries may be missed on initial presentation,[13,19,21] so it is imperative that the treating physician has a good knowledge of subtle radiologic findings. If percutaneous fixation is considered, it is a prerequisite that there is a thorough knowledge of the normal and abnormal radiologic findings at the Lisfranc joint complex.

Initial evaluation begins with simple radiography that generally consists of non–weight-bearing anteroposterior (AP), internal rotation oblique and lateral radiographs.

In many situations, the injury is obvious, but initial radiographs may be normal, as reported by Nunley and Vertollo,[41] who found that 50% of athletes with significant midfoot injuries had normal non–weight-bearing radiographs.

In patients with subtle abnormalities on non–weight-bearing films (**Fig. 1**), or in patients with a high clinical suspicion of midfoot injury, weight-bearing radiographs are

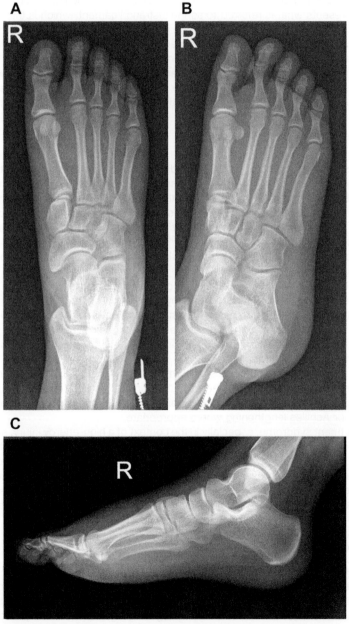

Fig. 1. Initial non–weight-bearing AP (*A*), oblique (*B*), and lateral (*C*) radiographs showing subtle malalignment of the bases of the first and second metatarsals consistent with Lisfranc injury.

advised.[42] A standing AP with both feet on a single cassette should be obtained along with a weight-bearing lateral radiograph looking for any displacement of the TMT joint complex (**Fig. 2**) or flattening of the longitudinal arch as well as dorsal displacement at the second TMT joint. A comparison weight-bearing lateral radiograph may also be of benefit.[14,43]

Important relationships of normal alignment are as follows:

1. On the AP radiograph, the lateral margins of the first TMT and medial margins of the second[44] and third[45] TMT articulations should align almost perfectly.
2. On the 30° oblique radiograph, the lateral margins of the middle cuneiform and second metatarsal base and the lateral cuneiform and third metatarsal base should align.[46] The fourth TMT articulation is more variable but should be within 2 mm to 3 mm.[44,45,47]
3. On the weight-bearing lateral radiograph, there should be no step-off at the dorsal margins of the TMT joints,[42] the talometatarsal angle should be less than 10°,[22] and

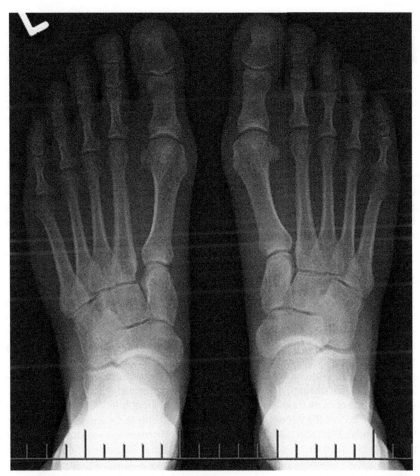

Fig. 2. Weight-bearing radiographs of both feet showing an increased gap between the bases of the first and second metatarsals and malalignment between the intermediate cuneiform and second metatarsal base due to subtle ligamentous Lisfranc injury on the left side. The alignment is normal on the right side.

the plantar surface of the medial cuneiform should be dorsal to the plantar aspect of the fifth metatarsal base.[43]

The most frequent and reliable indicator of Lisfranc injury is malalignment at the second TMT articulation, with lateral step-off at the second metatarsal base with respect to the middle cuneiform, which is best seen on the AP radiograph.[44] Diastasis of 2 mm or more indicates instability.[22,41,48] Additionally, another common pathognomonic finding is the fleck sign, which is an avulsion seen at the base of the second metatarsal described by Myerson and colleagues.[22]

The authors also look closely at the first TMT joint, noting any subtle subluxation of the joint that requires reduction at the time of surgery.

Other radiologic modalities that may be used in the evaluation of Lisfranc injury include stress radiographs, radionuclide bone scan, CT scanning, and MRI. Each has its own role in evaluating Lisfranc injuries; however, in the authors' practice, plain radiographs and CT scanning are usually sufficient to make the diagnosis and plan treatment.

Stress views may allow demonstration of instability in the context of normal radiographs or subtle abnormalities.[6,8,48,49] During surgery the authors often obtain a stress view with fluoroscopy to confirm and document the diagnosis and check the reducibility of the injury and suitability or otherwise of percutaneous treatment. A combination of pronation and abduction forces are commonly required, but adduction may also be necessary to demonstrate instability in the first ray.[48]

CT scanning accurately depicts osseous anatomy and articular alignment,[50] and CT with simulated weight bearing may be particularly helpful.[51] Fractures and TMT joint malalignment[50,52,53] are more readily visualized on CT scans (**Fig. 3**) than radiographs. The use of intraoperative 3-D CT scanning to assess reduction is an exciting prospect that is becoming more readily available, but the authors have not as yet used it routinely.

MRI depicts excellent soft tissue anatomy[46] compared with CT, although it is not routinely used in the authors' institution. MRI has been shown to reliably depict the anatomy of the TMT joint complex.[50,54,55] Sagittal sequences are useful for cross-referencing and assessing dorsal TMT joint ligaments. Oblique long-axis images optimally visualize the interosseous lisfranc and plantar TMT ligaments.

CLASSIFICATION

In 1909, Quenu and Kuss[56] published a classification scheme based on their column and spatula concept, dividing injuries into 3 types – homolateral (all metatarsals displacing in the same direction at their bases), isolated (subluxation of 1 or 2 metatarsal bases in 1 direction while the others remain enlocated), and divergent (displacement of metatarsal bases in different directions).

Later, Hardcastle and colleagues,[2] in 1982, described a similar classification based on Quenu and Kuss, dividing injuries into 3 types – A (complete incongruity with complete displacement of all metatarsal bases), B (partial incongruity with one or more of the metatarsal bases displaced), and C (divergent similar to Quenu and Kuss[56]).

More recently, Myerson and colleagues[22] (**Fig. 4**) modified Hardcastle and colleagues' classification to divide type B injuries into B1 and B2, where metatarsal bases may be displaced medially or laterally respectively. Type C (divergent) injuries were also divided into C1 and C2 based on partial or total incongruity, respectively.

Although these classifications are useful in delineating the nature of Lisfranc injuries, the authors do not apply them directly in decision making with regard to percutaneous treatment.

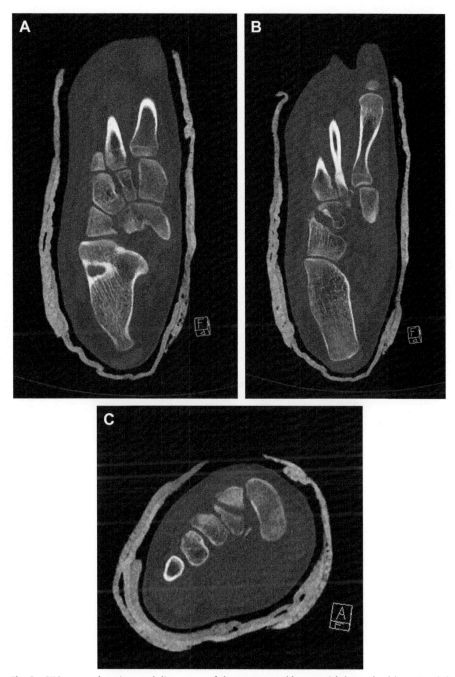

Fig. 3. CT images showing malalignment of the metatarsal bases with lateral subluxation (*A*) and a small avulsion fragment of the Lisfranc ligament (*B, C*) at the base of the second metatarsal.

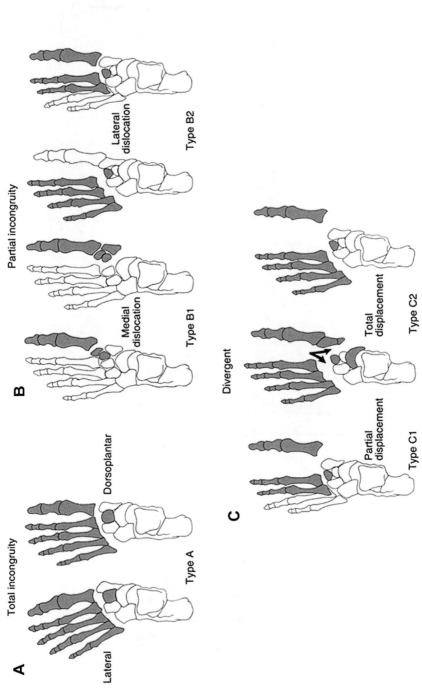

Fig. 4. Myerson classification of Lisfranc injuries. (A) Type A injuries, with total incongruity, involve displacement of all five metatarsal bases with or without fracture. These injuries are often referred to as "homolateral". (B) Type B injuries, with partial incongruity, are where one or more of the articulations at the metatarsal bases remain intact. B1 represents medial dislocation while B2 represents lateral dislocation. (C) Type C are divergent injuries with partial (C1) or total (C2) displacement. (From Myerson MS, Fisher RT, Burgess AR, et al. Fracture dislocations of the tarsometatarsal joints: end results correlated with pathology and treatment. Foot Ankle 1986;6(5):225–42; with permission.)

TREATMENT

In general, best results with treatment of Lisfranc injuries are obtained with anatomic reduction and internal fixation,[7,19,25,57,58] where outcomes have been shown to be correlated with accuracy of reduction.[4,18] In general, any radiographic abnormality (detailed previously) may be an indication of instability and the need for surgical intervention.

The surgical options for management of Lisfranc injuries include closed reduction and percutaneous fixation with wires and/or screws,[17] open reduction and internal fixation,[8–13,15,59–62] and primary arthrodesis.[9,11,15,60]

Traditionally, open anatomic reduction and internal fixation and primary arthrodesis have been advocated for the treatment of most unstable injuries and several studies have proved the efficacy of both of these treatment modalities.[8–13,15,59–62] Arthrodesis has been shown to have slightly favorable outcomes in patients with purely ligamentous injuries, with patients achieving slightly higher levels of function.[9,11,60] Also, Henning and colleagues[9] showed a lower rate of further surgical procedures and associated complications with primary arthrodesis; however, the long-term effects of early arthrodesis have not been fully evaluated. Adjacent joint degeneration is an area of potential concern after primary arthrodesis.

Although closed reduction and cast immobilization may have been an acceptable treatment method in the past, the authors do not believe there is a place in contemporary treatment for this method because reduction is often lost.[7] Closed nonsurgical treatment may be considered for patients with minimal ambulatory ability, an insensate foot, or preexisting arthritic conditions.[14] Other relative indications for closed, nonsurgical treatment may include substantial comorbidities precluding anesthesia or patients who decline surgery despite recommendations.

There is not much written about the outcomes of closed reduction and percutaneous fixation nor are there agreed indications for it. Perceived advantages of this treatment include less soft tissue dissection and disruption of the soft tissue envelope, a shorter operating time, the ability to perform surgery at an earlier stage, shorter hospital stay, earlier mobilization, and fewer wound complications. Potential drawbacks include technical difficulties and the inability to achieve a perfect anatomic reduction. It is the authors' opinion, however, that if an anatomic reduction cannot be achieved by closed means, then open reduction should be mandatory.

Kadakia and Myerson[63] have described their technique of closed reduction and percutaneous fixation, indicating that a thorough understanding of intraoperative radiography is imperative to achieving anatomic reduction. Recommendations for conversion to open reduction included greater than 2 mm of residual TMT joint displacement or more than 15° of persistent talo–first metatarsal angulation after attempts at closed reduction.

Perugia and colleagues[17] reported the largest independent series of medium-term outcomes of closed treatment with percutaneous screw fixation in 42 patients and noted that accuracy of reduction correlated well with overall outcome and also that outcomes in pure ligamentous injuries were inferior to those with fracture-dislocations. They also agreed with the published guidelines of Myerson and colleagues[22] on conversion to open reduction.

THE AUTHORS' INDICATIONS

Not all Lisfranc injuries are appropriate for this technique. First and foremost, the authors believe that an anatomic reduction must be achievable. If an anatomic reduction is not achievable, the authors routinely convert to open reduction.

The authors' relative indications include:

1. Injuries with obvious bony avulsions and minor displacement
2. Skeletally immature patients with open physes
3. Patients with a compromised soft tissue envelope
4. Low-energy injuries in the athletic population

Injury patterns that are more suitable for this technique include Myerson types A, B1, and B2. The type C patterns of injury are usually too unstable to be able to achieve anatomic reduction percutaneously.

The subtle injuries with Lisfranc ligament avulsion fractures and minor displacement are considered ideal because eventually fracture healing results in a well maintained reduction of the deformity. When fracture fragments are blocking reduction, an open approach is usually required unless the fragments can be moved out of the way percutaneously.

In open Lisfranc injuries, open reduction and internal fixation are often possible through the open wound; however, in some circumstances, percutaneous fixation can be used to augment open reduction, such as for the lateral column joints.

The authors do not believe that this technique should be used in primary ligamentous injuries with marked displacement or when there is anything less than anatomic reduction.

TECHNIQUE

The patient is positioned supine on the operating table. The procedure is performed under thigh tourniquet control and antibiotic prophylaxis. A small wedge is placed under the ipsilateral buttock to internally rotate the limb (**Fig. 5**). Standard sterile preparation of the limb is undertaken with the limb draped high up to the tourniquet.

An image intensifier is used to verify displacement or instability at the TMT joints. An understanding of the images required to assess the pattern of injury is imperative. An AP image with simulated weight bearing of the foot is obtained to assess the first and second TMT joints. An abduction force is used to assess the degree of instability. A 30° oblique view is then used to assess the third TMT joint and the fourth and fifth metatarsal-cuboid joints. If necessary, a 45° or 60° oblique view can be used to further assess the fourth and fifth joints (**Fig. 6**).

Once instability or displacement are confirmed, closed reduction is attempted, most often in lateral homolateral injuries by fully adducting and plantar flexing the first

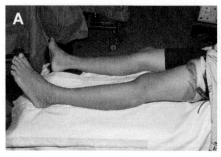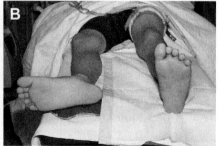

Fig. 5. Patient positioning for percutaneous treatment of Lisfranc injuries with a support under the ipsilateral hip (A) to allow the foot to sit in a neutral position (B).

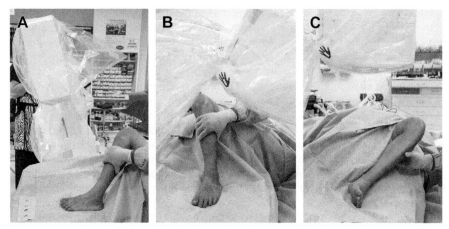

Fig. 6. Positioning of the leg to allow proper assessment of the reduction using the C-arm on AP (*A*), 30° oblique (*B*), and lateral (*C*) views.

metatarsal into an anatomic position (**Fig. 7**). Achievement of an anatomic reduction of the first ray is confirmed radiographically prior to proceeding.

Reduction commences from the medial column and then proceeds laterally. The first TMT joint is reduced with adduction and plantarflexion. A percutaneous

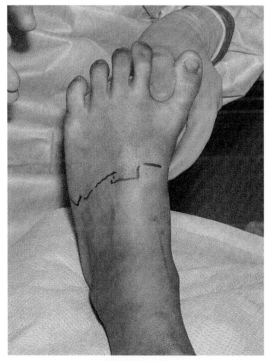

Fig. 7. The TMT joint location can be palpated and marked. Reduction begins with the first ray, which is adducted and plantarflexed slightly to fully reduce the deformity. Medial pressure over the medial cuneiform helps with the reduction.

longitudinal incision is made on the lateral side of the extensor hallucis longus tendon 2 cm distal to the joint. A 1.6 mm Kirschner (K)-wire is inserted retrograde across the first TMT joint while the joint is held manually reduced (**Fig. 8**) with this maneuver of adduction and plantarflexion. AP and lateral radiographs are obtained to check the reduction of the joint.

Once this is confirmed, the second TMT joint is reduced by making a direct medial percutaneous incision adjacent to the medial cuneiform and another incision along the lateral aspect of the second MT base just distal to the second TMT joint. Through these 2 incisions, a medium or large pointed reduction clamp is used to reduce the second MT to the medial cuneiform in the direction of the Lisfranc ligament (**Fig. 9**). The reduction is again confirmed with the use of AP and lateral fluoroscopy with simulated weight bearing to ensure the TMT joint axis is anatomically aligned. Attention is also paid to the talus–first metatarsal angle in both planes, which should be orthogonal.

A 30° oblique image of the foot is used to confirm reduction of the third TMT and the fourth and fifth metatarsal-cuboid joints. Once anatomic reduction is confirmed, the first through third TMT joints are stabilized with percutaneous retrograde screws or K-wires in children (**Fig. 10**). These screws are all inserted in a positional mode as opposed to a compression mode.

The authors routinely place a 4-mm cortical screw across the first TMT joint through the same incision used for the temporary K-wire. This is followed by a 3.5-mm screw inserted adjacent to the percutaneous clamp in the medial cuneiform.

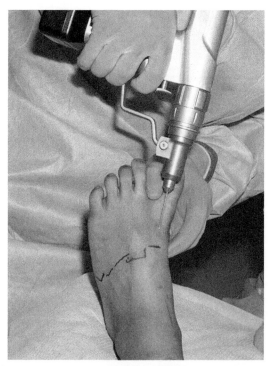

Fig. 8. A small stab incision is made 2 cm distal to the TMT joint and a K-wire inserted across the first TMT joint with the joint reduced. The position of the K-wire and the reduction are checked using the C-arm.

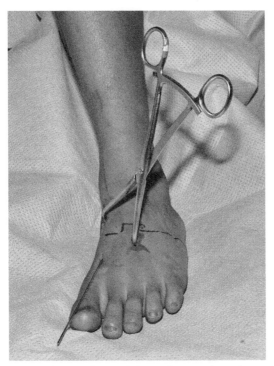

Fig. 9. A stab incision is made over the medial cuneiform and another at the lateral base of the second metatarsal and a medium or large reduction clamp used to reduce the base of the second metatarsal onto the medial cuneiform. The reduction is checked carefully using the C-arm.

This screw runs from the medial cuneiform to the second metatarsal base (**Fig. 11**). Then a single 3.5-mm cortical screw is used across the second and third TMT joints through 2 separate percutaneous incisions 2 cm distal to the second and third TMT joints (**Fig. 12**).

When the instability pattern involves the medial intercuneiform joint, a reduction clamp can be placed across the cuneiforms and a percutaneous screw placed from the medial cuneiform across to the intermediate or lateral cuneiform bone to hold the reduction.

If instability is detected in the fourth and fifth TMT joints, the authors prefer to use smooth K-wires to stabilize these joints rather than screws to preserve the integrity of these important joints as much as possible. If K-wires are used in these circumstances, they are removed in the outpatient clinic after 6 weeks.

Some surgeons prefer to use cannulated screws for fixation and these have the advantage that they can be placed directly over the K-wires, but the screws can compress normal articular cartilage, and the authors prefer to use solid static screws to hold the reduction and avoid cartilage compression.

All wounds are closed with simple skin sutures (**Fig. 13**) and patients are placed into a below-knee split plaster of Paris cast. The authors keep patients touch-down weight bearing for 6 weeks and routinely check wounds and change the plaster to a below-knee fibreglass cast after 2 weeks. At the 6-week mark, patients are transitioned into a walking boot and progressively increase their weight bearing over the next 6 weeks

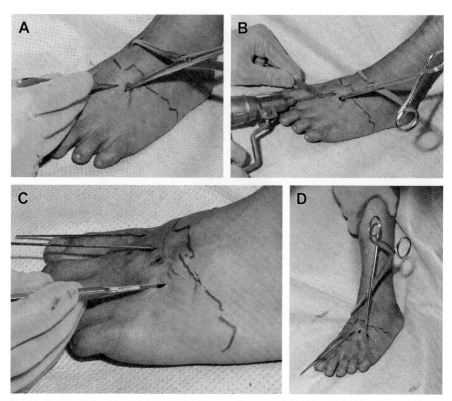

Fig. 10. Sequential wires are then placed across the second (*A, B*) and third metatarsal bases. The clamp can be moved more laterally to reduce the third metatarsal base (*C, D*).

until the 12-week mark when full weight bearing is allowed (**Fig. 14**). Ankle and subtalar joint range-of-motion exercises are performed during this time.

Hardware is usually left in place until at least 6 months when it is removed as an elective procedure. Hardware removal is normally achieved simply by using the scars

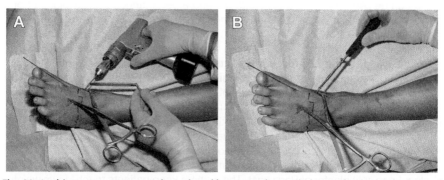

Fig. 11. In this case, a screw was then placed between the medial cuneiform and the base of the second metatarsal at an oblique angle (*A, B*). This screw should cross the facet between the medial cuneiform and base of second metatarsal without entering the TMT joints. This screw stabilizes the Lisfranc ligament.

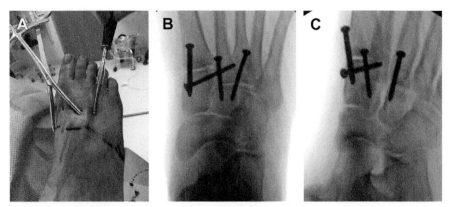

Fig. 12. Another case showing percutaneous placement of a third TMT joint screw (A) and the AP (B) and 30° oblique (C) intraoperative imaging.

from the initial surgery and dissecting bluntly down to the screw heads, which are normally palpable under the skin (**Fig. 15**). If the fourth and fifth metatarsal-cuboid joints are stabilized with percutaneous K-wires, then, as discussed, these are removed in clinic at the 6-week mark (**Fig. 16**).

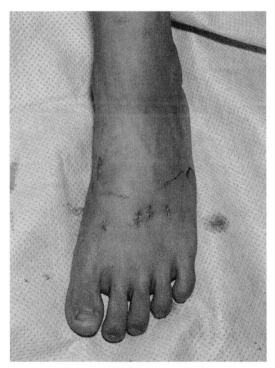

Fig. 13. In this case, in an adolescent with open growth plates, wires and a single Lisfranc screw were used as definitive fixation. The wires were buried under the skin, which was closed with simple skin sutures and later removed after 8 weeks.

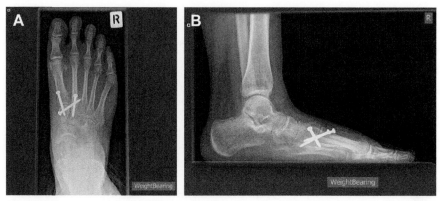

Fig. 14. Follow-up weight-bearing AP (*A*) and lateral (*B*) radiographs showing the configuration of screws at the Lisfranc joint complex after percutaneous fixation of the first and second rays.

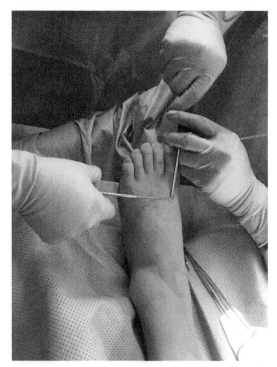

Fig. 15. Screw removal can be accomplished percutaneously through the old scars. The screw heads are usually palpable and easily removed or fluoroscopy can be used to find the screw heads if necessary.

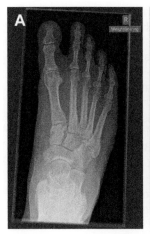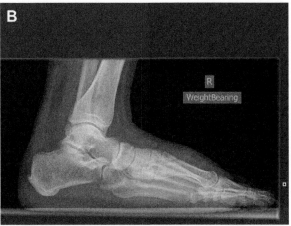

Fig. 16. Weight-bearing AP (*A*) and lateral (*B*) radiographs 9 months after a Lisfranc injury treated percutaneously showing maintenance of anatomic reduction after screw removal.

SUMMARY

The authors have used this technique in a few suitable patients and have been generally satisfied with the results, although long-term follow-up is not yet available. No patient so far has lost reduction or required an arthrodesis as a secondary procedure.

The authors emphasize that not all Lisfranc injury patterns are suitable for percutaneous fixation and this is an area that needs to be more clearly defined. Obtaining an anatomic reduction is paramount to the success of treatment, and this has been borne out by most long-term studies analyzing the results of Lisfranc injuries.[4,18] In the authors' experience, an anatomic reduction is usually achievable by closed means other than in the grossly unstable injury types. If an anatomic reduction is not obtainable, then open reduction is mandatory.

Future developments may include a better understanding of the indications for these techniques as well as more precise ability to assess intraoperative reduction and fixation of the injuries with new imaging techniques.

REFERENCES

1. Cassebaum WH. Lisfranc fracture-dislocations. Clin Orthop Relat Res 1963;30: 116–29.
2. Hardcastle PH, Reschauer R, Kutscha-Lissberg E, et al. Injuries to the tarsometatarsal joint: incidence, classification and treatment. J Bone Joint Surg Br 1982; 64(3):349–56.
3. Welck MJ, Zinchenko R, Rudge B. Lisfranc injuries. Injury 2015;46(4):536–41.
4. Thompson MC, Mormino MA. Injury to the tarsometatarsal joint complex. J Am Acad Orthop Surg 2003;11:260–7.
5. Stavlas P, Roberts CS, Xypnitos FN, et al. The role of reduction and internal fixation of Lisfranc fracture-dislocations: a systematic review of the literature. Int Orthop 2010;34(8):1083–91.
6. Aronow MS. Treatment of the missed Lisfranc injury. Foot Ankle Clin 2006;11(1): 127–42.
7. Myerson MS. The diagnosis and treatment of injury to the tarsometatarsal joint complex. J Bone Joint Surg Br 1999;81(5):756–63.

8. Arntz CT, Veith RG, Hansen ST. Fractures and fracture-dislocations of the tarso-metatarsal joint. J Bone Joint Surg Am 1988;70:173–81.

9. Henning JA, Jones CB, Sietsema DL, et al. Open reduction internal fixation versus primary arthrodesis for Lisfranc injuries: a prospective randomized study. Foot Ankle Int 2009;30:913–22.

10. Kuo RS, Tejwani NC, Digiovanni CW, et al. Outcome after open reduction and internal fixation of Lisfranc joint injuries. J Bone Joint Surg Am 2000;82-A:1609–18.

11. Ly TV, Coetzee JC. Treatment of primarily ligamentous Lisfranc joint injuries: primary arthrodesis compared with open reduction and internal fixation. A prospective, randomized study. J Bone Joint Surg Am 2006;88:514–20.

12. Rajapakse B, Edwards A, Hong T. A single surgeon's experience of treatment of Lisfranc joint injuries. Injury 2006;37:914–21.

13. Rammelt S, Schneiders W, Schikore H, et al. Primary open reduction and fixation compared with delayed corrective arthrodesis in the treatment of tarsometatarsal (Lisfranc) fracture dislocation. J Bone Joint Surg Br 2008;90(11):1499–506.

14. Watson TS, Shurnas PS, Denker J. Treatment of Lisfranc joint injury: current concepts. J Am Acad Orthop Surg 2010;18:718–28.

15. Mulier T, Reynders P, Dereymaeker G, et al. Severe Lisfrancs injuries: primary arthrodesis or ORIF? Foot Ankle Int 2002;23:902–5.

16. Ruedi TP, Buckley RE, Moran CG. AO philosophy and evolution. In: Ruedi TP, Buckley RE, Moran CG, editors. AO principles of fracture management, 2nd expanded edition. New York: AO Publishing; Thieme; 2007. p. 1–7.

17. Perugia D, Basile A, Battaglia A, et al. Fracture dislocations of Lisfranc's joint treated with closed reduction and percutaneous fixation. Int Orthop 2003;27: 30–5.

18. Richter M, Wipperman B, Krettek C, et al. Fractures and fracture dislocations of the midfoot: occurrence, causes and long term results. Foot Ankle Int 2001;22: 392–8.

19. Desmond EA, Chou LB. Current concepts review: Lisfranc injuries. Foot Ankle Int 2006;27(8):653–60.

20. Mantas JP, Burks RT. Lisfranc injuries in the athlete. Clin Sports Med 1994;13(4): 719–30.

21. Van Rijn J, Dorleijn DM, Boetes B, et al. Missing the Lisfranc fracture: a case report and review of the literature. J Foot Ankle Surg 2012;51(2):270–4.

22. Myerson MS, Fisher RT, Burgess AR, et al. Fracture dislocations of the tarsometatarsal joints: end results correlated with pathology and treatment. Foot Ankle 1986;6(5):225–42.

23. Tarczynska M, Gaweda K, Dajewski Z, et al. Comparison of treatment results of acute and late injures of the lisfranc joint. Acta Orthop Bras 2013;21(6):344–6.

24. Hatem SF, Davis A, Sundaram M. Your diagnosis? Midfoot sprain: Lisfranc ligament disruption. Orthopaedics 2005;28(1):2, 75–7.

25. Myerson MS, Cerrato RA. Current management of tarsometatarsal injuries in the athlete. J Bone Joint Surg Am 2008;90(11):2522–33.

26. Wiley JJ. The mechanism of tarsometatarsal joint injuries. J Bone Joint Surg Br 1971;53(3):474–82.

27. Scolaro J, Ahn J, Mehta S. Lisfranc fracture dislocations. Clin Orthop Relat Res 2011;469(7):2078–80.

28. Komenda GA, Myerson MS, Biddinger KR. Results of arthrodesis of the tarsometatarsal joints after traumatic injury. J Bone Joint Surg Am 1996;78(11):1665–76.

29. Goosens M, De Stoop N. Lisfranc's fracture-dislocations: Etiology, radiology, and results of treatment. A review of 20 cases. Clin Orthop Relat Res 1983;176: 154–62.

30. Sarrafian S. Synesmology. In: Sarrafian SK, editor. Anatomy of the foot and ankle: descriptive, topographic, functional. 2nd edition. Philadelphia: Lippincott; 1993. p. 204–7.

31. de Palma L, Santucci A, Sabetta SP, et al. Anatomy of the Lisfranc joint complex. Foot Ankle Int 1997;18(6):356–64.

32. Solan MC, Moorman CT III, Miyamoto RG, et al. Ligamentous restraints of the second tarsometatarsal joint: a biomechanical evaluation. Foot Ankle Int 2001; 22(8):637–41.

33. Panchbhavi VK, Molina D 4th, Villarreal J, et al. Three-dimensional, digital, and gross anatomy of the Lisfranc ligament. Foot Ankle Int 2013;34(6):876–80.

34. Johnson A, Hill K, Ward J, et al. Anatomy of the lisfranc ligament. Foot Ankle Spec 2008;1(1):19–23.

35. Ross G, Cronin R, Hauzenblas J. Plantar ecchymosis sign: a clinical aid to diagnosis of occult Lisfranc tarsometatarsal injuries. J Orthop Trauma 1996;10(2): 119–22.

36. Davies MS, Saxby TS. Intercuneiform instability and the "gap" sign. Foot Ankle Int 1999;20(9):606–9.

37. Ashworth MJ, Davies MB, Williamson DM. Irreducible Lisfranc's injury: the "toe up" sign. Injury 1997;28(4):321–2.

38. Karaindros K, Arealis G, Papanikolaou A, et al. Irreducible Lisfranc dislocation due to interposition of the tibialis anterior tendon: case report and literature review. Foot Ankle Surg 2010;16(3):e68–71.

39. Curtis MJ, Myerson M, Szura B. Tarsometatarsal joint injuries in the athlete. Am J Sports Med 1993;21(4):497–502.

40. Fakhouri AJ, Manoli A 2nd. Acute foot compartment syndromes. J Orthop Trauma 1992;6(2):223–8.

41. Nunley JA, Vertullo CJ. Classification, investigation, and management of midfoot sprains: Lisfranc injuries in the athlete. Am J Sports Med 2002;30(6):871–8.

42. Gupta RT, Wadhwa RP, Learch TJ, et al. Lisfranc injury: imaging findings for this important but often-missed diagnosis. Curr Probl Diagn Radiol 2008;37:115–26.

43. Faciszewski T, Burks RT, Manaster BJ. Subtle injuries of the Lisfranc joint. J Bone Joint Surg Am 1990;72(10):1519–22.

44. Foster SC, Foster RR. Lisfranc's tarsometatarsal fracture-dislocation. Radiology 1976;120(1):79–83.

45. Norfray JF, Geline RA, Steinberg RI, et al. Subtleties of Lisfranc fracture-dislocations. AJR Am J Roentgenol 1981;137:1151–6.

46. Hatem SF. Imaging of Lisfranc injury and midfoot sprain. Radiol Clin N Am 2008; 46:1045–60.

47. Goiney RC, Connell DG, Nichols DM. CT evaluation of tarsometatarsal fracture-dislocation injuries. AJR 1985;144:985–90.

48. Kaar S, Femino J, Morag Y. Lisfranc joint displacement following sequential ligament sectioning. J Bone Joint Surg Am 2007;89:2225–32.

49. Coss HS, Manos RE, Buoncristiani A, et al. Abduction stress and AP weightbearing radiography of purely ligamentous injury in the tarsometatarsal joint. Foot Ankle Int 1998;19:537–41.

50. Preidler KW, Peicha G, Lajtai G, et al. Conventional radiography, CT, and MR imaging in patients with hyperflexion injuries of the foot: diagnostic accuracy in the

detection of bony and ligamentous changes. AJR Am J Roentgenol 1999;173: 1673–7.

51. Seybold JD, Coetzee JC. Lisfranc injuries: when to observe, fix or fuse. Clin Sports Med 2015;34:705–23.

52. Haapamaki V, Kiuru M, Koskinen S. Lisfranc fracture-dislocation in patients with multiple trauma: diagnosis with multidetector computed tomography. Foot Ankle Int 2004;25:614–9.

53. Lu J, Ebraheim NA, Skie M, et al. Radographic and computed tomographic evaluation of Lisfranc dislocations: a cadaver study. Foot Ankle Int 1997;18:351–5.

54. Preidler KW, Brossman J, Daenen B, et al. Tarsometatarsal joint: anatomic details on MR images. Radiology 1996;199:733–6.

55. Preidler KW, Brossman J, Daenen B, et al. MR imaging of the tarsometatarsal joint: analysis of injuries in 11 patients. AJR 1996;267:1217–22.

56. Quenu E, Kuss G. Etude sur les luxations du metatarse (luxations metatarsotarsiennes) du diastasis entre le 1er et le 2e metatarsien. Rev Chir 1909;39:281–336, 720–91, 1093–134.

57. Hunt SA, Ropiak C, Tejwani NC. Lisfranc joint injuries: diagnosis and treatment. Am J Orthop 2006;35:376–85.

58. Loveday D, Robinson A. Lisfranc injuries. Br J Hosp Med 2008;69:399–402.

59. Perez Blanco R, Rodriguez Merchan C, Canosa Sevillano R, et al. Tarsometatarsal fractures and dislocations. J Orthop Trauma 1988;2:188–94.

60. Sheibani-Rad S, Coetzee JC, Givenas MR, et al. Arthrodesis versus ORIF for Lisfranc fractures. Orthopedics 2012;35(6):e868–73.

61. Tan YH, Chin TW, Mitra AK, et al. Tarsometatarsal (Lisfranc's) injuries – results of open reduction and internal fixation. Ann Acad Med Singapore 1995;24:816–9.

62. Teng AL, Pinzur MS, Lomasney L, et al. Functional outcome following anatomic restoration of tarsal-metatarsal fracture dislocation. Foot Ankle Int 2002;23:922–6.

63. Kadakia AR, Myerson MR. Percutaneous reduction and internal fixation of the Lisfranc fracture-dislocation. In: Scuderi GR, Tria AJ, editors. Minimally invasive surgery in orthopaedics. New York: Springer; 2010. p. 371–6.

Syndesmosis Stabilisation: Screws Versus Flexible Fixation

Matthew C. Solan, FRCS(Tr&Orth)[a,b,*], Mark S. Davies, FRCS(Tr&Orth)[a],
Anthony Sakellariou, FRCS(Tr&Orth)[b]

KEYWORDS

- Ankle • Syndesmosis • Injury • TightRope

KEY POINTS

- There is a wide variety of ankle injuries involving the distal tibiofibular syndesmosis.
- Appreciation of the injury severity and type of instability should guide treatment.
- Fixation of posterior malleolar fractures restores considerable stability to the syndesmosis, so additional fixation between the tibia and the fibula may not be required.
- Flexible fixation may not be sufficiently rigid where axial instability (shortening) is marked.

INTRODUCTION

Orthopedic and trauma surgery is not short of situations where there is controversy regarding the optimum management. The treatment of ankle syndesmosis injuries is certainly an example where practice varies widely and where there are many questions that are still not satisfactorily answered. These can be grouped into categories:

How are subtle injuries best identified and classified?
Which injuries require stabilization?
What type of stabilization is best?
Should hardware be removed routinely and, if so, when?

This article focuses on the second and third of these 4 categories.

Disclosure Statement: Drs M.C. Solan and A. Sakellariou run a Training Fellowship with support from Zimmer-Biomet; M.C. Solan is a member of the Zimmer-Biomet Speakers Bureau. Dr M.S. Davies has nothing to disclose.
[a] London Foot and Ankle Centre, Hospital of St John and St Elizabeth, 60 Grove End Road, London NW8 9NH, UK; [b] Surrey Foot and Ankle Clinic, Mount Alvernia Hospital, Harvey Road, Guildford, Surrey, GU1 3LX, UK
* Corresponding author.
E-mail address: Matthewsolan1@aol.com

Foot Ankle Clin N Am 22 (2017) 35–63
http://dx.doi.org/10.1016/j.fcl.2016.09.004
1083-7515/17/© 2016 Elsevier Inc. All rights reserved.

Foot and Ankle Clinics has published 8 articles relating to the injured syndesmosis since 2000.[1–8] These are all well worth reading and, in the interests of avoiding duplication, some of the introductory paragraphs in this paper are relatively brief.

Obviously, one more review publication will not clear up all the questions that practicing surgeons face, but in this article we aim to provide an up to date and logical approach to the injured syndesmosis and look particularly at when fixation is required (and when it is not), as well as the role of flexible suture–button devices as opposed to traditional screw stabilization.

ANATOMY AND BIOMECHANICS

The ankle mortise is formed by the distal tibia and fibula. The precise relationship between these 2 bones is critical for function of the ankle joint.[9,10] This is maintained by the ligaments of the distal tibiofibular joint and the interosseous membrane. If the relationship is disturbed, then there is potential for instability of the talus within the mortise.

The "Rule of Threes"

The ankle joint has 3 surgically important groups of ligaments. Each can be considered to have 3 components (**Fig. 1**):

1. The lateral ligament group includes the anterior talofibular ligament, the posterior talofibular ligament, and the calcaneofibular ligament.
2. Medially, the deltoid has both a superficial and 2 deep parts (anterior and posterior).
3. Although more complex classifications have been described, it is sufficient, from the point of view of surgical anatomy, to think of the syndesmosis as also comprising 3 structures: the anterior inferior tibiofibular ligament (AITFL), the interosseous ligament, and the posterior inferior tibiofibular ligament (PITFL).

The syndesmotic ligaments ensure that the 3 facets of the distal tibiofibular joint are aligned. The joint can then function properly and move in 3 planes as well as rotating (potentially, after fracture, around 3 axes).

Ankle dorsiflexion has been shown to result in proximal and posterior translation as well as external rotation of the fibula. When the ankle is subjected to external rotation

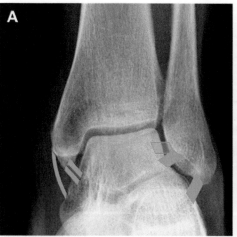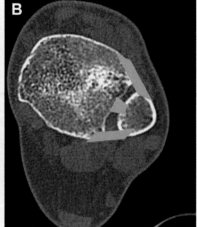

Fig. 1. (*A, B*) Anatomy of the ankle mortise.

forces, then, along with external rotation of the fibula, there is associated posterior and medial translation.

There are 3 eponymous bony fragments that are important. An AITFL injury may lead to an avulsion fracture, from either the tibia or the fibula, rather than ligament disruption. These avulsion fractures are named Tillaux-Chaput (tibial avulsion) or Wagstaff-LeFort (fibular avulsion) fractures. They are relatively rare beyond adolescence[11] but in children, the Salter-Harris type III Tillaux fracture is classically seen. Injury to the PITFL complex in adults more commonly involves the bony attachment, producing a posterior malleolus (PM) fracture (Volkmann fragment) of variable size. Where there is a posterior malleolar fracture, it has been shown in MRI studies that the PITFL is always intact. There is no eponym for a posterior fibula avulsion of the PITFL attachment (see **Fig. 1**).

PATHOMECHANICS

There are 3 common situations in which the syndesmosis is compromised: pronation external rotation fractures, supination external rotation fractures, and purely ligamentous injuries.

Pronation External Rotation Fractures

Pronation injuries (Weber C fibula fractures) are those that are most commonly associated with syndesmosis injury (**Fig. 2**). Because these injuries start on the medial side of the ankle, with the deltoid ligament under tension, there is joint instability as soon as the syndesmosis is disrupted (pronation external rotation [PER] stage 2). The fibula fracture (Stage 3) may be just above the level of the syndesmosis, in the fibular diaphysis, or, more proximal, at the fibula neck (Maisonneuve fracture). The Lauge-Hansen classification is far from perfect,[12] but remains a useful tool in the analysis of ankle injuries.[13] Fracture dislocations are the most unstable variant and have been shown to have a worse prognosis, owing to articular surface damage, even when the subsequent syndesmosis reduction is good.[14] A study from the Hospital for Special Surgery in New York found that the rate of syndesmosis malreduction in PER injuries was 40%, whereas it was 18% in injuries where the supinated foot is subject to an external rotation force (SER).[15] They recommend heightened awareness of the potential for malreduction in PER-type fractures.

Supination External Rotation Fractures

The most common ankle injuries are, when classified according to the Lauge-Hansen system, SER injuries (**Fig. 3**). In these circumstances, the lateral structures are in tension and therefore injured first. Stage I is rupture of the lower part of the AITFL. Next an oblique fibula fracture, typically "at the level of the syndesmosis" (Weber B). A small proportion of Weber C fractures are, however, also supination injuries.[16] The amount of AITFL that remains intact is variable and, with it, the potential for syndesmosis instability varies as well. Syndesmosis instability is more prevalent in SER injuries than is widely believed, as Stark and colleagues[17] demonstrated. Their study found that 39% of SER fractures with deltoid ligament rupture showed diastasis on stress testing. Intraoperative stress testing of all Weber B fractures has been recommended. Randomised studies show, however, no advantage in terms of patient outcome if syndesmosis screw fixation is used as an adjunct for cases where examination under anesthesia shows syndesmosis widening. In a properly randomized clinical trial, 140 patients with SER4 fractures were subjected to a standardized stress test after fixation of the fibula. If the syndesmosis widened by at least 2 mm, subjects were randomized

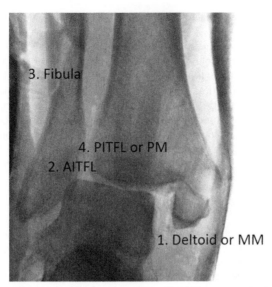

Fig. 2. Lauge-Hansen pronation external rotation 1 to 4. AITFL, anterior inferior tibiofibular ligament; MM, medial malleolus; PITFL, posterior inferior tibiofibular ligament; PM, posterior malleolus.

to either single screw syndesmosis fixation or to no additional treatment. Seventeen percent of the whole cohort exhibited positive findings during stress testing. These cases were randomized to syndesmosis screw or no additional fixation. At medium term follow-up (an average of 4 years), there were no clinical or radiologic (including MRI) differences between the 2 groups.[18–20]

Purely Ligamentous Injuries

Syndesmotic ligament injury can occur in other circumstances, not included in either the Weber or the Lauge-Hansen classification systems **(Fig. 4)**.[21] Forced dorsiflexion of the ankle may produce an AITFL tear without significant deltoid injury. This

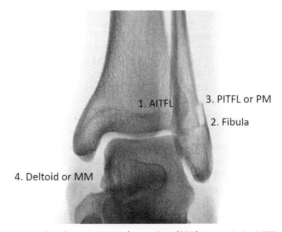

Fig. 3. Lauge-Hansen supination – external rotation (SER) types 1–4. AITFL, anterior inferior tibiofibular ligament; MM, medial malleolus; PITFL, posterior inferior tibiofibular ligament; PM, posterior malleolus.

mechanism does not fit neatly into the Lauge-Hansen classification and yet is a relatively common sports injury. The West Point Grading system[22,23] is the best known method for classifying stability after purely ligamentous injury to the syndesmosis. This system however, predates the availability of routine MRI scanning and does not, arguably, contain a sufficient number of "grades." In particular, the West Point grade 2 injury of "latent instability" is a heterogeneous group.

DEGREES OF INSTABILITY

When considering the mechanisms discussed, it should be appreciated that the degree of ankle instability is greatly variable. At one end of the injury spectrum is an AITFL sprain in an otherwise stable ankle joint, whereas at the other extreme, is a fracture–dislocation of the ankle with a high fibula fracture. The former is, at worst, subtly unstable with forced external rotation of the foot. The latter is unstable in all directions (**Fig. 5**). When considering the type of syndesmosis stabilization that is required, it is essential to ascertain the extent of the instability. Only then can a logical approach to stabilizing the ankle mortise be achieved.

Zones of Injury

When distilled down to basic components, the stability of the ankle mortise depends on 3 zones of injury:

Structures on the medial side (medial malleolus or deltoid ligament),
The syndesmosis (ligaments and their bony attachments), and
The fibula (fracture level and pattern).

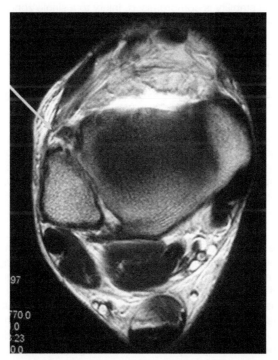

Fig. 4. MRI scan of an anterior inferior tibiofibular ligament tear without medial injury (hyperdorsiflexion injury; *arrow*).

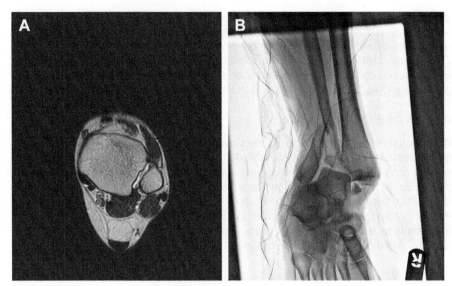

Fig. 5. (*A*) Stable anterior inferior tibiofibular ligament sprain (minimal rotational instability) versus (*B*) fracture dislocation (multiple planes of instability).

The order in which these 3 structures are injured varies according to the mechanism of injury. Pronation injuries begin with damage to the medial zone. In supination injuries, the medial structures are the final part to be damaged. When more than 1 zone is injured, then stability is compromised. Injury to a single zone does not render the ankle unstable.

Fracture Patterns

With Weber C (or Pronation External Rotation [PER]) injuries all 3 zones are involved. Weber type B fractures occur as the second stage of SER injuries. Two zones are involved in lower grades of SER injury, 3 zones once the medial side (SER4, last to be injured) is involved.

Ligament Injuries

With purely ligamentous damage, an athlete who sustains a rotation injury causing AITFL sprain is very likely to have an injury to the deltoid ligament also (2 zones). However, if the AITFL sprain was caused through a hyperdorsiflexion injury, then the medial side can be relatively spared (only 1 zone affected).

MISSED INJURY

Injury to the ankle that results in a widened ankle mortise and incongruent tibiotalar joint leads to abnormal mechanics, joint degeneration, pain, swelling, and reduced function. It is disappointing that so many injuries are still misdiagnosed. Swelling above the level of the malleoli should prompt a thorough assessment to ensure that the syndesmosis is not injured. There is no single clinical test that is sufficiently reliable to diagnose syndesmosis injury, and plain radiographic measurements to assess the position of the fibula relative to the tibia are unreliable. The threshold for axial imaging should therefore be low. Emergency department radiographs should, if radiographs of a very swollen ankle show no fractures of the malleoli, be extended to include the whole fibula. This will prevent a Maisonneuve fracture being missed (**Fig. 6**).

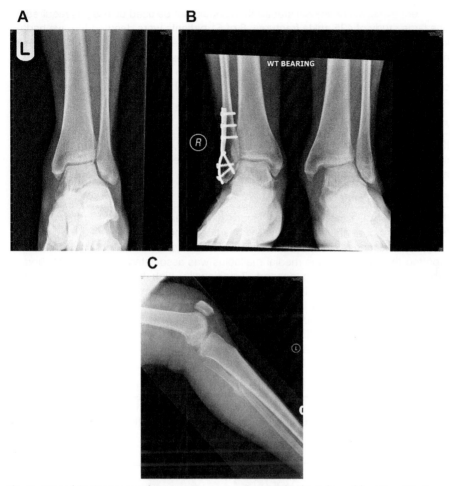

Fig. 6. Missed Maisonneuve fracture, presenting late with tibiotalar subluxation (*B*). Proximal Xray (*C*) shows the fibula fracture that is not evident on the inadequate radiograph taken at the time of injury (*A*).

SURGICAL STRATEGY

Restoring bony anatomy and strength is more reliable than ligament repair and should be the primary consideration when planning surgical reconstruction of ankle fractures. Ideally, all 3 zones should be addressed but, if there is a very high fibula fracture or if there is no medial malleolar (MM) fracture, this is difficult to achieve.

Judicious Use of Syndesmosis Hardware

The published literature shows that patients with ankle fractures where syndesmosis hardware has been used, fare less well than those with fractures where such fixation was not used.[24] In the absence of a controlled study, where injury severity is matched, it is difficult to be sure whether the syndesmosis hardware (or associated slower rehabilitation) directly causes a poor result or whether there is selection bias. It may be that only the more severe injuries were treated with syndesmosis stabilization. A randomized, controlled study to answer this question would be difficult to undertake.

Nevertheless, syndesmosis stabilization should not be used unless it is required. In one large study of 425 ankle fractures, 8 of 51 patients were deemed to have had no indication for the syndesmosis screws that were used.[25] Syndesmosis hardware is, however, appropriate for a proportion of ankle injuries. When it is required, a syndesmosis screw should be used properly, engaging both cortices of the fibula and then 1 or 2 cortices of the tibia. Two radiographic views should be taken in the operating room to check screw placement (**Fig. 7**).

Fibula and Medial Zone Fixation

If medial and fibula zone fractures are both stabilised, then the likelihood of additional syndesmosis fixation being required is reduced. Every opportunity to fix the medial and fibula zone fractures should be taken.

Fixation of the Fibula

It was shown by Chissell and Jones[26] more than 20 years ago that the further the fibula fracture lies above the level of the syndesmosis, the greater the need for position screw stabilization of the tibiofibular joint in Weber type C fractures. The same study reported that fixation of the medial malleolus was associated with less likelihood of syndesmosis fixation being needed. Traditionally, high fibula fractures have not been fixed, with a reliance instead placed on position screw(s) for the syndesmosis alone. However, fractures in the middle and distal thirds of the bone are readily amenable to surgical stabilization and this is extremely worthwhile. Once fixed, both length and rotation of the fibula are restored precisely. The fibula fixation prevents shortening and provides resistance to lateral, anteroposterior (AP) and rotational displacement.

Medial Side

In SER injuries, an unstable SER4 can be rendered (much more) stable by fixation of the MM fracture alone. This is particularly true where the MM is a large fragment. A

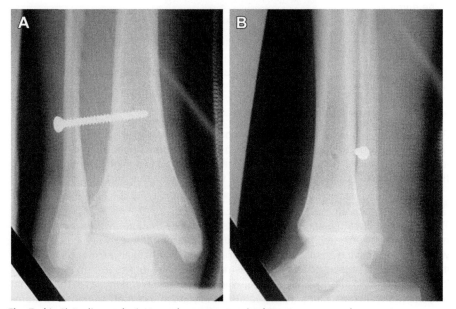

Fig. 7. (A, B) Radiographs in two planes are required to assess screw placement.

small MM fracture (anterior colliculus fracture) is associated with injury to the posterior part of the deep deltoid ligament. When the MM fragment is relatively small, fixation is not only more demanding technically but, because of the associated deltoid injury, the resultant stability is also less complete. Converting an SER4 to an SER2 by fixation of the (large) MM fracture is a useful strategy if, for example, lateral soft tissues mean that fibula fixation is relatively contraindicated. Conceptually, once the MM is fixed, the injury is then stable. Tornetta and colleagues[27] showed that, if the medial malleolus is fixed first and the ankle then subjected to an external rotation stress test before fibula fixation, the ankle is seen to be stable with no talar shift. This is not true when the MM only involves the anterior colliculus, because of the associated rupture of the posterior part of the deep deltoid ligament. In PER injuries, a large, well-fixed medial malleolus fracture ensures that the talus is well-positioned beneath the tibial plafond. Deltoid ligament disruption, instead of medial malleolus fracture, means that there is greater reliance on fibula zone and syndesmosis zone fixation for stability. Deltoid ligament repair in these circumstances is logical, but how much strength is restored by suturing the damaged deltoid is not well-understood. Laboratory studies have demonstrated that deltoid and AITFL repair is initially as strong as a single syndesmosis screw.[28] However, further clinical studies are required before this technique is widely adopted.

Syndesmosis Zone

Tillaux or Wagstaff fracture
Avulsion fractures of the AITFL attachment sites are a surgical bonus. The opportunity to reduce and fix them should be welcomed. Anatomic restoration will ensure that the length, rotation, and AP displacement of the fibula are perfect. Tillaux fractures are, however, more common in children[29] and only rarely seen in conjunction with posterior malleolar fractures.[11]

Posterior malleolus fixation
The surgical "generalist" is often reluctant to reduce and fix a PM fracture. "It's less than 25% of the articular surface" is perhaps the most widely used excuse for not fixing this important component of ankle fractures. There is no evidence in the literature to support this assumption. The statement misses the important point regarding the PITFL, which is intact where there is a PM fracture, just as the AITFL is intact with a Tillaux fracture. Fixation of the PM ensures, via the PITFL, that the fibula is restored to its anatomic length. Furthermore, the PITFL provides 70% of the strength of the syndesmosis according to laboratory studies.[30,31] Clinical studies have shown that fixing the PM is as effective as screw fixation of the syndesmosis, when postoperative computed tomography (CT) scans and 12-month outcome scores are reviewed.[32] There is, therefore, a very strong argument for reducing and fixing the PM fracture, irrespective of the extent of articular surface involvement, whether this is 5%, 25%, or 35%. Sadly, even when the fracture is treated surgically, there is an inexplicable tendency to try to "lag the body onto the small fragment" with a percutaneous screw from the front of the tibia into the PM fragment.[33] This technique defies all the principles of fracture fixation and adequate reduction is seldom achieved. Familiarity with the posterolateral approach to the ankle[34] is all that is required to allow a buttress plate or PA lag screw to secure the Volkmann fragment. Once the PM is reduced and fixed then length, antero-posterior (AP) and medio-lateral (ML) position and rotation of the fibula are correct. If the fibula has been internally fixed too then, despite AITFL and interosseous ligament injury, the syndesmosis is likely to show no widening on stress testing. The bony versus ligamentous nature of any medial zone injury determines

whether this contributes to overall construct stability or not. Where MM stabilisation is possible, along with fibula and PM fixation, the construct is highly stable and a syndesmosis position screw unlikely to confer any extra advantage.

Open Technique for Syndesmosis Reduction

Malreduction of the syndesmosis is associated with poor outcome (**Fig. 8**).[35] AP displacement is hard to detect on radiographs. Intraoperative 3-dimensional imaging has been advocated,[36] but is not available routinely[37] and does not always serve to reduce the incidence of malreduction.[38] Shortening of the fibula is poorly tolerated but still commonly seen.[39] If Tillaux or PM fractures are reduced and fixed, then the fibular position will be restored more accurately. However, even when the syndesmosis injury includes bony avulsion fractures, proper reduction of the distal tibiofibular joint is difficult to be certain about.[37] Standard fluoroscopy is unreliable.[40] Until validated fluoroscopic measurements are proven to be reliable or, intraoperative CT scanning becomes commonplace, surgeons should have a low threshold for visualizing the inferior tibiofibular joint with an anterolateral incision to check reduction.[41] Sagi and colleagues,[35] in a study using CT and clinical follow-up at a minimum of 2 years from fracture fixation, showed that this strategy produces significant improvements in the reduction of the syndesmosis.

Checking for Adequacy and Maintenance of Reduction

Plain radiologic parameters are not accurate for either the diagnosis of syndesmosis injury or for confirming reduction intraoperatively. Postoperative plain radiographs will not, therefore, show whether the surgical treatment has achieved proper reduction. For assessing reduction postoperatively, CT scans should be routinely used,[42] although which measurements are the most reliable is debated.[43] There are published protocols for doing this with a minimum of radiation.[44] The advantages of routinely using postoperative CT to promote better outcomes and to inform personal surgical reflection are well worth the time and costs involved.[41]

Warner and colleagues[45] studied 155 ankle fractures requiring syndesmosis fixation and used a variety of indices to quantify reduction, compared with the normal contralateral ankle, with CT scans. The mean displacement measurements ranged from 1.32 to 1.88 mm, according to which measurement technique was used. Malrotation averaged 5.75°. The clinical scores did not correlate with the degree of malreduction. This casts doubt on the importance of perfect reduction. However, this cohort of patients

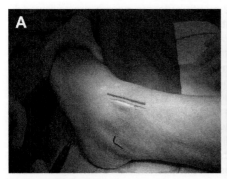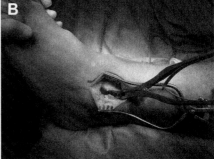

Fig. 8. (A, B) Exposure for open syndesmosis reduction.

all had relatively well-reduced syndesmoses and clinical scores were, at a minimum of 12 months, relatively short term.

FLEXIBLE STABILIZATION OF THE SYNDESMOSIS
Problems with Screw Fixation

When screws are used to manage syndesmosis instability, the small amount of normal physiologic motion between the tibia and the fibula is abolished. This allows the syndesmotic ligaments to heal. The screw may then be removed with a small second surgical procedure, or left to fatigue and eventually break under the repetitive strain that movement induces when the ankle is loaded. Opinions vary with regard to screw removal[46–55] and this topic is not discussed further.

Open Reduction and Internal Fixation: Reduction Before Fixation

When trying to choose between rigid screw fixation, or a Tightrope (Arthrex, Naples, Fl) or similar device, it is important to remember that this decision means nothing, in terms of eventual outcome, if the syndesmosis is not reduced properly. Accurate reduction of the fibula should restore length and rotation, but this is not always achieved (**Fig. 9**). The AP and ML position of the fibula at the incisura also needs addressing. Intraoperative fluoroscopy is not a reliable way to judge this, although recent studies are helping to standardize measurements.[56] Radiologic studies outside of the operating room have shown that more than 3 mm of displacement is needed before detection on plain films. Intraoperative CT scans are not available widely. Fixation of a PM or Tillaux fracture "guarantees" that the fibula is in the right place.

Is Anything Needed at All?

As emphasized already, there are good reasons to avoid "unnecessary" fixation of the syndesmosis. Also, fixation between the tibia and the fibula can be associated with poor outcomes. Rehabilitation will probably take longer, not least because a second

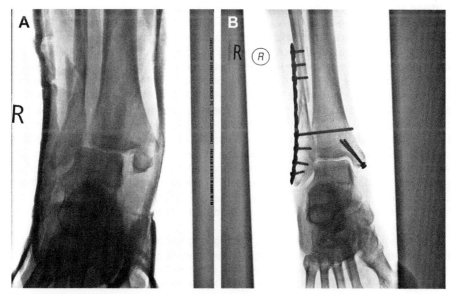

Fig. 9. (A, B) Fibula fracture inadequately reduced.

operation may be required to remove the hardware. If the hardware is not removed electively, it may require removal later, if it becomes prominent or broken.

It was the combined issues of hardware removal and the abolition of physiologic motion at the tibiofibular joint, caused by screw fixation, that led to the development of flexible options. The device in most common use is the TightRope. This is a modified suture button that uses a fiber wire suture to provide stability to the syndesmosis. Similar devices have been used to stabilize acromioclavicular ligament injuries, Lisfranc ligament disruption,[57] and, more controversially, to close the intermetatarsal angle in hallux valgus correction.[58] This list of uses of the device is not exhaustive.

Flexible System

The first publication regarding the TightRope system for the fixation of the tibiofibular joint was in 2003.[59] The aim was to restore stability to the syndesmosis without abolishing physiologic motion. It was postulated that this low-profile hardware would not need to be removed. The cadaver study showed that TightRope and screw fixation had equivalent resistance to external rotation torque.

There are earlier reported examples of flexible syndesmosis stabilisation,[60] but the Tightrope device is the product most widely used and investigated. It is elegant in design, easy to use and for some surgeons it has become an indispensable part of their "toolkit".

Laboratory Studies

Laboratory tests other than the originators' study have also shown that resistance to external rotation and widening of the syndesmosis is good. Ebramzadeh and colleagues[61] compared the TightRope with ZipTight and screw constructs in a cadaveric study and concluded that all 3 methods provided sufficient stability to resist the loads expected within a cast. Only 1 study shows that the TightRope is less effective than screw fixation at maintaining reduction of the syndesmosis.[62] The same study found that load to failure was higher when compared with screw fixation. Screw construct failure, owing to fibula fracture, may have been influenced by low bone mineral density in the cadaver specimens. In a different study, cyclical loading of paired specimens showed that the TightRope allowed more sagittal plane movement than intact specimens. Screw fixation reduced the measured motion when compared with intact ankles.[63]

As is true in all areas of orthopedic surgery, "strong enough is strong enough" and the temptation to always use the very strongest construct should be avoided. A Weber type B fibula fracture does not routinely require a low contact dynamic compression plate to buttress the fracture or to neutralize the forces remaining after lag screw fixation, since a one-third tubular plate is sufficiently strong for these purposes. Biomechanical testing of the syndesmosis has shown that, when paired specimens are tested with a cyclical loading regimen, 2 quadricortical screws are just as effective as a locked plate construct (2 screws passing through a locked plate and then through 4 cortices). Because the plate-augmented construct had a higher load to failure (in external rotation) the authors concluded that the plate augmentation was "better," but this laboratory difference is unlikely to have any clinical relevance.[64] The costs of a locked plate and screw system compared with 2 nonlocking screws was not discussed.

There are no biomechanical studies investigating the use of 2 TightRopes, although this is a method used in clinical practice. Sometimes, surgeons use 1 TightRope and 1 screw (**Fig. 10**). When the screw is removed, the TightRope ensures no late widening of the syndesmosis. Whether this is really the best of both worlds or just a reflection of the level of confusion surrounding this topic is not clear.

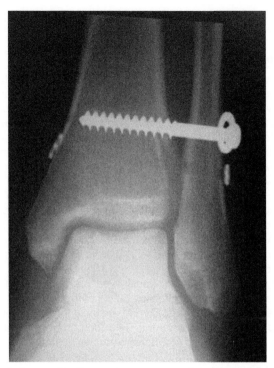

Fig. 10. Hybrid technique, reflecting controversy over screw vs tightrope fixation.

Clinical cohort studies

Early case series of clinical outcomes using the TightRope instead of screw fixation showed promising results. A comparative series from the developer found rapid recovery and the need for no implant removal in 16 patients compared with a (nonrandomized) control group who had screw fixation. CT scans were used to confirm that reduction was maintained 3 months after surgery.[65]

Cottom and colleagues[66] reviewed 25 cases at an average of 10.8 months from surgery. Clinical scores and plain radiograph analysis were both considered to be more than satisfactory. The same group later published results in 37 patient in whom 64 tightropes were used to treat a wide range of syndesmosis injuries, including 4 Maisonneuve fractures.[67] It is not clear whether this larger group included longer follow-up of the initial cohort of patients or not. Low complication rates and infrequent implant removal (6.25%) were reported, although 19% experienced knot irritation.

A small study from 2015 compared 2 cohorts of injuries, 17 with a single 4 cortices screw and 15 with TightRope fixation. They noted statistically better dorsiflexion and plantarflexion movement in the TightRope group but no difference in American Orthopaedic Foot and Ankle Society (AOFAS) scores.[68]

Systematic review

In 2012, Scheppers published a systematic review of the literature pertaining to the use of the TightRope. Relevant studies from 2000 to 2011 were included. The implant removal rate was 10% for those treated with the TightRope and 51.9% with screw fixation. The AOFAS scores were not different between the 2 groups. In their concluding comments, the authors noted the need for more uniform outcome reporting methods and a need for cost-effectiveness studies.[69]

Randomized Controlled Trials

Recent comparative studies, including randomized controlled trials, have also shown that the TightRope is as effective as screw fixation. Kortekangas and colleagues[70] used intraoperative and postoperative CT scans in patients randomized to either Tightrope (n = 21) or single screw fixation (n = 22). The radiologic findings are confused, owing to the effect of foot position on the CT appearances intraoperatively. This limits the usefulness of the study. At the 2-year follow-up, no clinical differences were evident between the groups.

A multicenter level 2 study randomized 32 patients to dynamic and 36 to static syndesmosis fixation. Implant failure and loss of syndesmosis reduction was statistically higher in the screw group (3.5-mm screw, 4 cortices). The Olerud-Molander scores were significantly better in the TightRope group at 12 months, but not at earlier review. Conversely, AOFAS scores were statistically better at 3 months but not with later reviews. The authors conclude that flexible fixation is advantageous, but the clinical score paradox should be noted.[71]

Another level 2 study, with 23 participants in each group, compared flexible with rigid stabilization methods.[72] A single slice CT of both ankles was used to assess reduction postoperatively. More than 20% of the screw fixation groups were considered to be malreduced, versus 0% for the TightRope group. Clinical results did not differ though, at a mean follow-up of 2.5 years (range, 1.5–3.5)

Complications and Reoperation Rates

Complications can occur with any surgical procedure and the original hope that the TightRope would completely remove the need for secondary surgery has not been realized. Complication rates are low, but several issues have been noted.[67,73] Case reports of infection[74] and prominent washers were soon followed by published technique tips for easy removal of the device.[75] Studies of the local anatomy have shown that the saphenous vein and nerve are at risk and a small medial incision rather than percutaneous placement of the tibial washer is recommended to ensure that the washer sits against bone without soft tissue (or saphenous vein and nerve) interposition.[76–78] In a large series of TightRope stabilizations, Storey and colleagues[73] reviewed 102 cases. At the short-term follow-up (3 months), the authors found that 8 implants had been removed, mostly for infection or painful osteolysis.

Although there are no specific studies investigating the rate of complications with the "Knotless TightRope," this modification of the device (since 2012 in the UK) does mean less subcutaneous irritation from the fiber wire knot on the fibula side. Anecdotally, the rate of implant removal has been lower since this modification was introduced. This modification does not, however, address anecdotal reports of soft tissue irritation on the medial side. Slim patients in particular complain of prominence of the washer/button that becomes noticeable once the swelling has totally subsided at about 1 year after surgery.

Critical Analysis of the Literature and Future Research

Clinical series include a range of different fracture patterns, with widely differing degrees of instability. None of the existing biomechanical studies focus on proximal migration of the fibula. It is, therefore, difficult to be sure that flexible fixation of the syndesmosis is suitable for all situations.

If there is a very high (Maisonneuve) fibula fracture then plating the bone is generally considered to be impractical. If all the distal (medial and syndesmosis) elements of the injury are ligamentous, then the situation is extremely unstable until the tibiofibular alignment is restored surgically. The fixation chosen needs to be capable of resisting AP displacement, widening, rotation, and shortening of the fibula.

If the fibula fracture has been plated accurately, then there is no risk of fibula shortening. Biomechanical studies have shown that the TightRope affords good stability of the syndesmosis, but testing regimens have all focused on lateral translation and rotation of the distal fibula. A flexible device, under sufficient tension, would be expected to provide adequate resistance to lateral movement. With the distal fibula properly reduced in the incisura of the distal tibia, then the same tension could reasonably be expected to provide resistance to external rotation. Laboratory tests have not, however, explored specifically whether the TightRope prevents the shortening of the fibula that may accompany injuries where the fibula fracture is not reduced and fixed. Intuitively, to resist this vertical displacement, screw fixation engaging all 4 cortices of the fibula and tibia would be expected to provide more strength than other constructs. Three cortex fixation may easily loosen with "windscreen wiping" of the screws in the relatively soft metaphyseal bone of the distal tibia. Flexible fixation might also be expected to be less strong than 4 cortex screw fixation in this respect. Currently, the literature does not address the question of whether the TightRope is strong enough in these most unstable situations. Specific studies to investigate this question are needed before flexible fixation can be recommended in cases where the fibula may shorten.

Cost Analysis

Critics of the TightRope device hold that it is expensive. It is "much cheaper than a second operation to routinely remove a screw" counter the enthusiasts. Of course, some surgeons leave screws in place in the expectation that they will, once weight-bearing commences, eventually break allowing dynamization of the inferior tibiofibular joint. Also, some TightRopes are eventually removed because of discomfort. Rates of reoperation for failure of fixation would also need to be factored in to a meaningful cost analysis.

EXAMPLES AND CASES
Anterior Inferior Tibiofibular Ligament Nonoperative Treatment

This young sportsman presented after a rugby injury. He was pushing in a ruck, with the ankle in full dorsiflexion, when sudden pain was accompanied by "something snapping" (**Fig. 11**). He required analgesia at the side of the pitch and attended the emergency department. Radiographs showed no fracture. A removable walking boot and crutches were provided. Ten days later, he attended for specialist review. Tenderness was maximal over the AITFL and stressing this, with an external rotation force, reproduced pain. There were no medial sided signs of tenderness, swelling, or bruising. Radiographs were unremarkable.

An MRI showed rupture of the AITFL and partial injury to the deep deltoid ligament.

This combination represents a West Point grade 2 "gray area" injury. MRI suggested that instability may become evident under load, with injury to 2 zones. To determine whether there was "latent instability" of the syndesmosis, an ultrasound stress test was performed.[79] Even under maximum manual external rotation stress, the syndesmosis and the deltoid were sufficiently stable that there was no talar shift or sign of syndesmosis opening. The local tenderness was improving. Nonoperative management was therefore advised.

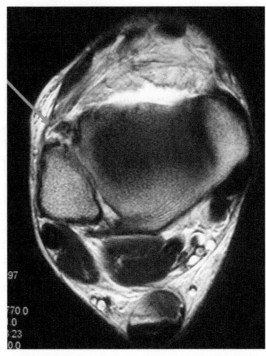

Fig. 11. Anterior inferior tibiofibular ligament rupture (*arrow*): non-operative treatment.

Discussion

The deep deltoid injury, restricted to the anterior portion, was not severe enough to produce instability so, in functional terms, this represents a single zone injury. A recent study has shown that delayed return to sport is strongly associated with those AITFL injuries where there is deltoid ligament injury as well. Further studies are needed to evaluate different management options for AITFL sprains with different degrees of deltoid injury. At the present time, we advise dynamic ultrasound stress testing as an additional investigation if an MRI shows any damage to the deep deltoid ligament.[80]

Anterior Inferior Tibiofibular Ligament and Deltoid: Stabilization

A 21-year-old athlete sustained a twisting injury of his ankle during training. He was unable to bear weight and the swelling and bruising extended well above the level of the malleoli (**Fig. 12**). His MRI showed complete rupture of the AITFL and significant bone bruising in the PM, with suspicion of PITFL involvement. There was injury to the deep deltoid ligament as well. Examination under anesthetic and arthroscopy revealed syndesmosis widening. Stabilisation was performed using flexible fixation.

Discussion

The combined syndesmosis and deltoid ligament injury rendered this ankle unstable. This was not evident on plain radiographs. MRI alone may not be sufficient to determine accurately the functional integrity of the posterior part of the deep deltoid ligament. Whether fluoroscopy, arthroscopy, or dynamic ultrasound imaging is the best and most cost-effective means of assessing whether fixation is required is an important area for future research.

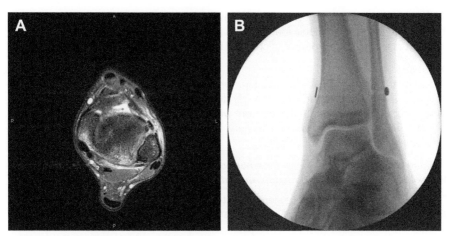

Fig. 12. (*A*, *B*) Anterior inferior tibiofibular ligament and deltoid: stabilization.

Supination - External Rotation Type 2: Stable, Non-operative

SER type 2 injuries, once proven to be stable, do not require operative fixation (**Fig. 13**). A whole article could be written about the best way to ascertain whether a Weber type B fracture without MM fracture is stable or unstable. The current best

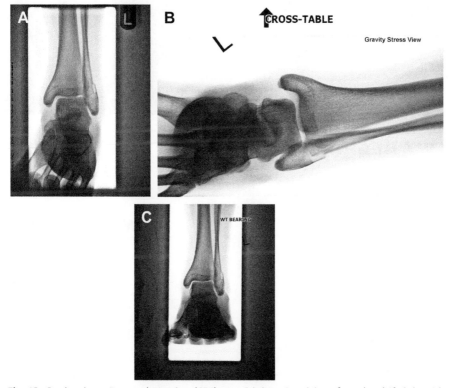

Fig. 13. Supination – External rotation (*SER*) type 2 injury. Suspicious for talar shift (*A*). Wide clear space medially with gravity stress view (*B*) yet weight bearing view shows excellent alignment (*C*). Sufficiently stable to be managed non-operatively.

practice, in these authors' opinion, is to have a proper weight bearing radiograph of the ankle. If, under physiologic load, there is no talar shift then there is sufficient deltoid ligament competence to permit successful nonoperative management.

Discussion

This patient's ankle had, on initial radiographs, a widened medial clear space. A gravity stress view was "positive," but the literature has shown this to be an oversensitive assessment of instability.[81] A subsequent weight-bearing radiograph proved satisfactory and he was managed without surgery. With the medial side functionally competent, this injury affects 2 zones only.

Supinated Foot Subjected to an External Rotation Force Type 4 with a Posterior Malleolus Fracture: Open Reduction and Internal Fixation

This horse rider sustained a trimalleolar fracture dislocation with deltoid ligament injury (**Fig. 14**). Three zones are involved. Two antiglide plates were used to buttress the

A

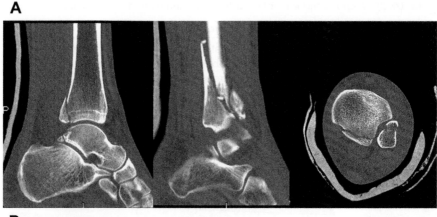

B

WT BEARING

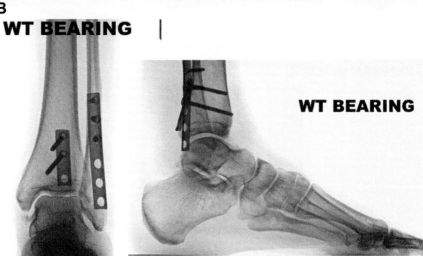

WT BEARING

Fig. 14. Supination–external rotation injury (*SER*) type 4 with posterior malleolus (*PM*) fracture (*A*). Open reduction and internal fixation, through a posterolateral approach. Antiglide plates restore stability (*B*). Note no distal screws required.

fibula and the PM fractures. There was no instability of the syndesmosis on stress testing. She progressed to full weight bearing after 2 weeks and (against medical advice!) was back in the saddle 6 weeks after injury.

Discussion

When a Weber type B injury has a PM fracture then there is posterolateral instability. If only the fibula fracture is fixed, then the combined AITLF and PITFL (attached to the PM fragment) injuries mean that the syndesmosis may be unstable, depending on the medial zone injury. By fixing the PM fracture, the function of the PITFL is restored and with this the syndesmosis is restored to 70% of its strength.

Pronation External Rotation Injury with Medial Malleolus and Tillaux Fracture

This high-energy fracture is unusual in that there are a greater number of bony than ligamentous components in the syndesmosis zone of injury (**Fig. 15**). Fixation of these allows accurate restoration of both fibula length and rotation. Accurate plating of the fibula shaft has been achieved.

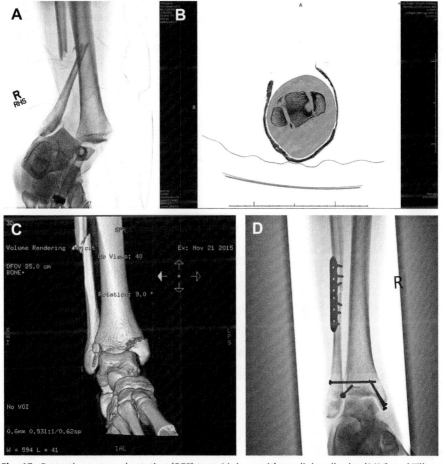

Fig. 15. Pronation external rotation (*PER*) type 4 injury, with medial malleolus (*MM*) and Tillaux fracture (*A–C*). Fibula length and rotation restored with open reduction and internal fixation. Medial malleolus and Tillaux fractures fixed as well. Diastasis screw could have been omitted (*D*).

Discussion

The operating surgeon elected to add a syndesmosis screw. With Tillaux fixation serving to supplement the open reduction and internal fixation of the fibula, there is a strong argument that, in this case, the additional syndesmotic stabilization did not need to be rigid, because flexible fixation would neutralize the lateral displacement and rotation forces. Because a large MM fracture was also present (allowing the medial zone to be stabilized), syndesmosis positioning hardware may not even have been needed at all.

Pronation External Rotation Injury, Open Reduction and Internal Fixation Fibula

This sports injury was stabilized by fibula fixation (**Fig. 16**). The fracture was relatively low but, nevertheless, stress testing intraoperatively showed widening of the distal tibiofibular joint. Although this was relatively mild, additional fixation was chosen, in part because of the large size of the patient and because of the degree of comminution of the fibula.

Discussion

In terms of zones of injury, fixation of the fibula at this level means that the likelihood of syndesmosis fixation being needed is low. With the medial zone being ligamentous and not bony, residual instability was evident at EUA. In an equivalent injury, with MM fracture instead, the situation after restoration of the bony anatomy may have been much more stable than that in the current example and

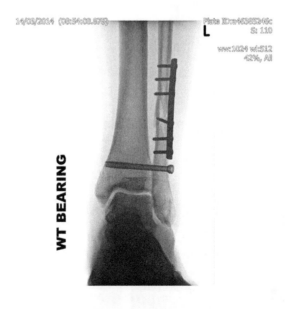

Fig. 16. Pronation external rotation (*PER*) type 4 injury, with deltoid ligament disruption. Very large patient, so despite dynamic compression plate (*in bridging mode*) fixation of the fibula an additional diastasis position screw was used. In the presence of a reduced and fixed medial malleolus fracture the diastasis screw would not have been required.

so either flexible fixation or no positioning hardware could then have been considered.

Pronation External Rotation, Fibula Fracture, and Deltoid Ligament Injury

This patient returned from a holiday abroad where a cycling accident had led to a tri-malleolar ankle fracture (**Fig. 17**). Deltoid repair had been undertaken, along with open reduction and internal fixation of the fibula. Plain radiographs were suspicious for re-sidual displacement of the syndesmosis.

Discussion

A CT scan showed a degree of residual displacement of the fibula; however, the patient declined revision surgery. The scope for improvement was modest because the displacement is not severe. At medium term clinical follow-up, function was good. The patient (aged 54) has returned to both tennis and skiing.

Pronation External Rotation, High Fibula

This young man suffered a high-energy injury (**Fig. 18**). The very high fibula fracture was reduced and fixed with excellent restoration of both length and rotation. There were no PM or MM fractures to repair and so 2 position screws, each through 4 cortices, were used. The postoperative CT scan showed that the fibula was properly restored to its position in the incisura.

Discussion

Plating a fibula fracture at this level requires a large surgical exposure, but allows ac-curate restoration of fibula length and rotation. Open reduction of the syndesmosis ensured that the distal fibula was accurately positioned before fixation. Rigid fixation was chosen. Had there been an MM fracture instead of the deltoid injury, then Tight-Rope fixation would have been selected.

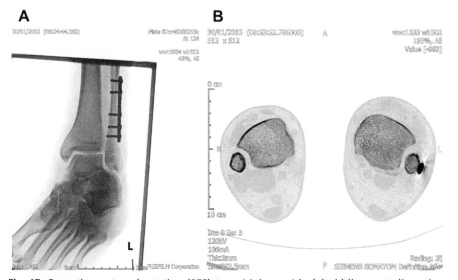

Fig. 17. Pronation external rotation (*PER*) type 4 injury, with deltoid ligament disruption. Fixation with strong bridging plate of the fibula fracture and deltoid ligament repair (*A*). CT scan shows only mild malreduction of the syndesmosis (*B*). The role of deltoid ligament repair remains poorly defined.

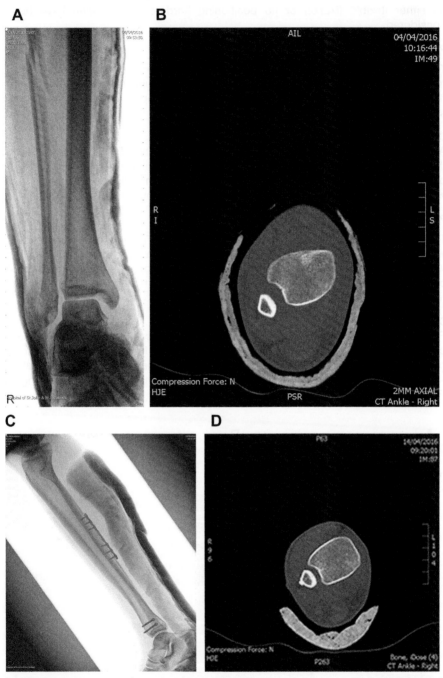

Fig. 18. Pronation external rotation (PER) type 4 injury, with proximal fibula fracture and deltoid disruption (*A, B*). Bridging plate for the fibula restores length and rotation and syndesmosis screws were selected to stabilise the syndesmosis after open reduction via an anterolateral approach (*C, D*).

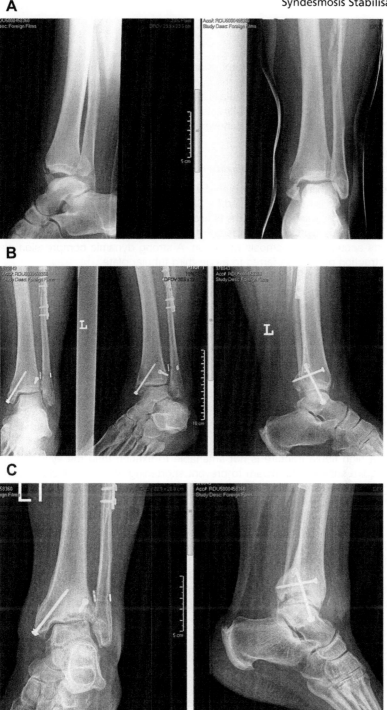

Fig. 19. Pronation external rotation (PER) type 4 injury, with medial malleolus (MM) fracture and posterior malleolus fracture (PM) (*A*). Malreduced fibula, single screw in MM and malreduced PM all indicate poor technique. The unique "2 cortex" utilisation of the Tightrope is not recommended (*B*). The inevitable consequence of poor surgical management of a high grade fracture is rapid onset of degenerative joint disease (*C*).

Good Theory, Poor Practice

This case exemplifies how important reduction is (**Fig. 19**). The surgical team began with the aim of reducing and fixing the fractures and stabilizing the syndesmosis. Unfortunately, the reduction of the fibula is incomplete; the PM has been fixed from front to back and is not reduced, the MM fracture may have been comminuted (no CT scan), and the TightRope placement was never going to help.

SUMMARY
Syndesmosis Reduction and Stabilization

Syndesmosis stabilization is associated with poor clinical outcomes. Stabilisation of the syndesmosis is not often needed for SER injuries, even if stress testing after fibula fixation reveals opening between the tibia and the fibula. Fixation of the fibula in Weber type C fractures, even in the middle one-third of the bone, affords improved stability and aids accurate syndesmosis reduction. A strong dynamic compression plate or reconstruction plate is preferred to a one-third tubular plate.

Syndesmosis stabilization is likely to be required in PER injuries without PM or MM fractures, but with bony injuries in the medial and syndesmosis zones there may be no added benefit in using distal tibiofibular joint hardware. The role of deltoid ligament repair is not well-understood. Accurate reduction of the syndesmosis is critical for good outcome. Open reduction improves accuracy. Postoperative CT scans should be used to check the position of the fibula relative to the tibia, and revision surgery considered if there is malreduction.

Rigid versus Flexible Fixation

Laboratory and clinical studies show that results using flexible fixation are equivalent to the outcomes using screws. Screw fixation should be considered in some circumstances:

- If a high fibula fracture is not amenable to fixation then the syndesmosis will require sufficient hardware to prevent shortening as well as resist widening or rotation. There is currently no evidence to determine whether or not flexible stabilization is sufficient in such cases.
- If, after fixation of the fibula, PM, and/or MM, there remains concern over stability of the inferior tibiofibular joint, then flexible stabilization will almost certainly suffice. Similarly, in purely ligamentous injury, with mild rotational instability only, flexible fixation has been shown to be strong enough. Surgeons can, in these situations, use either screws or flexible fixation with confidence. They must exercise their judgment on the economic arguments that surround implant cost versus a reduced "need" for hardware removal.

REFERENCES

1. Clanton TO, Paul P. Syndesmosis injuries in athletes. Foot Ankle Clin 2002;7(3): 529–49.
2. Espinosa N, Smerek JP, Myerson MS. Acute and chronic syndesmosis injuries: pathomechanisms, diagnosis and management. Foot Ankle Clin 2006;11(3): 639–57.
3. Jelinek JA, Porter DA. Management of unstable ankle fractures and syndesmosis injuries in athletes. Foot Ankle Clin 2009;14(2):277–98.
4. Mak MF, Gartner L, Pearce CJ. Management of syndesmosis injuries in the elite athlete. Foot Ankle Clin 2013;18(2):195–214.

5. Miller SD. Controversies in ankle fracture treatment. Indications for fixation of stable Weber type B fractures and indications for syndesmosis stabilization. Foot Ankle Clin 2000;5(4):841–51.vi.
6. Mosier-LaClair S, Pike H, Pomeroy G. Syndesmosis injuries: acute, chronic, new techniques for failed management. Foot Ankle Clin 2002;7(3):551–65.ix.
7. Pena FA, Coetzee JC. Ankle syndesmosis injuries. Foot Ankle Clin 2006;11(1): 35–50.viii.
8. Rammelt S, Zwipp H, Grass R. Injuries to the distal tibiofibular syndesmosis: an evidence-based approach to acute and chronic lesions. Foot Ankle Clin 2008; 13(4):611–33, vii–viii.
9. Golano P, Vega J, Perez-Carro L, et al. Ankle anatomy for the arthroscopist. Part II: role of the ankle ligaments in soft tissue impingement. Foot Ankle Clin 2006; 11(2):275–96, v–vi.
10. Hermans JJ, Beumer A, de Jong TA, et al. Anatomy of the distal tibiofibular syndesmosis in adults: a pictorial essay with a multimodality approach. J Anat 2010; 217(6):633–45.
11. Kose O, Yuksel HY, Guler F, et al. Isolated adult Tillaux fracture associated with Volkmann fracture: a unique combination of injuries-report of two cases and review of the literature. J Foot Ankle Surg 2016;55(5):1057–62.
12. Gardner MJ, Demetrakopoulos D, Briggs SM, et al. The ability of the Lauge-Hansen classification to predict ligament injury and mechanism in ankle fractures: an MRI study. J Orthop Trauma 2006;20(4):267–72.
13. Warner SJ, Garner MR, Hinds RM, et al. Correlation between the Lauge-Hansen classification and ligament injuries in ankle fractures. J Orthop Trauma 2015; 29(12):574–8.
14. Warner SJ, Schottel PC, Hinds RM, et al. Fracture-dislocations demonstrate poorer postoperative functional outcomes among pronation external rotation IV ankle fractures. Foot Ankle Int 2015;36(6):641–7.
15. Schottel PC, Berkes MB, Little MT, et al. Comparison of clinical outcome of pronation external rotation versus supination external rotation ankle fractures. Foot Ankle Int 2014;35(4):353–9.
16. Hinds RM, Schottel PC, Berkes MB, et al. Evaluation of Lauge-Hansen designation of Weber C fractures. J Foot Ankle Surg 2014;53(4):434–9.
17. Stark E, Tornetta P 3rd, Creevy WR. Syndesmotic instability in Weber B ankle fractures: a clinical evaluation. J Orthop Trauma 2007;21(9):643–6.
18. Kortekangas TH, Pakarinen HJ, Savola O, et al. Syndesmotic fixation in supination-external rotation ankle fractures: a prospective randomized study. Foot Ankle Int 2014;35(10):988–95.
19. Pakarinen H. Stability-based classification for ankle fracture management and the syndesmosis injury in ankle fractures due to a supination external rotation mechanism of injury. Acta Orthop Suppl 2012;83(347):1–26.
20. Pakarinen HJ, Flinkkila TE, Ohtonen PP, et al. Syndesmotic fixation in supination-external rotation ankle fractures: a prospective randomized study. Foot Ankle Int 2011;32(12):1103–9.
21. Lauge-Hansen N. Fractures of the ankle. V. Pronation-dorsiflexion fracture. AMA Arch Surg 1953;67(6):813–20.
22. Gerber JP, Williams GN, Scoville CR, et al. Persistent disability associated with ankle sprains: a prospective examination of an athletic population. Foot Ankle Int 1998;19(10):653–60.
23. Hopkinson WJ, St Pierre P, Ryan JB, et al. Syndesmosis sprains of the ankle. Foot Ankle 1990;10(6):325–30.

24. Egol KA, Pahk B, Walsh M, et al. Outcome after unstable ankle fracture: effect of syndesmotic stabilization. J Orthop Trauma 2010;24(1):7–11.
25. Weening B, Bhandari M. Predictors of functional outcome following transsyndesmotic screw fixation of ankle fractures. J Orthop Trauma 2005;19(2): 102–8.
26. Chissell HR, Jones J. The influence of a diastasis screw on the outcome of Weber type-C ankle fractures. J Bone Joint Surg Br 1995;77(3):435–8.
27. Tornetta P 3rd. Competence of the deltoid ligament in bimalleolar ankle fractures after medial malleolar fixation. J Bone Joint Surg Am 2000;82(6):843–8.
28. Schottel PC, Baxter J, Gilbert S, et al. Anatomic ligament repair restores ankle and syndesmotic rotational stability as much as syndesmotic screw fixation. J Orthop Trauma 2016;30(2):e36–40.
29. Pesl T, Havranek P. Rare injuries to the distal tibiofibular joint in children. Eur J Pediatr Surg 2006;16(4):255–9.
30. Gardner MJ, Brodsky A, Briggs SM, et al. Fixation of posterior malleolar fractures provides greater syndesmotic stability. Clin Orthop Relat Res 2006;447: 165–71.
31. Beumer A, van Hemert WL, Swierstra BA, et al. A biomechanical evaluation of the tibiofibular and tibiotalar ligaments of the ankle. Foot Ankle Int 2003;24(5): 426–9.
32. Miller AN, Carroll EA, Parker RJ, et al. Posterior malleolar stabilization of syndesmotic injuries is equivalent to screw fixation. Clin Orthop Relat Res 2010;468(4): 1129–35.
33. Bottlang M, Schemitsch CE, Nauth A, et al. Biomechanical concepts for fracture fixation. J Orthop Trauma 2015;29(Suppl 12):S28–33.
34. Tornetta P 3rd, Ricci W, Nork S, et al. The posterolateral approach to the tibia for displaced posterior malleolar injuries. J Orthop Trauma 2011;25(2):123–6.
35. Sagi HC, Shah AR, Sanders RW. The functional consequence of syndesmotic joint malreduction at a minimum 2-year follow-up. J Orthop Trauma 2012;26(7): 439–43.
36. Franke J, von Recum J, Suda AJ, et al. Intraoperative three-dimensional imaging in the treatment of acute unstable syndesmotic injuries. J Bone Joint Surg Am 2012;94(15):1386–90.
37. Franke J, von Recum J, Suda AJ, et al. Predictors of a persistent dislocation after reduction of syndesmotic injuries detected with intraoperative three-dimensional imaging. Foot Ankle Int 2014;35(12):1323–8.
38. Davidovitch RI, Weil Y, Karia R, et al. Intraoperative syndesmotic reduction: three-dimensional versus standard fluoroscopic imaging. J Bone Joint Surg Am 2013; 95(20):1838–43.
39. Sinha A, Sirikonda S, Giotakis N, et al. Fibular lengthening for malunited ankle fractures. Foot Ankle Int 2008;29(11):1136–40.
40. Marmor M, Hansen E, Han HK, et al. Limitations of standard fluoroscopy in detecting rotational malreduction of the syndesmosis in an ankle fracture model. Foot Ankle Int 2011;32(6):616–22.
41. Miller AN, Carroll EA, Parker RJ, et al. Direct visualization for syndesmotic stabilization of ankle fractures. Foot Ankle Int 2009;30(5):419–26.
42. Gardner MJ, Demetrakopoulos D, Briggs SM, et al. Malreduction of the tibiofibular syndesmosis in ankle fractures. Foot Ankle Int 2006;27(10):788–92.
43. Knops SP, Kohn MA, Hansen EN, et al. Rotational malreduction of the syndesmosis: reliability and accuracy of computed tomography measurement methods. Foot Ankle Int 2013;34(10):1403–10.

44. Kotwal R, Rath N, Paringe V, et al. Targeted computerised tomography scanning of the ankle syndesmosis with low dose radiation exposure. Skeletal Radiol 2016; 45(3):333–8.

45. Warner SJ, Fabricant PD, Garner MR, et al. The measurement and clinical importance of syndesmotic reduction after operative fixation of rotational ankle fractures. J Bone Joint Surg Am 2015;97(23):1935–44.

46. Clanton TO, Matheny LM, Jarvis HC, et al. Quantitative analysis of torsional stiffness in supplemental one-third tubular plate fixation in the management of isolated syndesmosis injuries: a biomechanical study. Foot Ankle Int 2013;34(2): 267–72.

47. Dattani R, Patnaik S, Kantak A, et al. Injuries to the tibiofibular syndesmosis. J Bone Joint Surg Br 2008;90(4):405–10.

48. Jordan TH, Talarico RH, Schuberth JM. The radiographic fate of the syndesmosis after trans-syndesmotic screw removal in displaced ankle fractures. J Foot Ankle Surg 2011;50(4):407–12.

49. Kaftandziev I, Spasov M, Trpeski S, et al. Fate of the syndesmotic screw–Search for a prudent solution. Injury 2015;46(Suppl 6):S125–9.

50. Manjoo A, Sanders DW, Tieszer C, et al. Functional and radiographic results of patients with syndesmotic screw fixation: implications for screw removal. J Orthop Trauma 2010;24(1):2–6.

51. Schepers T. To retain or remove the syndesmotic screw: a review of literature. Arch Orthop Trauma Surg 2011;131(7):879–83.

52. Schepers T, van der Linden H, van Lieshout EM, et al. Technical aspects of the syndesmotic screw and their effect on functional outcome following acute distal tibiofibular syndesmosis injury. Injury 2014;45(4):775–9.

53. Song DJ, Lanzi JT, Groth AT, et al. The effect of syndesmosis screw removal on the reduction of the distal tibiofibular joint: a prospective radiographic study. Foot Ankle Int 2014;35(6):543–8.

54. Tucker A, Street J, Kealey D, et al. Functional outcomes following syndesmotic fixation: a comparison of screws retained in situ versus routine removal - Is it really necessary? Injury 2013;44(12):1880–4.

55. van Vlijmen N, Denk K, van Kampen A, et al. Long-term results after ankle syndesmosis injuries. Orthopedics 2015;38(11):e1001–6.

56. Summers HD, Sinclair MK, Stover MD. A reliable method for intraoperative evaluation of syndesmotic reduction. J Orthop Trauma 2013;27(4):196–200.

57. Brin YS, Nyska M, Kish B. Lisfranc injury repair with the TightRope device: a short-term case series. Foot Ankle Int 2010;31(7):624–7.

58. Kayiaros S, Blankenhorn BD, Dehaven J, et al. Correction of metatarsus primus varus associated with hallux valgus deformity using the arthrex mini tightrope: a report of 44 cases. Foot Ankle Spec 2011;4(4):212–7.

59. Thornes B, Walsh A, Hislop M, et al. Suture-endobutton fixation of ankle tibiofibular diastasis: a cadaver study. Foot Ankle Int 2003;24(2):142–6.

60. Seitz WH Jr, Bachner EJ, Abram LJ, et al. Repair of the tibiofibular syndesmosis with a flexible implant. J Orthop Trauma 1991;5(1):78–82.

61. Ebramzadeh E, Knutsen AR, Sangiorgio SN, et al. Biomechanical comparison of syndesmotic injury fixation methods using a cadaveric model. Foot Ankle Int 2013;34(12):1710–7.

62. Forsythe K, Freedman KB, Stover MD, et al. Comparison of a novel FiberWire-button construct versus metallic screw fixation in a syndesmotic injury model. Foot Ankle Int 2008;29(1):49–54.

63. Klitzman R, Zhao H, Zhang LQ, et al. Suture-button versus screw fixation of the syndesmosis: a biomechanical analysis. Foot Ankle Int 2010;31(1):69–75.

64. Gardner R, Yousri T, Holmes F, et al. Stabilization of the syndesmosis in the Maisonneuve fracture–a biomechanical study comparing 2-hole locking plate and quadricortical screw fixation. J Orthop Trauma 2013;27(4):212–6.

65. Thornes B, Shannon F, Guiney AM, et al. Suture-button syndesmosis fixation: accelerated rehabilitation and improved outcomes. Clin Orthop Relat Res 2005;(431):207–12.

66. Cottom JM, Hyer CF, Philbin TM, et al. Treatment of syndesmotic disruptions with the Arthrex Tightrope: a report of 25 cases. Foot Ankle Int 2008;29(8): 773–80.

67. Rigby RB, Cottom JM. Does the Arthrex TightRope(R) provide maintenance of the distal tibiofibular syndesmosis? A 2-year follow-up of 64 TightRopes(R) in 37 patients. J Foot Ankle Surg 2013;52(5):563–7.

68. Seyhan M, Donmez F, Mahirogullari M, et al. Comparison of screw fixation with elastic fixation methods in the treatment of syndesmosis injuries in ankle fractures. Injury 2015;46(Suppl 2):S19–23.

69. Schepers T. Acute distal tibiofibular syndesmosis injury: a systematic review of suture-button versus syndesmotic screw repair. Int Orthop 2012;36(6): 1199–206.

70. Kortekangas T, Savola O, Flinkkila T, et al. A prospective randomised study comparing TightRope and syndesmotic screw fixation for accuracy and maintenance of syndesmotic reduction assessed with bilateral computed tomography. Injury 2015;46(6):1119–26.

71. Laflamme M, Belzile EL, Bedard L, et al. A prospective randomized multicenter trial comparing clinical outcomes of patients treated surgically with a static or dynamic implant for acute ankle syndesmosis rupture. J Orthop Trauma 2015;29(5): 216–23.

72. Naqvi GA, Cunningham P, Lynch B, et al. Fixation of ankle syndesmotic injuries: comparison of tightrope fixation and syndesmotic screw fixation for accuracy of syndesmotic reduction. Am J Sports Med 2012;40(12):2828–35.

73. Storey P, Gadd RJ, Blundell C, et al. Complications of suture button ankle syndesmosis stabilization with modifications of surgical technique. Foot Ankle Int 2012; 33(9):717–21.

74. Hong CC, Lee WT, Tan KJ. Osteomyelitis after TightRope((R)) fixation of the ankle syndesmosis: a case report and review of the literature. J Foot Ankle Surg 2015; 54(1):130–4.

75. Bayer T, McKenna J. Technical tips for the removal of TightRope ankle syndesmosis fixation. Foot Ankle Surg 2015;21(3):214–5.

76. Naqvi GA, Shafqat A, Awan N. Tightrope fixation of ankle syndesmosis injuries: clinical outcome, complications and technique modification. Injury 2012;43(6): 838–42.

77. Pirozzi KM, Creech CL, Meyr AJ. Assessment of anatomic risk during syndesmotic stabilization with the suture button technique. J Foot Ankle Surg 2015; 54(5):917–9.

78. Willmott HJ, Singh B, David LA. Outcome and complications of treatment of ankle diastasis with tightrope fixation. Injury 2009;40(11):1204–6.

79. Mei-Dan O, Carmont M, Laver L, et al. Standardization of the functional syndesmosis widening by dynamic U.S examination. BMC Sports Sci Med Rehabil 2013;5:9.

80. Calder JD, Bamford R, Petrie A, et al. Stable versus unstable grade II high ankle sprains: a prospective study predicting the need for surgical stabilization and time to return to sports. Arthroscopy 2016;32(4):634–42.
81. Dawe EJ, Shafafy R, Quayle J, et al. The effect of different methods of stability assessment on fixation rate and complications in supination external rotation (SER) 2/4 ankle fractures. Foot Ankle Surg 2015;21(2):86–90.

Late Treatment of Syndesmotic Injuries

Michael P. Swords, DO[a],*, Andrew Sands, MD[b], John R. Shank, MD[c]

KEYWORDS

- Syndesmosis • Late fixation • Ankle • Malunion • Fibula

KEY POINTS

- Syndesmotic injuries may be subtle and difficult to diagnose.
- Malalignment at the syndesmosis may result in decreased function, pain, and arthritis.
- Late reconstruction of the syndesmosis should be considered in cases of malreduction.

Ankle fractures are one of the more common fractures treated by orthopedic surgeons. Normal function of the ankle requires appropriate alignment and stability for function. Ankle fractures include a broad spectrum of injury, including stable patterns as well as severe fracture dislocations; 23% of ankle fractures are reported to have a syndesmotic injury.[1] Operatively treated fractures are, by definition, less stable and are associated with a higher rate of injury to the syndesmosis, with reports as high as 39% to 45%.[2,3] Despite the frequency of these injuries, accurate diagnosis, reliable treatment methods, and restoration of normal anatomic relationships continue to prove challenging. High rates of malreduction continue to be seen in operative treatment of syndesmotic injuries. Strategies and surgical techniques for late treatment of syndesmotic injuries are reviewed.

The osseous anatomy of the distal tibia and fibula and associated ligaments is referred to collectively as the syndesmosis. The anterolateral (Chaput) tubercle of the tibia, the anterior (Wagstaffe) tubercle of the distal fibula, and the incisura fibularis are all important osseous contributions to the syndesmosis. The shape of the incisura is not consistent and may be concave or shallow concave.[4] The relationship between the distal tibia and fibula at the syndesmotic region is also variable.[5,6] The anterior

Swords is a consultant for DePuy Synthes, Pacira and Acelity. Sands is a consultant for DePuy Synthes.
[a] Orthopedic Surgery, Sparrow Hospital, Michigan Orthopedic Center, 2815 South Pennsylvania Avenue, Suite 204, Lansing, MI 48910, USA; [b] Foot and Ankle Surgery, Downtown Orthopedic Associates, AO Foot and Ankle Expert Group, Weill Cornell Medical College, 170 William Street, New York, NY 10038, USA; [c] Department of Orthopedic Surgery, Colorado Center of Orthopaedic Excellence, 2446 Research Pkwy, #200, Colorado Springs, CO 80920, USA
* Corresponding author.
E-mail address: Foot.trauma@gmail.com

Foot Ankle Clin N Am 22 (2017) 65–75
http://dx.doi.org/10.1016/j.fcl.2016.09.005
1083-7515/17/© 2016 Elsevier Inc. All rights reserved.

inferior tibiofibular ligament (AITFL) spans from the anterolateral tubercle of the tibia and attaches to the anterior tubercle of the fibula. The posterior inferior tibiofibular ligament (PITFL) travels from the posterior malleolus to attach along the posterior tubercle of the fibula. The interosseous membrane is located between the tibia and fibula spanning nearly the entirety of the lower leg. The interosseous tibiofibular ligament (IOL) is found in the distal 1 cm of the lower leg and is contiguous with the interosseous membrane. As the number of ligaments that are sectioned increases, the ankle has more instability.[7] In a study performed by section-specific ligaments, Ogilvie-Harris and colleagues[8] found that the AITFL provided 35%; the transverse tibiofibular ligament, or deep portion of the PITFL, 33%; the IOL 22%; and the PITFL 9% of the overall stability. A second sectioning study resulted in significant syndesmotic widening occurring only after the IOL was sectioned.[9]

Injury to the syndesmosis may occur from fracture, ligament injury, or both.

Late presentation and need for delayed reconstruction may occur in a variety of clinical scenarios. Unrecognized syndesmotic injury and resulting instability may result in long-term pain and disability. All injuries about the ankle should be treated in a diligent manner to try to prevent missing a syndesmotic injury. In a successive series of patients reporting to a tertiary center for ankle arthrodesis, 20.3% had significant widening of the ankle mortise.[10] Biomechanical studies have shown that small amounts of deformity can result in alteration of ankle function; 1 mm to 2 mm of lateral translation, shortening of more than 2 mm, and malunion resulting in more than 5° of external rotation of the distal fibula are all associated with generating abnormal pressure distribution at the ankle.[11–13] As a result of these findings, reconstruction is recommended for cases with malreduction. Malreduction may occur at the time of ankle fracture fixation. This malreduction may occur in fixation of the lateral malleolus (**Fig. 1**), reducing the fibula in the incisura fibularis, or both (**Fig. 2**). Finally, late fixation may be necessary in cases where either the hardware has broken resulting in instability or, in some cases, when the surgeon removes the hardware prior to adequate healing of the syndesmosis so late widening occurs.

Isolated malleolar fractures with syndesmotic injury have been reported to have worse functional outcome (Short Musculoskeletal Function Assessment Questionnaire [SMFA]) at 1 year than patients who had a malleolar fracture without syndesmotic injury.[14] In a recent study, Sagi and colleagues[15] reported worse outcomes at 2 years on both the SMFA and Olerud-Molander ankle score in patients with syndesmotic malreduction, as confirmed by CT, than patients with an anatomic reduction. Weening and Bhondari[16] have shown that improved SMFA and Olerud- Molander scores were predicted by anatomic reduction of the syndesmosis on radiographic assessment.

Patients with syndesmotic malreduction complain of ankle pain. They often report that since the time of injury the ankle has never felt right. Syndesmosis malreduction must be evaluated in individuals with persistent disability or pain after an ankle injury (**Fig. 3**). Surgical treatment of syndesmotic malreduction is performed ideally before significant ankle arthritis is present. In the presence of advance arthritis, ankle arthrodesis or ankle arthroplasty should be considered as reconstruction options. The goal is to restore normal anatomic alignment, resulting in improved function, ideally prior to development of arthritis.

SURGICAL TECHNIQUE

All patients require a thorough clinical examination of both the affected and nonaffected ankle. Complete imaging requires CT examination as well as weight-bearing ankle radiographs (**Fig. 4A–C**).

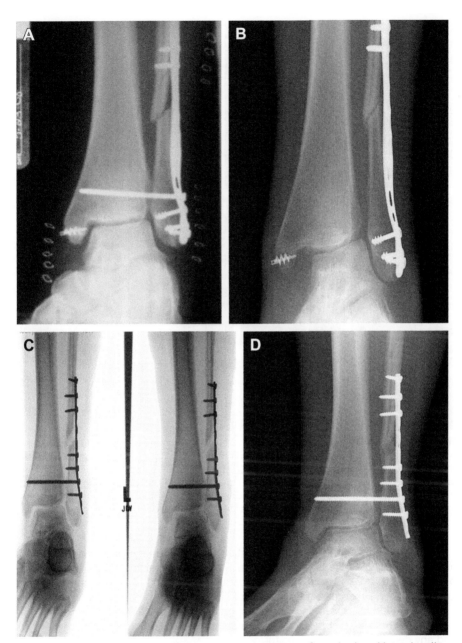

Fig. 1. (*A*) Demonstrates an immediate postoperative image of a malreduced lateral malleolus fracture with an attempt at syndesmotic fixation. A suture anchor has been used to attempt to reduce the medial clear space. (*B*) The 6-month image after syndesmotic fixation has been removed and the medial clear space has increased. (*C*) The patient was treated with fibular osteotomy to correct alignment and lengthen the fibula and revision of syndesmotic fixation. (*D*) Final image demonstrates a well-aligned lateral malleolus with restoration of normal syndesmotic relationship.

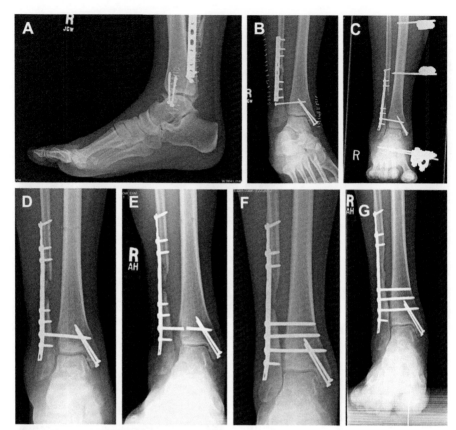

Fig. 2. (*A*) lateral and (*B*) mortise radiograph of a university-age woman who fell hiking in Africa. She was treated with excision of comminution of the fibula and fixation. The fibula is short and the syndesmosis is malreduced. (*C, D*) She was treated with revision fixation, including (*C*) external fixation (*D*) lengthening of her fibula, bone grafting, and revision of syndesmosis. (*E*) The fibula went on to nonunion. (*F*) Revision bonegrafting and placement of additional syndesmotic fixation was performed (*G*) resulting in union.

After a patient is anesthetized, true mortise and lateral images are obtained of both ankles and saved on the fluoroscopy unit. The contralateral images are used if comparison images are needed to assess reduction. The range of motion of both ankles is assessed and recorded. Many patients have chronic pain and may guard when examined in the clinical setting so it is important to re-evaluate motion when the patient is anesthetized to obtain a clear understanding of the range of motion of the ankle and any deficits that may be present.

The patient is placed in the supine position with a bump under the ipsilateral hip. If, based on the preoperative CT scan, it is necessary to approach the posterior aspect of the syndesmosis, it is important to position the patient for improved access by using a larger bump. The leg is elevated on a positioning pillow to facilitate intraoperative imaging. A longitudinal incision is made down the lateral aspect of the fibula. Dissection is carried down to fibula. If any old syndesmotic or fibular fixation is present, it is removed. Care is taken to look for, and protect, the superficial peroneal nerve because the position of the nerve is variable.

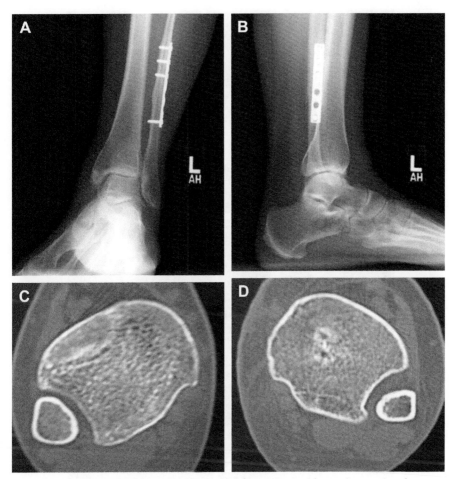

Fig. 3. (*A*) Mortise and (*B*) lateral radiograph of a patient with continue pain after open reduction and internal fixation of lateral malleolus. The radiographs show good alignment of the fibula. CT scan demonstrates abnormal position of the fibula in the incisura when comparing (*C*) the contralateral side to (*D*) the injured side. These findings can be subtle and are best seen on CT scan.

Dissection is carried over the front of the fibula. The syndesmotic region is often full of posttraumatic scar tissue and may require débridement over approximately the distal 6 cm to 8 cm. Initially, dissection occurs over the fibula anteriorly and soft tissue is removed, allowing the placement of a lamina spreader approximately 5 cm to 6 cm above the ankle joint (**Fig. 4**E). After the lamina spreader is placed, débridement continues distally toward the distal tibiofibular articulation. The lamina spreader is gradually moved distal to assist with exposure. Bone is often present and may consist of generalized posttraumatic ossification of the syndesmotic region or bone fragments from the initial injury. The incisura region is débrided carefully to prevent injury to the articular cartilage found on the corresponding articular facets at the distal tibiofibular articulation (**Fig. 4**F). Osteophyte formation is common in the late reconstruction setting. It may be present on the distal tibia, distal fibula, or both. The presence and location of osteophytes are determined from the preoperative CT scan. Osteophytes

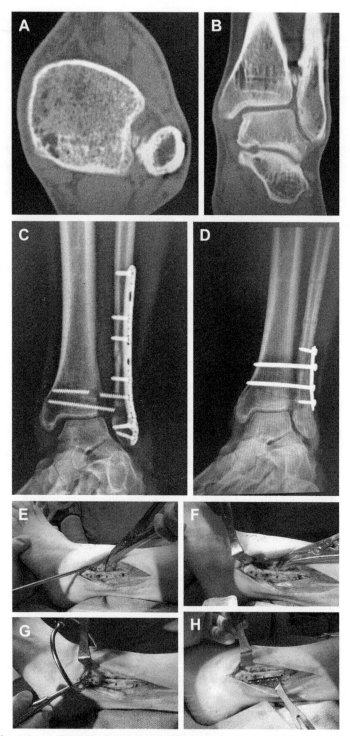

Fig. 4. (*A*) Axial and (*B*) coronal CT scans and (*C*) mortise radiograph of a patient presenting for evaluation of continued pain after an ankle injury (*C*) radiograph of a patient presenting

may be present posteriorly or anteriorly off either the fibula or tibia, if translational mal-reduction in the sagittal plane is present, or in the syndesmotic region itself. The osteo-phytes need to be carefully removed with an osteotome. The syndesmosis is débrided carefully all the way down to the ankle joint until the articular cartilage of the talar dome is visible when looking distally between the fibula and tibia. A pituitary rongeur is help-ful for this portion of the procedure (**Fig. 5**A). Fluoroscopy may be used as the débride-ment of the syndesmotic region approaches the ankle joint to confirm position and prevent accidental injury to the talar articular cartilage (**Fig. 5**B). Occasionally, the inci-sion may need to be lengthened distally to remove any osteophytes present at the anterior ankle level extending off the anterolateral aspect of the tibia or off the fibula.

After the syndesmotic region is clean of all impediments of reduction, the ankle joint is addressed. An anteromedial ankle arthrotomy is made just medial to the anterior tibialis (**Fig. 5**C). The ankle joint capsule is opened sharply. Most patients have exten-sive scarring within the ankle joint. A thorough arthrolysis is performed removing any soft tissue obstruction in the medial gutter as well as across the anterior aspect of the ankle. Any osteophytes or loose ossific densities are removed (**Fig. 5**D). Patients often have diminished dorsiflexion at presentation, which may be a result of intra-articular pathology, such as scar tissue or osteophytes, generalized posttraumatic scarring af-ter injury, or equinus contracture. With the presence of osteophytes and scar tissue, it is difficult to assess for the presence or absence of a contracture, so they must be removed to allow for a more accurate assessment.

Obvious malunions of the fibula are then addressed to re-establish normal length and alignment of the fibula. Malunions may include shortening, angular, or rotational deformities in isolation or combination. Angular deformities are easiest to correct whereas rotation deformities prove the most difficult to accurately restore, partly due to the inability to adequately assess with standard fluoroscopy.[17]

The fibula is a straight bone and should appear straight on all radiographs. Angular deformity is corrected by osteotomy. Osteotomy type depends on the amount and type of correction necessary. Closing wedge osteotomies should be avoided due to the potential for shortening. Oblique osteotomies may be used for restoration of length alignment and rotation through a single cut if made in the correct plane.[18]

Restoring length may be difficult and surgical tricks include accurately placing the plate on the distal segment and using a push screw proximal to the plate to assist with length. A bicortical drill hole is made 3 mm to 4 mm proximal to the plate. The depth is measured using a measuring device; 6 mm are added to the measurement to allow the screw to remain prominent on the near cortex. A lamina spreader is then used to push the screw and plate apart, increasing the length of the fibula. Once appropriate length is achieved, the proximal end of the plate is secured to the fibula. Caution is necessary to avoid introducing an angular deformity while distracting

---

for evaluation of continued pain after an ankle injury. The syndesmosis is poorly aligned and ossific debris is noted in the incisura. (*D*) Alignment was corrected by repeat fixation of the syndesmosis including thorough de'bridement of the syndesmosis. (*E*) Surgical views demon-strate the fibular hardware has been removed and a lamina spreader is placed between the fibula and tibia. The syndesmotic area is cleaned out using a pituitary rongeur. (*F*) The syn-desmotic region is cleared of scar tissue and the fibula is mobile. (*G*) The fibula is carefully reduced under direct visualization and a clamp is placed from the tip of the fibula to the tip of the medial malleolus following the transmalleolar axis. (*H*) Final fixation consists of 4.0 cortical screws placed through a plate. The screws follow the trajectory of the reduction clamp and are placed through a plate to prevent potential loss of reduction if a fracture were to occur through one of the screw holes from prior fixation.

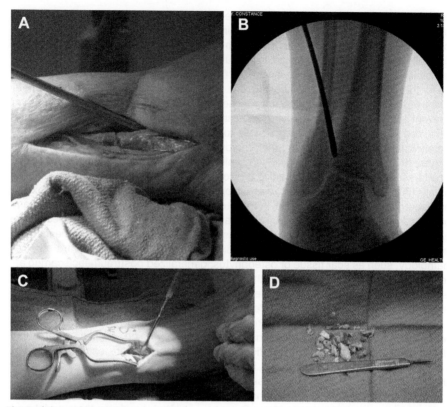

Fig. 5. (*A*) A pituitary rongeur is used to remove debris from the syndesmotic region all the way to the ankle joint. (*B*) Fluoroscopy may be used to determine location of pituitary and prevent injury to the ankle articular cartilage. (*C*) The medial gutter and ankle are débrided through a medial ankle arthrotomy. (*D*) Products of débridement of the incisura, medial gutter, and ankle in a revision syndesmosis case are seen.

with the lamina spreader. Several modern plating systems incorporate distraction devices and hole geometry, which may be used to help restore length. Small distractor systems may also be used. If a void is present, bone graft is required to fill the void.

After anatomic restoration of fibular alignment and stabilization, the fibula is reduced back into the incisura. This is done with direct visualization and can generally be performed with manual pressure. A pointed reduction clamp is then placed from the tip of the lateral malleolus to the tip of the medial malleolus, recreating the transmalleolar axis (**Fig. 4**G). A Kirschner wire is then placed above the level of anticipated syndesmotic fixation to prevent introduction of rotational deformity at the time of screw insertion. Prior to screw insertion, reduction is visually confirmed by looking at the relationship between the fibula and tibia. The mortise view is reviewed and a lateral view may be obtained and compared with the contralateral ankle to help evaluate the fibular position in the sagittal plane by assessing the distance from the posterior cortex of the fibula to the posterior cortex of the fibula. Fixation generally consists of 4.0 cortical screws through all 4 cortices. In later presentations, individuals with larger body habitus, or in cases of a greater amount of fibular lengthening, an additional screw or 2 should be considered. Screw trajectory should parallel the tip-to-tip axis of the reduction clamp.

In cases of chronic syndesmotic malposition without fibular malunion where fibular hardware is removed from the fibula, new fixation should be placed through a plate to avoid loss of fixation or fracture from occurring through the holes in the fibula left from the old fixation construct (**Fig. 4**D, H).

Postoperatively, patients are placed in a splint for 2 weeks and then in a fracture boot for the remainder of treatment. Non–weight bearing is maintained for 6 weeks. Screws are left in indefinitely and are only removed if the lateral hardware proves symptomatic and typically after a minimum of a year. The hardware is maintained in a majority of patients.

Prior studies of late reconstruction of the syndesmosis are limited. Most report descriptions of a surgical technique or consist of a small series of patients. Outland,[19] in 1943, suggested placing bone graft through drill holes in the tibia and fibula above the ankle joint. Mullis and Salis[20] reported on a mix of acute and chronic cases of syndesmotic widening treated with lag screw fixation with good results. Beals and Manoli[21] reported on a single patient who presented 6 months after repair of an ankle fracture with daily pain and inability to return to preinjury activities. The patient had a lateral shift of his talus on mortise examination with a healed well and aligned fibula fracture. The patient was treated with débridement of the syndesmotic region and medial gutter and then stabilized with a single 6.5-mm syndesmotic screw. Postoperatively the patient was non–weight bearing for 3 months and had screw removal performed at 7 months. He had a full return to all function, with significant improvement in his American Orthopaedic Foot and Ankle Society (AOFAS) score to normal.[21]

Harper[22] reported on a series of 6 patients who were treated for late widening of the syndesmosis after pronation external rotation injury (PER) stage 4 fractures. Four patients had operative fixation and 2 were treated with casting. Reconstruction was performed an average of 15 months after initial injury. Five patients were treated with repair of the syndesmosis with screw fixation and 1 patient was treated with an arthrodesis. Patients were followed for an average of 23 months. Immobilization, postoperative weight bearing, and screw removal were not standardized; 5 of 6 patients were satisfied or completely satisfied with their result. The dissatisfied patient with a poor outcome had loosening of his screw fixation, necessitating screw removal and recurrent widening at 12 weeks, and elected for no further treatment.

Ligamentous procedures have also been described for late repair of syndesmotic injuries. Grass and colleagues[23] reported on a technique using a split peroneus longus tendon to recreate the anterior and posterior tibial fibular ligaments and the interosseous ligament; 15 of 16 patients reported resolution of pain using this technique. Yasui and colleagues[24] reported on a technique advancing the AITFL using a gracilis tendon for chronic widening after pronation external rotation stage 4 fractures in 6 patients. All patients had an arthroscopy to confirm that posterior ligamentous stability was present. All patients had an improvement in AOFAS score.

Arthrodesis of the syndesmosis has also been reported as a salvage technique. Katznelson and colleagues[25] reported on a small series of patients treated for chronic ruptures of the syndesmosis by arthrodesis using a small rotated bone plug and a lag screw. Pena and Coetzee[26] advocated arthrodesis in patients greater than 6 months from injury. At the time of arthrodesis, the syndesmotic area may be débrided in an open or arthroscopic fashion.[27] van Dijk[28] described using a bone block for arthrodesis in 9 patients with symptoms greater than 6 months with good/excellent results achieved in all and most able to return to sports. Concern exists that arthrodesis of the syndesmosis may alter normal joint biomechanics. Additionally, malreduction of the syndesmosis is a known risk with acute repair of the syndesmosis. Anatomic reduction of the syndesmosis is likely even more difficult in chronic cases after the opposing surfaces have been prepared for arthrodesis. There are a few cases of arthrodesis for late reconstruction of the syndesmosis in the literature. Generally, all report good results. Isolated syndesmosis arthrodesis is a viable option for late reconstruction where arthritic change is present in the syndesmosis and in cases of other means of reconstruction not possible due to posttraumatic deformity to the area.

Normal syndesmosis anatomy is crucial for ankle function. All efforts should be made to restore normal anatomy and stability at the time of injury. Chronic syndesmotic injury and malreduction should be considered when evaluating patients with persistent pain and disability after injury. Late reconstruction should be performed if chronic syndesmotic abnormality is present.

REFERENCES

1. Purvis GD. Displaced, unstable ankle fractures: classification, incidence, and management of a consecutive series. Clin Orthop Relat Res 1982;(165):91–8.
2. Tornetta P 3rd, Axelrod TW, Sibai TA, et al. Treatment of the stress positive ligamentous SE4 ankle fracture: incidence of Syndesmotic injury and clinical decision making. J Orthop Trauma 2012;26(11):659–61.
3. Stark E, Tornetta P 3rd, Creevy WR. Syndesmotic instability in Weber B ankle fractures: a clinical evaluation. J Orthop Trauma 2007;21(9):643–6.
4. Elgafy H, Semann HB, Blessinger B, et al. Computed tomography of normal distal tibiofibular Syndesmosis. Skeletal Radiol 2010;39(6):559–64.
5. Hermans JJ, Beumer A, de Jong TA, et al. Anatomy of the distal tibiofibular syndesmosis in adults: a pictorial essay with a multimodality approach. J Anat 2010; 217(6):633–45.
6. Nault ML, Hebert-Davies J, LaFlamme GY, et al. CT scan assessment of the syndesmosis: a new reproducible method. J Orthop Trauma 2013;27(11):638–41.
7. Xenos JS, Hopkinson WJ, Mulligan ME, et al. Evaluation of the ligamentous structures, methods of fixation, and radiographic assessment. J Bone Joint Surg Am 1995;77(6):847–56.
8. Ogilvie-Harris DJ, Reed SC, Hedman TP. Disruption of the ankle Syndesmosis: biomechanical study of the ligamentous restraints. Arthroscopy 1994;10(5):558–60.
9. Bachmann L, Seifert C, Zwipp H. Experimental and clinical diagnosis of ankle injuries with the Syndesmosis spreader. In: Schmidt R, Benesch S, Lipke K, editors. Chronic ankle instability. Ulm (Germany): Libri; 2000. p. 235–8.
10. Grass R, Herzmann K, Biewener A, et al. Injuries of the distal tibiofibular Syndesmosis. Unfallchirurg 2000;103:520–32 [in German].
11. Ramsey PL, Hamilton W. Changes in the tibiotalar area of contact caused by lateral talar shift. J Bone Joint Surg Am 1976;58:356–7.
12. Zindrick MR, Hopkins DE, Knight GW, et al. The effects of lateral talar shift upon the biomechanics of the ankle joint. Orthopaedic Trans 1985;9:332–3.
13. Thordarson DB, Motamed S, Hedman T, et al. The effect of fibular malreduction on contact pressures in an ankle fracture malunion model. J Bone Joint Surg Am 1997;79(12):1809–15.
14. Egol KA, Pahk B, Walsh M, et al. Outcome after unstable ankle fracture: effect of Syndesmosis stabilization. J Orthop Trauma 2010;24(1):7–11.
15. Sagi HC, Shah AR, Sanders RW. The functional consequence of Syndesmotic joint malreduction at a minimum 2-year follow-up. J Orthop Trauma 2012;26(7): 439–43.
16. Weening B, Bhondari M. Predictors of functional outcome following transsyndesmotic screw fixation of ankle fractures. J Orthop Trauma 2005;19(2):102–8.

17. Marmor M, Hansen E, Han HK, et al. Limitations of standard fluoroscopy in detecting rotational malreduction of the Syndesmosis in an ankle fracture model. Foot Ankle Int 2011;32(6):616–22.
18. Sangeorzan BJ, Sangeorzan BP, Hansen ST, et al. Mathematically directed single-cut osteotomy for correction of tibial malunion. J Orthop Trauma 1989; 3(4):267–75.
19. Outland T. Sprains and separations of the inferior tibiofibular joint without important fracture. Am J Surg 1943;59:320–9.
20. Mullins J, Sallis J. Recurrent sprains of the ankle joint with diastasis. J Bone Joint Surg Br 1958;40-B(2):270–3.
21. Beals T, Manoli A. Late Syndesmosis reconstruction: a case report. Foot Ankle Int 1998;19:485–7.
22. Harper M. Delayed reconstruction and stabilization of the tibiofibular Syndesmosis. Foot Ankle Int 2001;22(1):15–8.
23. Grass R, Rammelt S, Biewener A, et al. Peroneus longus ligamentoplasty for chronic instability of the distal tibiofibular Syndesmosis. Foot Ankle Int 2003; 24(5):392–7.
24. Yasui Y, Takao M, Miyamoto W, et al. Anatomical reconstruction of the anterior inferior tibiofibular ligament for chronic dispruption of the distal tibiofibular Syndesmosis. Knee Surg Sports Traumatol Arthrosc 2011;19(4):691–5.
25. Katznelson A, Lin E, Militiano J. Ruptures of the ligaments about the tibio-fibular Syndesmosis. Injury 1983;15(3):170–2.
26. Pena FA, Coetzee JC. Ankle Syndesmosis injuries. Foot Ankle Clin 2006;11(1): 35–50, viii.
27. Espinosa N, Smerek JP, Myerson MS. Acute and chronic Syndesmosis injuries: pathomechanisms, diagnosis and management. Foot Ankle Clin 2006;11(3): 639–57.
28. van Dijk CN. Syndesmotic injuries. Tech Foot Ankle Surg 2006;5(1):34–7.

Calcaneal Fracture Management

Extensile Lateral Approach Versus Small Incision Technique

Nathan J. Kiewiet, MD[a],*, Bruce J. Sangeorzan, MD[b]

KEYWORDS

• Calcaneus fracture • Extensile lateral approach • Percutaneous fixation calcaneus

KEY POINTS

• Calcaneal fracture management continues to be an area of sustained interest.
• Extensile lateral approach to the calcaneus carries significant risks of wound complications and infection.
• Small incision techniques may reduce risks and improve recovery.
• Less invasive techniques have been shown to reduce risk of wound-healing complications.

INTRODUCTION

Intra-articular calcaneus fractures have long been a vexing problem for the treating orthopedic surgeon. First described by Malgaigne in 1843, calcaneus fractures were not consistently diagnosed until the development of radiography in the late 1890s. The most common tarsal bone fracture, calcaneal fractures currently account for approximately 2% of all fractures; displaced intra-articular fractures represent 60% to 75% of all calcaneal fractures.

Historically these fractures were treated nonoperatively; but over the past few decades, surgical fixation has become more prevalent. Cotton[1] identified the poor outcome associated with treatment without reduction and favored closed manipulation using a hammer to reduce the lateral wall and reimpact the fracture and suggested that open reduction is contraindicated. By the 1920s, Cotton[2] reported on his treatment of

Disclosures: The authors have nothing to disclose.
[a] Drisko, Fee, and Parkins Orthopedic Surgery, 19550 East 39th Street, Suite 410, Independence, MO 64057, USA; [b] Department of Orthopedics and Sports Medicine, Harborview Medical Center, University of Washington, 325 9th Avenue, Seattle, WA 98104, USA
* Corresponding author.
E-mail address: nkiewiet@dfportho.com

Foot Ankle Clin N Am 22 (2017) 77–91
http://dx.doi.org/10.1016/j.fcl.2016.09.013
1083-7515/17/© 2016 Elsevier Inc. All rights reserved.

healed malunions. He continued to endorse initial reduction in acute cases of calcaneal fractures to reduce the morbidity seen with malunions. In 1952, Essex-Lopresti[3] showed good results with open reduction through a lateral approach and stated that joint-depression fractures require formal open reduction with internal fixation. Operative management again fell into disfavor in the 1950s after Lindsay and Dewar[4] presented results that suggested primary subtalar fusions were being performed unnecessarily and that operative intervention of acute calcaneus fractures had many complications. Kitaoka and colleagues[5] evaluated gait analysis outcomes of 16 of 27 patients treated conservatively with casting. Most patients exhibited altered gait patterns, particularly on uneven ground, confirming nonoperative management led to at least some persistent functional impairment. Crosby and Fitzgibbons[6] reviewed their results of conservative management with casting. They showed good results of closed treatment of nondisplaced fractures and poor results of displaced fractures of the posterior facet based on computed tomography (CT) scans. They suggested operative treatment was indicated for displaced fractures of the posterior facet.

NONOPERATIVE VERSUS OPERATIVE MANAGEMENT

Several studies have been published comparing nonoperative and operative management, many with contradicting results. Jarvholm and colleagues[7] and Parmar and colleagues[8] compared operative versus nonoperative treatment and found no difference in clinical outcome and that problems associated with internal fixation did not justify operative management. There were several limitations to their studies making meaningful conclusions difficult to reach. Studies by Agren and colleagues[9] and Ibrahim and colleagues[10] reported no significant advantage to surgical management. Agren and colleagues[9] found that surgical intervention was associated with a higher risk of complications and no improvement in outcome measures with surgical management at 1 year. However, at an 8- to 12-year follow-up there was a trend toward better outcomes with regard to patient-reported visual analog scale (VAS) pain and function scores and better physical component of the 36-Item Short Form Health Survey (SF-36) scores in the operative group. These results did not reach significance. There was also an increased prevalence of radiographically documented posttraumatic subtalar arthritis in the nonoperative group; however, the need for secondary subtalar arthrodesis was not increased. Ibrahim and colleagues[10] showed no difference at a 15-year follow-up between surgical and nonsurgical management. On the other hand, studies by O'Farrell and colleagues,[11] Leung and colleagues,[12] and Crosby and Fitzgibbons[13] showed better results with surgical intervention. A randomized, prospective study by Thordarson and Krieger[14] compared operative versus nonoperative management for displaced fractures. This study showed statistically significant improvement in functional results and overall outcome in the surgically treated group, confirming that operative intervention could lead to improved outcomes. Buckley and colleagues[15] reported on a prospective, randomized controlled trial comparing operative versus nonoperative treatment of displaced intra-articular calcaneal fractures. Their results showed no significant difference in outcome measures, including SF-36 and VAS scores, between operative and nonoperative management. However, nonoperative treatment did result in a subtalar fusion rate for failed outcomes 6 times higher than the operative group.

SALVAGE OF CALCANEAL MALUNION

Nonoperative management of intra-articular calcaneus fractures increases the risk for malunion and posttraumatic subtalar arthrosis. Fractures left untreated result in significant displacement leading to altered morphology and function. The resultant morphology can adversely affect the function of the surrounding joints and soft tissues. Sequelae following nonoperative treatment of calcaneus fractures include loss of height, heel widening, subfibular and calcaneocuboid joint impingement, varus heel alignment, and posttraumatic subtalar arthrosis (**Fig. 1**).[4,5] Symptomatic complaints following calcaneal malunion may include lateral hindfoot pain due to subfibular impingement, anterior ankle pain due to loss of height resulting in a more horizontal talus and anterior ankle impingement, and pain due to posttraumatic arthrosis of the subtalar or calcaneocuboid joints. Functionally, the ankle, subtalar, and transverse tarsal joints can all be affected by calcaneal malunion.

The reconstructive procedures to correct calcaneal malunions are technically demanding and carry significant risks of complications as well. Distraction bone-block subtalar arthrodesis was originally described by Gallie[16] and modified by Carr and Benirschke[17] to help correct hindfoot alignment (**Fig. 2**). Stephens and Sanders[18] reported a CT-based classification system for calcaneal malunions based on the coronal CT images and a treatment protocol based on this classification system. Surgical treatment included lateral wall exostectomy with peroneal tenolysis for type I malunions, lateral wall exostectomy with peroneal tenolysis and distraction subtalar arthrodesis for type II malunions, and lateral wall exostectomy with peroneal tenolysis and distraction subtalar arthrodesis with calcaneal osteotomy for type III malunions. Clare and colleagues[19] then reported long-term results using this classification and treatment protocol. In their series, they treated 40 type II and III malunions with an initial fusion rate of 93%. Overall their protocol was shown to be effective at relieving pain, improving patient function, and reestablishing a plantigrade foot. They noted significant difficulty with restoring talocalcaneal height in type III nonunions; given the technical difficulties encountered, they concluded that patients with displaced intraarticular calcaneal fractures benefit from initial operative intervention. Radney and colleagues[20] reported their results for a series of patients who underwent subtalar arthrodesis for painful posttraumatic subtalar arthrosis. One group had been treated surgically initially and underwent an in situ subtalar fusion while the second group had been treated nonoperatively and developed a painful malunion, which was treated with distraction subtalar arthrodesis. Their results showed improved outcomes and fewer wound complications in patients undergoing subtalar fusion after originally being treated surgically with open reduction internal fixation compared with patients

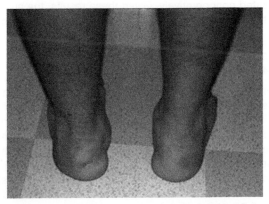

Fig. 1. Heel widening and varus alignment is noted at the left heel following nonoperative management of a calcaneus fracture.

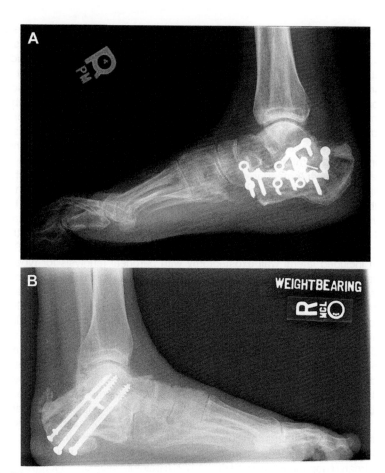

Fig. 2. (*A*) Lateral view of a calcaneal malunion with flattening of Bohler angle. (*B*) Lateral view following distraction bone block subtalar arthrodesis for salvage of calcaneal malunion.

originally being treated nonoperatively. Given these results, the authors recommend open reduction internal fixation of displaced calcaneal fractures when appropriate.

SURGICAL MANAGEMENT
Extensile Lateral Approach

Surgical management of intra-articular calcaneus fractures can be technically demanding with regard to reduction and fixation and also carries a high risk of complications.[9,10,21–25] The traditional extensile lateral approach for open reduction internal fixation of calcaneus fractures creates an L-shaped soft tissue flap that depends on the lateral calcaneal branch of the peroneal artery, which is vulnerable to injury during the extensile approach.[24–27] When the extensile lateral approach is inappropriately placed, the sural nerve is also in danger (**Fig. 3**). Although the extensile approach offers good visualization of the posterior facet for fracture reduction and direct access to the lateral wall, expertise is required to minimize high rates of complications with regard to wound healing and infection (**Fig. 4**).[21–23,28] Timing of surgical intervention is also important with regard to the extensile lateral approach. Surgeons must wait until soft tissue swelling and any blisters have resolved before proceeding with the extensile lateral approach. Once the calcaneal fracture is reduced, most investigators advocate for lag screw fixation of the posterior facet with placement of a neutralization plate on the lateral wall of the calcaneus (**Fig. 5**). Postoperatively, patients are allowed to begin working on range of motion once the incision is well healed. Weight bearing is commenced once there is adequate fracture healing, typically 2 to 3 months after surgery.

Small Incision Techniques

Recently, there has been increased interest in using less invasive surgical techniques for treating intra-articular calcaneus fractures. Less invasive techniques may reduce the risk of complications from surgical intervention and may allow for accelerated recovery following surgical intervention. Less invasive techniques can be reasonably used with displaced tongue-type fractures and joint-depression–type fractures with 2 fracture fragments of the posterior facet. Joint-depression–type fractures in patients with significant medical comorbidities may also benefit from fixation with less invasive techniques. Surgical timing is also important with regard to less invasive techniques. Less invasive techniques are more reliable when done within the first 2 weeks of injury when the fracture fragments are easily manipulated. Recent studies have shown promising results with less invasive techniques with regard to lower complication rates.

Limited-incision sinus tarsi techniques have been used to minimize the amount of soft tissue dissection while allowing for fracture reduction and stabilization. A distinct advantage to sinus tarsi approaches is the ability to directly visualize the posterior facet reduction, the anterolateral fragment at the anterior process, and the lateral wall. Kline and colleagues[29] reported on a series of 112 fractures treated either with an extensile lateral incision or a less invasive technique with a sinus tarsi approach. The investigators found significantly lower rates of wound complications and secondary surgery with the

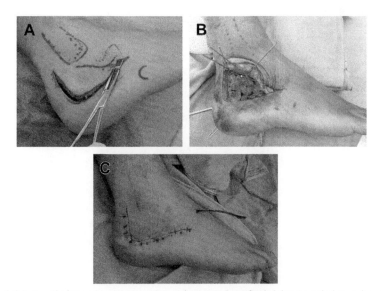

Fig. 3. (*A*) Extensile lateral incision with sural nerve identified. (*B*) Extensile lateral approach with Kirschner wire retraction in place. (*C*) Extensile lateral approach following closure.

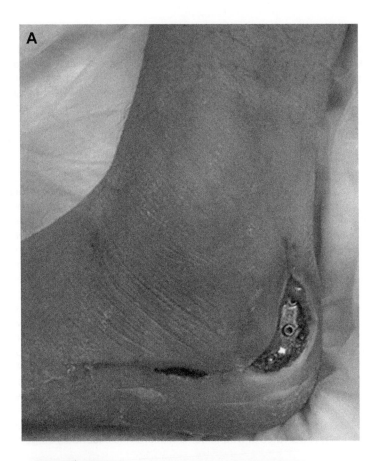

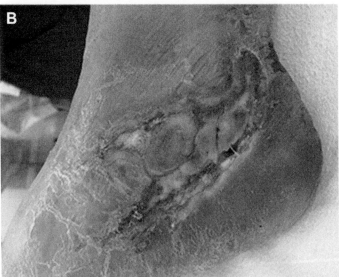

Fig. 4. (*A*) Wound necrosis at the apex of the extensile lateral approach with exposed hardware. (*B*) Extensive skin necrosis following the extensile lateral approach.

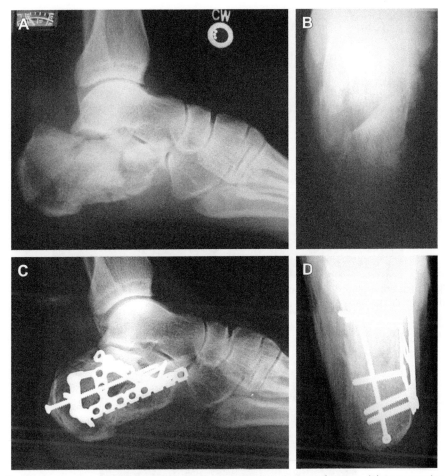

Fig. 5. (A) Preoperative lateral view of joint-depression calcaneus fracture. (B) Preoperative axial view of joint-depression calcaneus fracture. (C) Postoperative lateral view of joint-depression calcaneus fracture. (D) Postoperative axial view of joint-depression calcaneus fracture.

less invasive technique. Outcomes reported were similar between the two groups, and both techniques had a union rate of 100%. Xia and colleagues[30] reported on a randomized controlled trial of 117 calcaneus fractures comparing an extensile lateral approach with a limited sinus tarsi approach. Their study showed decreased surgical times and lower wound complications with the less invasive technique. Significantly higher Maryland Foot Scores were also found in the less invasive group.

SMALL INCISION FIXATION SURGICAL TECHNIQUE

The authors use a small incision technique for some displaced tongue-type fractures and joint-depression–type fractures without significant comminution of the posterior facet. During surgical intervention, patients are placed in the lateral decubitus position using a beanbag or alternative positioner with all bony prominences well padded (**Fig. 6**). The authors do place a thigh tourniquet, but this is not routinely used during

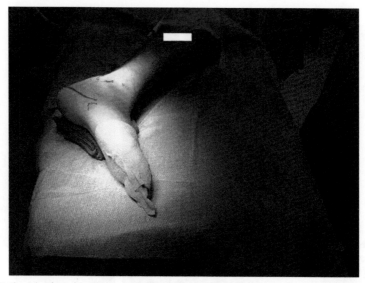

Fig. 6. Patient is placed in the lateral decubitus position on a beanbag with all bony prominences well padded.

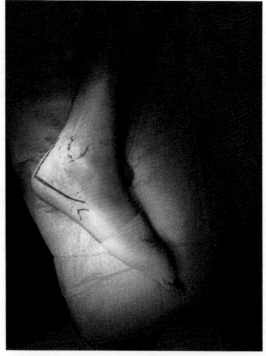

Fig. 7. Markings are made for the lateral extensile incision, and small incisions are made in line with the extensile incision.

the case unless there is substantial bleeding. The distal fibula and base of the fifth metatarsal are outlined, and the standard extensile lateral approach is outlined in case it is necessary to transition to this approach following an attempt at reduction through small incisions (**Fig. 7**). Fluoroscopy is brought in from the end of the bed so that lateral and axial images can be obtained (**Fig. 8**). Using fluoroscopy, a lateral image is obtained to mark the level of the displaced posterior facet fragment. A small subcentimeter incision is made in the skin at this level along the horizontal limb of the extensile lateral approach, and blunt dissection is carried out down to the lateral wall of the calcaneus. A second small incision is made at the posterior heel, and a 4.0- or 5.0-mm Schanz pin is placed posteriorly into the calcaneal tuberosity. With a tongue-type fracture, the Schanz pin is placed into the tongue fragment to assist in

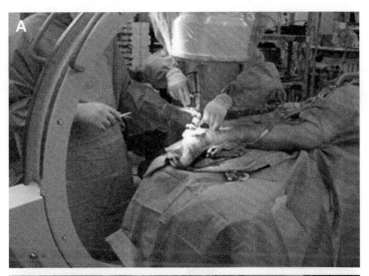

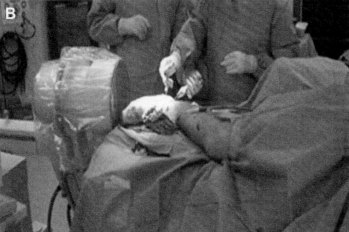

Fig. 8. (*A*) Fluoroscopy is brought in from the end of the bed to allow for obtaining a lateral view. (*B*) An axial view can also be obtained by bringing fluoroscopy in from the end of the bed.

reduction; with a joint-depression–type fracture, the Schanz pin is placed into the tuberosity to assist in reduction of the tuberosity fragment. A freer or arbeitsgemeinschaft fur osteosynthesefragen (AO) elevator is then inserted through the initial small incision on the horizontal limb to assist in reduction of the posterior facet

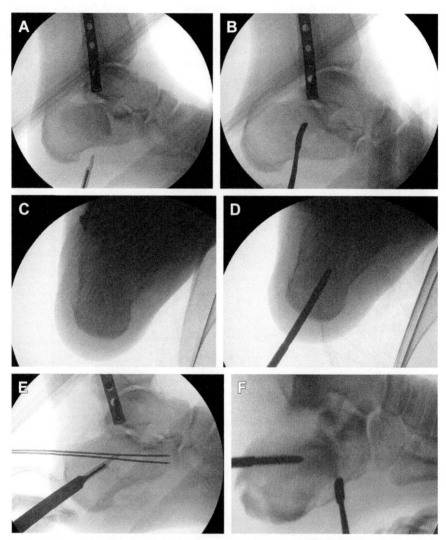

Fig. 9. (A) Site of the displaced posterior facet fragment is identified with fluoroscopy, and a subcentimeter incision is made in line with the plantar limb of the extensile lateral incision. (B) An elevator is inserted to reduce the displaced posterior facet fragment. (C) Axial view of a joint-depression calcaneus fracture before placement of a Schanz pin and reduction. (D) With joint-depression–type fractures, a Schanz pin is placed into the tuberosity fragment to assist in reduction of the tuberosity. (E) Once the posterior facet is reduced, 2 guidewires are placed just below the posterior facet and critical angle of Gissane. The knife blade is marking the posterior facet for placement of the lag screw across the posterior facet. (F) For tongue-type fractures, a Schanz pin is placed into the tongue fragment to assist in reduction.

fragment. The posterior facet fragment is reduced; joint-depression fractures, the tuberosity is reduced with a combination of distraction for length, rotation out of varus, and medialization. Once reduced, 2 guide pins or Kirschner wires are placed from the superior aspect of the calcaneal tuberosity beneath the posterior facet and critical angle of Gissane and into the anterior process of the calcaneus (**Fig. 9**). Adequate reduction and placement of guide pins are confirmed with fluoroscopic views,

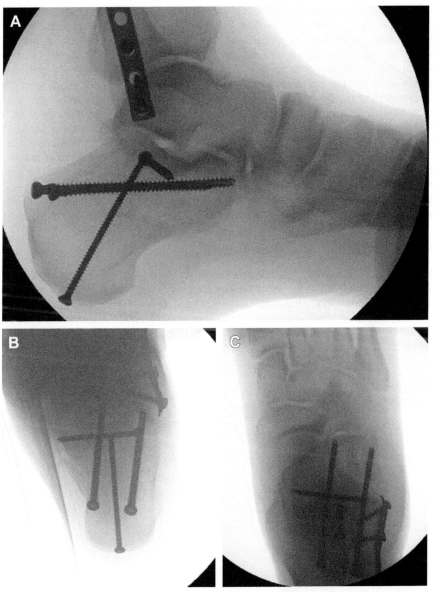

Fig. 10. (*A*) Lateral view with screws in place following small incision technique. (*B*) Axial view showing screw placement with small incision technique. (*C*) AP foot view showing screw placement with small incision technique.

including a lateral and axial view of the calcaneus, an AP view of the foot, and Broden views of the calcaneus to evaluate the posterior facet reduction. Once reduction is confirmed, the authors then proceed with placement of screws in the same path as the guidewires. The authors prefer to use cannulated 4.5- or 5.5-mm fully threaded screws. The lateral hindfoot is marked just plantar to the posterior facet using fluoroscopy, and a small incision is made in the skin with blunt dissection through the subcutaneous tissue down to the lateral calcaneus. A 3.5-mm cortical screw is then placed using lag technique across the posterior facet fracture fragment securing the lateral posterior facet fragment to the medial sustentaculum fragment and giving compression across the posterior facet fragment. A small incision is then made at the plantar aspect of the heel for placement of a 3.5-mm screw as a kickstand from the plantar aspect of the calcaneal tuberosity to just inferior to the posterior facet. In joint-depression–type fractures, the placement of 2 more 3.5-mm fully threaded screws from the plantar aspect of the tuberosity into the anterior process of the calcaneus may be warranted to assist in holding reduction of the tuberosity fragment. Fluoroscopy is used to obtain final lateral and axial views of the calcaneus, an anteroposterior (AP) view of the foot, and Broden views of the calcaneus to assure adequate reduction and good placement of hardware (**Fig. 10**). The incisions are closed with a 4-0 nylon suture (**Fig. 11**). The incisions are dressed, and patients are placed in a posterior splint or a tall controlled ankle motion (CAM) boot. Postoperatively, range-of-motion exercises are started either immediately or 1 to 2 weeks after surgery. Weight bearing is commenced at 6 to 8 weeks after surgery or when fracture healing seems adequate to begin weight bearing on follow-up radiographs.

EXTENSILE LATERAL VERSUS SMALL INCISION TECHNIQUE

The senior author and his colleagues have undertaken a prospective study evaluating the extensile lateral approach versus minimally invasive reduction and small fragment fixation for tongue-type calcaneus fractures. These data remain unpublished to date; however, their study showed a significant difference in length of hospital stay and time to weight bearing between the two groups. They also showed improved musculoskeletal function assessment (MFA) scores at 1 year in the small incision group (**Table 1**).

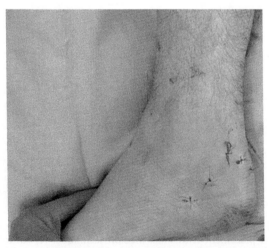

Fig. 11. Closed incisions used for small incision calcaneus fixation technique.

Table 1
Results of unpublished data from senior author comparing an extensile lateral approach with a small incision technique for tongue-type calcaneus fractures

	Small Incision	Extensile Lateral	Overall	P Value
Hospital stay (d)	1.6	3.7	2.8	<.001
Time to weight bearing (wk)	12.3	20.5	16.8	.03
Pain (VAS) (1–10)	2.6	3.1	2.9	NS
MFA scores (6 wk)	41.1	46.1	—	—
MFA scores (3 mo)	36.0	40.9	—	—
MFA scores (6 mo)	23.5	29.9	—	—
MFA scores (12 mo)	17.0	28.9	—	—

Abbreviation: NS, no significance.

SUMMARY

Treatment of displaced intra-articular calcaneus fractures has long been a controversial topic among orthopedic surgeons. Historically, nonoperative management was the treatment of choice; but over the past few decades, operative management has become more prevalent, with studies showing improved outcomes following surgical management.

Surgical intervention with an extensile lateral approach continues to be most prevalent; however, there is recent interest in less invasive techniques for fixation of displaced calcaneal fractures. The extensile lateral approach allows for direct visualization of the posterior facet reduction; however, it carries risks of wound-healing complications and infection. Less invasive techniques have been shown to have less wound-healing complications. Small incision techniques can be used for certain tongue-type fractures and for joint-depression fractures with minimal comminution. Joint-depression fractures with extensive posterior facet comminution are less amenable to small incision techniques. The authors allow for an accelerated recovery following fixation with a small incision technique in a hope to reduce the significance of loss of range of motion.

Studies have shown advantages to less invasive techniques recently, and unpublished data by the senior author and his colleagues show advantages with regard to hospital length of stay and time to weight bearing. Although the authors recognize these techniques may be a compromise between reducing the risks associated with the extensile lateral approach and accepting a possible imperfect reduction, they think that the benefits of the small incision techniques outweigh the drawbacks. Given the results of recent studies and the authors' experience, they do think that small incision techniques are a viable option for surgical management of specific calcaneus fracture types, including tongue-type calcaneal fractures and joint-depression fractures without significant comminution of the posterior facet.

REFERENCES

1. Cotton FJ. Fractures of the os calcis. Boston Med Surg J 1908;18:559–65.
2. Cotton FJ. Old os calcis fractures. Ann Surg 1921;74:294–303.
3. Essex Lopresti P. The mechanism, reduction technique, and results in fractures of the os calcis. Br J Surg 1952;39:395–419.
4. Lindsay WRN, Dewar FP. Fractures of the os calcis. Am J Surg 1958;95:555–76.
5. Kitaoka HB, Schaap EJ, Chao EY, et al. Displaced intra-articular fractures of the calcaneus treated non-operatively: clinical results and analysis of motion

and ground-reaction and temporal forces. J Bone Joint Surg Am 1994;76: 1531–40.

6. Crosby LA, Fitzgibbons T. Computerized tomography scanning of acute intra-articular fractures of the calcaneus. J Bone Joint Surg Am 1990;72:852–9.

7. Jarvholm U, Korner L, Thoren O, et al. Fractures of the calcaneus. Acta Orthop Scand 1984;55:652–6.

8. Parmar HV, Triffitt PD, Gregg PJ. Intra-articular fractures of the calcaneum treated operatively or conservatively: a prospective study. J Bone Joint Surg Br 1993;75: 932–7.

9. Agren PH, Wretenberg P, Sayed-Noor AS. Operative versus nonoperative treatment of displaced intra-articular calcaneal fractures: a prospective, randomized, controlled multicenter trial. J Bone Joint Surg Am 2013;95:1351–7.

10. Ibrahim T, Roswell M, Rennie W, et al. Displaced intra-articular calcaneal fractures: 15 year follow-up of a randomised controlled trial of conservative versus operative treatment. Injury 2007;38:848–55.

11. O'Farrell DA, O'Byrne JM, McCabe JP, et al. Fractures of the os calcis: improved results with internal fixation. Injury 1993;24:263–5.

12. Leung KS, Yuen KM, Chan WS. Operative treatment of displaced intra-articular fractures of the calcaneum: medium-term results. J Bone Joint Surg Br 1993; 75:196–201.

13. Crosby LA, Fitzgibbons TC. Open reduction and internal fixation of Type II intra-articular calcaneus fractures. Foot Ankle Int 1996;17:253–8.

14. Thordarson DB, Krieger LE. Operative vs. nonoperative treatment of intra-articular fractures of the calcaneus: a prospective randomized trial. Foot Ankle Int 1996;17:2–9.

15. Buckley R, Tough S, McCormack R, et al. Operative compared with non-operative treatment of displaced intra-articular calcaneal fractures: a prospective, randomized, controlled multicenter trial. J Bone Joint Surg Am 2002;84:1733–44.

16. Gallie WE. Subastragalar arthrodesis in fractures of the os calcis. J Bone Joint Surg Am 1943;25:731–6.

17. Carr JB, Benirschke SK. Subtalar distraction bone block fusion for late complications of os calcis fractures. Foot Ankle 1988;9:81–6.

18. Stephens HM, Sanders R. Calcaneal malunions: results of a prognostic computed tomography classification system. Foot Ankle Int 1996;17:395–401.

19. Clare MP, Lee WE 3rd, Sanders RW. Intermediate to long-term results of a treatment protocol for calcaneal fracture malunions. J Bone Joint Surg Am 2005;87: 963–73.

20. Radney CS, Clare MP, Sanders RW. Subtalar fusion after displaced intra-articular calcaneal fractures: does initial operative treatment matter? J Bone Joint Surg Am 2009;91:541–6.

21. Gardner MJ, Nork SE, Barei DP, et al. Secondary soft tissue compromise in tongue-type calcaneus fractures. J Orthop Trauma 2008;22(7):439–45.

22. Gougoulias N, Khanna A, McBride DJ, et al. Management of calcaneal fractures: systematic review of randomized trials. Br Med Bull 2009;92:153–67.

23. Swanson SA, Clare MP, Sanders RW. Management of intra-articular fractures of the calcaneus. Foot Ankle Clin 2008;13(4):659–78.

24. Cavadas PC, Landin L. Management of soft tissue complications of the lateral approach for calcaneal fractures. Plast Reconstr Surg 2007;120(2):459–66.

25. Bibbo C, Ehrlich DA, Nguyen HM, et al. Low wound complication rates for the lateral extensile approach for calcaneal ORIF when the lateral calcaneal artery is patent. Foot Ankle Int 2014;35(7):650–6.

26. Gould N. Lateral approach to the os calcis. Foot Ankle 1984;4(4):218–20.
27. Benirschke SK, Sangeorzan BJ. Extensive intraarticular fractures of the foot. Surgical management of calcaneal fractures. Clin Orthop Relat Res 1993;292: 128–34.
28. Abidi NA, Dhawan S, Gruen GS, et al. Wound-healing risk factors after open reduction and internal fixation of calcaneal fractures. Foot Ankle Int 1998; 19(12):856–61.
29. Kline AJ, Anderson RB, Davis WH, et al. Minimally invasive technique versus an extensile lateral approach for intra-articular calcaneal fractures. Foot Ankle Int 2013;34(6):773–80.
30. Xia S, Lu Y, Wang H, et al. Open reduction and internal fixation with conventional plate via L-shaped lateral approach versus internal fixation with a percutaneous plate via a sinus tarsi approach for calcaneal fractures: a randomized controlled trail. Int J Surg 2014;12(5):475–80.

Early Fixation of Calcaneus Fractures

Michael P. Swords, DO[a],*, Phillip Penny, DO, MA[b]

KEYWORDS

- Calcaneus • Early fixation • Sinus tarsi • Fracture dislocation • Tuberosity avulsion
- Open calcaneus fractures

KEY POINTS

- Early fixation of fracture-dislocations of the calcaneus should be considered to avoid contracture of soft tissues.
- Calcaneal tuberosity avulsion fractures are a surgical emergency and should be stabilized early to prevent skin breakdown of the posterior soft tissues.
- Early fixation of calcaneus fractures in hospitalized patients is often possible.
- Small incision or sinus tarsi approaches can be used for many calcaneus fractures, and reduction is less difficult when performed early.
- Open calcaneus fractures require early debridement and irrigation. Immediate internal fixation of open fractures may be considered with small incision or sinus tarsi techniques.

INTRODUCTION

Optimal management of calcaneus fractures has been an area of great interest and continues to be a subject of debate. Numerous reports have documented improved outcomes and patient satisfaction with operative fixation of calcaneus fractures compared with nonoperative management.[1–5] Nonoperatively managed patients have a 6 times greater risk of requiring subtalar arthrodesis when compared with those who have had operative management.[6] Furthermore, it has been shown that fixation of displaced, intra-articular calcaneus fractures is associated with a reduced radiographic prevalence of posttraumatic arthritis.[7] Complication rates associated with the extensile lateral approach has led to the interest in less invasive techniques to treat calcaneus fractures, including percutaneous and small incision techniques. These less invasive techniques have led to lower wound complication rates and have paved the way for early fixation of many calcaneus fractures.[8–10] Early fixation of calcaneal

Dr Swords is a consultant for DePuy Synthes, Pacira, and Acelity.
[a] Orthopedic Surgery, Michigan Orthopedic Center, Sparrow Hospital, 2815 South Pennsylvania Avenue, Suite 204, Lansing, MI 48910, USA; [b] Department of Orthopedic Surgery, Mclaren Greater Lansing, 401 West Greenlawn Avenue, Lansing, MI 48910, USA
* Corresponding author.
E-mail address: foot.trauma@gmail.com

fractures is a requirement in calcaneal tuberosity avulsion fractures and is a treatment option for the management of fracture-dislocations of the calcaneus, select hospitalized patients, and open and closed fractures treated with small incision or sinus tarsi approaches. Early treatment of these injuries is reviewed.

HINDFOOT FRACTURE-DISLOCATIONS

A rare variant of the intra-articular fracture involves fracture of the posterior facet into 2 parts with associated dislocation of most of the posterior facet superior and lateral. This fracture pattern is seen in a small percentage of Sanders IIC fractures. As the fracture dislocates laterally, the peroneal tendons dislocate from the superior peroneal retinaculum. A fracture of the fibula will often be present. This fracture will consist of either an avulsion-type injury of the superior peroneal retinaculum or an impaction injury of the distal fibula from the lateral dislocation of the calcaneus (**Fig. 1**A–D).

In this fracture pattern the lateral portion of the posterior facet is contiguous with the entire lateral portion of the calcaneus, making surgical treatment of this fracture pattern by a standard extensile approach extremely difficult. These fractures are classified as Sanders IIC fractures with an associated dislocation. This fracture pattern benefits from early reduction of the dislocation and stabilization. Delayed treatment of this injury is difficult because of contracture of the lateral soft tissues and peroneal tendons, which occur from the superior and lateral dislocation. Reduction of the dislocation increases in difficulty if treated in a delayed manner. If patients' overall condition or soft tissues preclude early treatment, the dislocation should be reduced and an external fixator used for temporary stabilization.

A direct lateral approach for treatment of calcaneus fractures has been described and extends from the tip of the fibula and runs parallel to and slightly superior to the peroneal tendons and along the sinus tarsi (**Fig. 1**E).[11] This incision can be extended to create a dislocation approach, allowing fixation of both the calcaneus fracture dislocation as well as the peroneal/fibula injury.[12] The dissection follows the normal course of the peroneal tendons allowing visualization of the dislocated lateral articular fragment and tuberosity from above. Care is taken to avoid injuring the peroneal tendons, which are dislocated anteriorly. After the fracture line is cleaned of hematoma, the lateral portion of the calcaneus including the tuberosity and most of the posterior facet is reduced under the talus. A Schanz pin placed in the tuberosity may assist reduction. A pointed reduction clamp may be placed through a small medial incision along the sustentaculum to assist in reduction of the fracture (**Fig. 1**F). In most cases fixation consists of simple lag screws (**Fig. 1**G, H). The peroneals are relocated after the calcaneus fixation is complete. The dislocated peroneals are repaired either with rigid fixation, if the injury includes enough bone to allow fixation, or with sutures if it is a pure retinaculum injury. Delayed treatment of this injury is difficult because of the contracture of the lateral soft tissues and peroneal tendons, which occur from the superior and lateral dislocation.

CALCANEAL TUBEROSITY AVULSION FRACTURES

Posterior calcaneal tuberosity fractures represent 1% to 3% of all calcaneal fractures.[13] Although these fractures are extra-articular tongue or beak fractures, it is crucial to understand at the time of initial assessment that the timing of treatment of these injuries varies from most calcaneus fractures (**Fig. 2**). The most common cause of these fractures is a violent pull from the gastrocnemius-soleus complex coupled with foot in dorsiflexion. This injury is usually associated with a low-energy fall or sudden push-off from standing in diabetic or osteoporotic patients.[14] Gross displacement of the superior margin of the calcaneal tuberosity will often create soft tissue necrosis

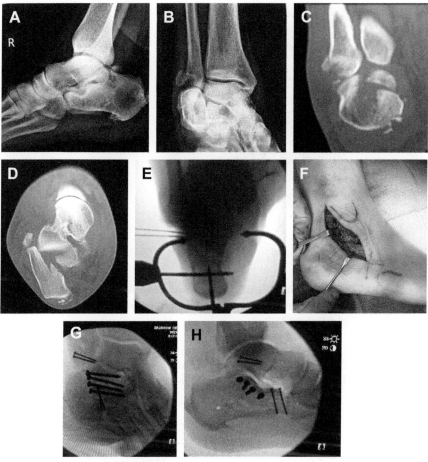

Fig. 1. A man involved in a head-on motor vehicle collision resulting in a fracture dislocation pattern. (*A*) Overlap of the subtalar joint. (*B*) The lateral portion of the calcaneus is dislocated under the fibula resulting in fracture to the fibula. (*C, D*) Coronal and axial computed tomography cuts demonstrating dislocation of the lateral portion of the posterior facet. (*E*) A large clamp may be inserted to assist in reduction. (*F*) A dislocation approach was used following the peroneal tendons. (*G, H*) Fixation was achieved using simple lag screws.

to the posterior soft tissues and can result in catastrophic complications if not treated acutely (**Fig. 3**). Initial treatment should consist of splinting the foot in maximal plantar flexion. This treatment will bring the foot up to the avulsed fragment reducing the amount of displacement and decreasing the amount of deformity on the posterior aspect of the heel. Excess padding should be placed under the splint around the posterior of the foot to avoid additional pressure on the soft tissues overlying the fracture fragment. Tuberosity avulsion fractures of the calcaneus represent a surgical urgency, if not a true surgical emergency. A delay in treatment is associated with greater risk of posterior soft tissue complications (**Fig. 4**). Fractures with greater displacement and fractures occurring in smokers carry increased risk.[15,16] Although there is general agreement regarding the urgency in reducing and stabilizing these fracture patterns, the method of fixation is a topic of debate. Current treatment strategies include

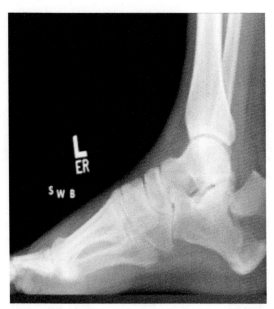

Fig. 2. A calcaneal beak fracture or posterior tuberosity avulsion fracture in an elderly woman who tripped while walking.

fragment excision in very-low-demand patients; open reduction with screws, plates, or suture anchors; percutaneous fixation; and suture fixation through bony tunnels. Locking plate fixation may be of benefit as this injury often occurs in osteoporotic patients (**Fig. 5**).[17]

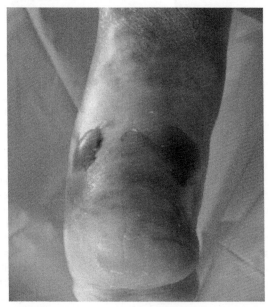

Fig. 3. Blistering and swelling of the posterior soft tissues from internal pressure from the displaced fracture fragment.

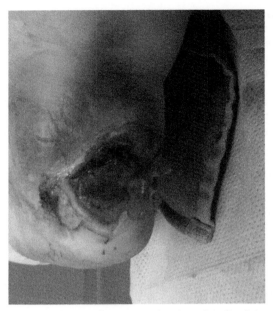

Fig. 4. Full-thickness necrosis in a patient presenting 2 weeks after injury.

The incision should be placed laterally along the vertical limb of the extensile lateral approach. Hematoma is removed from the fracture interval. The posterior superior aspect is reduced using a Schanz pin in the displaced fracture fragment or alternatively using reduction clamps. The foot is placed in maximal plantar flexion to assist

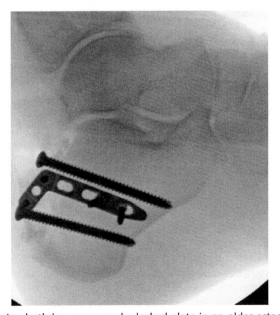

Fig. 5. Fixation using both lag screws and a locked plate in an older osteoporotic patient.

reduction. Suture may by placed in the Achilles to further assist in reduction. Care must be taken to avoid iatrogenic comminution of the fracture fragment. After surgical fixation is completed, the foot should be splinted in slight plantar flexion to reduce deforming forces from the gastrocnemius soleus complex. The need for a concomitant gastrocnemius recession procedure or Achilles lengthening is controversial. Intrinsic muscle tightness of the gastrocnemius is a risk factor for the development of these fracture patterns and may contribute to fixation failure if not addressed surgically.[18] Although the method of fixation for these injuries varies, there is consensus that this fracture pattern requires emergent or urgent surgical treatment to avoid soft tissue complications.

HOSPITALIZED PATIENTS

Admission to the hospital is a relative indication for early operative fixation of calcaneus fractures. Traditionally, patients with calcaneal fractures are treated initially with application of a bulky splint, pain control, and discharge instructions to keep their foot elevated to allow for resolution of soft tissue swelling. At home, patient compliance with elevation instructions may be less for a variety of reasons. In the home environment patients often are responsible for a greater share of their basic needs. Toileting, meals, bathing, and dressing may all require patients to elevate the extremity to a lesser extent then ideal. Additionally, patients will need to travel to and from the outpatient clinic to assess the swelling.

Patients may be admitted to the hospital for pain control after the initial traumatic injury, medical comorbidities, or polytrauma. Closer supervision of hospitalized patients ensures compliance with elevation. The hospital staff is able to assist patients in bathing, dressing, and many other daily tasks. Compliance with nicotine cessation is also easier to monitor. Intermittent pneumatic pedal compression devices have been shown to lead to a significant progressive decrease in the foot volume in the first 48 hours after application.[19] Because of these factors the resolution of soft tissue swelling may be much quicker in hospitalized patients. These patients should be monitored closely as early fixation is possible for many fractures in this patient population.

MINIMALLY INVASIVE TECHNIQUES: THE SINUS TARSI APPROACH

Percutaneous and/or mini-open approaches for the operative management of calcaneus fractures are becoming more popular for fixation of intra-articular fractures. For these techniques to be successful they must be performed at the earliest time that the soft tissues will allow so fracture fragments will still be mobile, generally within the first 1 to 2 weeks after injury. Current less invasive approaches include open reduction and internal fixation through a sinus tarsi approach, limited-incision open reduction internal fixation (ORIF), percutaneous screw placement, arthroscopic-assisted reduction, and, most recently, intramedullary nailing.[20] The extensile lateral approach has been associated with significant complications, including infection in as high as 20% of cases and wound complications in as many as 37% of cases.[21,22] Smaller incision techniques may reduce complications and result in shorter operative times when compared with traditional extensile lateral approaches.[23] Smokers and patients with medical comorbidities may also benefit from smaller incision techniques, as they are at increased risk for complications with lateral extensile approaches.

Similar to fractures treated by a lateral extensile approach, restoration of the overall bony morphology of the calcaneus is the goal of small incision techniques. A thorough knowledge of the 3-dimensional calcaneal anatomy and open reduction maneuvers is a prerequisite for good results with less invasive techniques.

Tongue-type patterns and more simple 2-part articular fractures are generally amenable to treatment via a sinus tarsi approach. With increased surgeon experience, a wider range of fractures may be treated in this manner. This approach combines the tissue-friendly concepts of percutaneous fixation with the benefit of direct visualization of the posterior facet, critical angle, and anterior process, which is essential to obtain an anatomic reduction and improved outcome.[24] A randomized controlled trial of 117 operatively treated calcaneus fractures demonstrated shorter operative times, lower wound complication rates, and higher Maryland Foot Scores in patients treated using a sinus tarsi approach as compared with a lateral extensile approach.[25] A second trial comparing the lateral extensile approach with the sinus tarsi approach in 112 calcaneus fractures demonstrated lower wound complications and a lower reoperation rate using a sinus tarsi approach.[26] Yeo and colleagues,[27] in a retrospective review comparing lateral extensile and sinus tarsi approaches for Sanders type II and type III fractures, found similar clinical and radiographic outcomes with a lower rate of wound healing complications. Weber and colleagues[28] compared extensile lateral approach with a limited incision approach in patients with Sanders type II or III fractures and found equivalent functional outcomes and anatomic reduction in both groups. The group using the less invasive technique had shorter surgical times and no cases of hematoma, wound breakdown, or sural nerve symptoms. Future prospective randomized series are needed to determine the precise indications as well as the short- and long-term outcomes of each specific technique.

Sinus Tarsi Operative Technique

Patients are positioned in a lateral position with the injured extremity up and at the end of the table. Care is taken to pad the peroneal nerve on the down leg. Two small towels are folded and placed just proximal to the malleoli to allow the foot to invert improving visualization into the subtalar joint. A 3- to-4 cm incision is placed along the critical angle of Gissane. Sinus tarsi adipose tissue and hematoma are removed with a small rongeur, pituitary, or suction to improve visualization. An elevator is used to elevate the peroneal tendons off the lateral aspect of the calcaneus and the lateral wall. The lateral subtalar joint capsule may be released, if necessary, sharply with a knife from inside the joint using care to avoid injuring the peroneal tendons. A Schanz pin is placed in the lateral aspect of the calcaneal tuberosity. Two Kirschner (K) wires are placed from the calcaneal tuberosity just inside the medial wall up to, but not across, the fracture (**Fig. 6D**). The lateral articular fragment of the posterior facet is dis-impacted from the body of the calcaneus using an elevator. An elevator is then passed under the leading edge of the lateral margin of the posterior facet and follows the fracture line out the medial side of the calcaneus (**Fig. 6E**). The medial wall is reduced by lifting the elevator, resulting in dis-impaction and manipulation of the medial portion of the posterior facet. At the same time, the Schanz pin is used to distract and rotate the tuber out of varus. Once successful, the 2 previously placed K wires are advanced across the fracture to maintain reduction of the medial wall (**Fig. 6F**). This reduction recreates appropriate height and alignment. The lateral fragments are then reduced to the medial fragment under direct visualization and held with additional K wires. After the posterior facet is reduced, the anterior process is addressed. Any fracture lines extending through the anterior process are reduced and held with additional K wires. Once the anterior process reduction is completed, additional K wires are inserted through the skin into the anterior process. The anterior process is then reduced to the posterior facet at the critical angle and the wires are advanced. Reduction is then confirmed both radiographically and with direct visualization (**Fig. 6G**). A small plate is then placed on the lateral side of the calcaneus just below the critical angle.

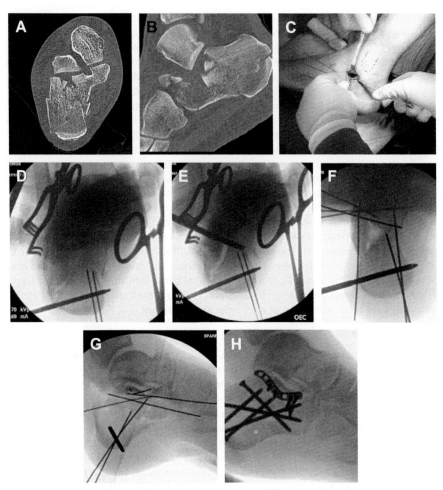

Fig. 6. (*A*) Coronal and (*B*) sagittal computed tomography scan demonstrates a comminuted calcaneus fracture due to a fall (*A, B*). (*C*) A sinus tarsi approach was used for fixation. (*D*) A Schanz pin and K wires are placed to assist with reduction. (*E*) An elevator is used to assist in reduction of the medial wall restoring height. (*F*) The K wires are advanced when reduction of the medial wall is achieved. (*G, H*) Provisional and final fixation of this comminuted injury using the sinus tarsi approach.

Plate position is confirmed by fluoroscopy, and then screws are inserted through the plate. If additional compression of the articular fragments is required, lag technique is used. This plate will provide fixation of the posterior facet to the anterior process and maintain the reduction at the critical angle. Independent 4.0-mm screws are then inserted from the calcaneal tuberosity to complete the fixation construct. Two screws are placed just inside the medial wall to replace the previously inserted wires and maintain the height and alignment of the tuberosity relative to the posterior facet. It is crucial to maintain 2 points of fixation along the medial wall to avoid loss of reduction. A screw is directed from central aspect of the tuberosity to the most anterior and distal portion of the anterior process. A final screw is placed from the posterior aspect of the tuberosity passing just under the critical angle into the anterior process (**Fig. 6**H).

An additional screw, or 2, may be required from the posterior superior ridge of the calcaneus to the plantar cortex in tongue pattern injuries or injuries with displacement of the plantar cortex. After final images are obtained, the towels are moved distal to the malleolus to allow the weight of the leg to help evert the foot to assist with wound closure. Patients are placed in a removable brace; range of motion is instituted when the wound is stable, typically by 7 to 14 days.

OPEN FRACTURES OF THE CALCANEUS

Open calcaneus factures represent high-energy injuries associated with significant soft tissue compromise.[29] Current literature estimates the rate of open calcaneus fractures to be between 1% and 10% and complication rates as high as 67%.[30] Most commonly the wound that occurs in conjunction with an open calcaneus fracture is located on the medial side of the foot. The location of the medial wound may facilitate both irrigation and debridement as well as an opportunity to reduce the medial wall. Limited fixation may be placed either medially or axially from the tuberosity. Early fixation through a minimally invasive lateral approach is preferred because most of the soft tissue stripping has occurred on the medial side. Many open calcaneus fractures can be treated with immediate ORIF through limited incisions. However, laterally based traumatic wounds are historically poor prognostic indicators and are best managed with a staged protocol.[31] In addition, type III open fractures should be

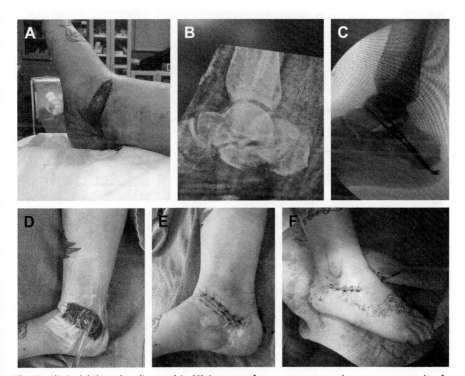

Fig. 7. Clinical (A) and radiographic (B) images of a severe open calcaneus as a result of a motor vehicle accident. They medial wall was reduced through the open wound and held with temporary wires (C). An incisional negative pressure dressing was used after closing the medial wound (D). Edema had improved (E), and the fracture was repair by a sinus tarsi approach 6 days after injury (F).

treated with a staged protocol because of the risk of wound complications and deep infection.[29] However, recent evidence supports immediate fixation of severe open calcaneus factures when the medial wound can be closed with a vacuum-assisted device and the fracture pattern allows for treatment with a minimally invasive, laterally based incision.[32]

Open Fracture Operative Technique

Patients are initially placed supine on the operative table. The medial wound is addressed with appropriate surgical debridement and copious irrigation. The primary fracture line exiting the medial wall may be reduced through the open wound and provisional wire fixation placed through a small incision at the calcaneal tuberosity The wires are bent and cut just under the skin (**Fig. 7**). The medial wound is closed if amenable. If the wound cannot be closed primarily, a vacuum assisted closure (VAC) dressing is applied. Providing restoration of height and width through the medial wound allows for more rapid resolution of soft tissue swelling. If swelling is minimal or moderate, patients are placed in a lateral position and immediate fixation of the fracture is performed through a sinus tarsi approach as previously described (**Fig. 8**). If patients are unstable or soft tissue swelling is prohibitive, the procedure is concluded

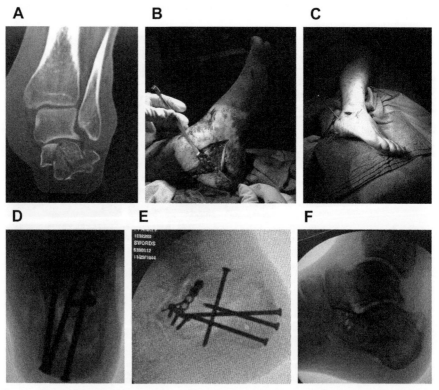

Fig. 8. Computed tomography (A) and clinical images (B) of an open calcaneus fracture from a 10-ft fall. After appropriate debridement of the open fracture, the medial wound was closed and the patient underwent immediate repair of the fracture by a sinus tarsi approach (C). Axial (D) and lateral (E) images demonstrate anatomic reconstruction with fixation present. The hardware was removed 3 years after injury (F).

and definitive fixation is performed in a delayed fashion (see **Fig. 7**).[29] By obtaining provisional reduction, restoring alignment at the time of debridement, applying negative pressure wound therapy, and treating these fractures with a sinus tarsi approach, staged procedures may be done safely at an earlier time than required with traditional extensile lateral approaches.

SUMMARY

The management of calcaneus fractures continues to evolve. Historically these fractures were treated almost universally in a delayed fashion. Early surgical treatment is necessary in select fractures. With less invasive fixation techniques, many calcaneus fractures may be considered for early surgical fixation. Surgeon experience is required to obtain optimal results.

REFERENCES

1. Sanders R, Fortin P, DiPasquale T, et al. Operative treatment in 120 displaced intra-articular calcaneal fractures: results using a prognostic computed tomography scan classification. Clin Orthop Relat Res 1993;290:87–95.
2. Thordarson DB, Krieger LE. Operative vs. nonoperative treatment of intra-articular fractures of the calcaneus: a prospective randomized trial. Foot Ankle Int 1996;17(1):2–9.
3. O'Farrell DA, O'Byrne JM, McCabe JP, et al. Fractures of the os calcis: improved results with internal fixation. Injury 1993;24:263–5.
4. Leung KS, Yuen KM, Chan WS. Operative treatment of displaced intra-articular fractures of the calcaneum: medium-term results. J Bone Joint Surg Br 1993; 75:196–201.
5. Crosby LA, Fitzgibbons TC. Open reduction and internal fixation of type II intra-articular calcaneus fractures. Foot Ankle Int 1996;17:253–8.
6. Buckley R, Tough S, McCormack R, et al. Operative compared with non-operative treatment of displaced intra-articular calcaneal fractures: a prospective, randomised, controlled multicentre trial. J Bone Joint Surg Am 2002;84:1733–4.
7. Agren PH, Wretenberg P, Sayed-Noor AS. Operative versus nonoperative treatment of displaced intra-articular calcaneal fractures: a prospective, randomized, controlled multicenter trial. J Bone Joint Surg Am 2013;95(15):1351–7.
8. DeWall M, Henderson CE, McKinley TO, et al. Percutaneous reduction and fixation of displaced intraarticular calcaneus fractures. J Orthop Trauma 2010;24(8): 466–72.
9. Kikuchi C, Charlton TP, Thordarson DB. Limited sinus tarsi approach for intraarticular calcaneus fractures. Foot Ankle Int 2013;34(12):1689–94.
10. Rammelt S, Amlang M, Barthel S, et al. Percutaneous treatment of less severe intra-articular calcaneal fractures. Clin Orthop Relat Res 2010;468(4):983–90.
11. Geel CW, Flemister AS. Standardized treatment of intra-articular calcaneal fractures using an oblique lateral incision and no bone graft. J Trauma 2001;50:1083–9.
12. Rammelt S, Zwipp H. Fractures of the calcaneus: current treatment strategies. Acta Chir Orthop Traumatol Cech 2014;81:177–96.
13. Beavis RC, Rourke K, Court-Brown C. Avulsion fracture of the calcaneal tuberosity: a case report and literature review. Foot Ankle Int 2008;29(8):863–6.
14. Hedlund LJ, Maki DD, Griffiths HJ. Calcaneus fractures in diabetic patients. J Diabetes Complications 1998;12:81–7.
15. Gardner MJ, Nork SE, Barei DP, et al. Secondary soft tissue compromise in tongue-type calcaneus fractures. J Orthop Trauma 2008;22(7):439–45.

16. Hess M, Booth B, Laughlin RT. Calcaneal avulsion fractures: complications from delayed treatment. Am J Emerg Med 2008;26(2):254.e1-4.

17. Swords M, Marsh R. Operative treatment of osteoporotic calcaneus fractures. Tech Foot Ankle Surg 2007;12(1):7–14.

18. DiGiovanni CW, Langer P. The role of isolated gastrocnemius and combined Achilles contractures in the flatfoot. Foot Ankle Clin 2007;12(2):363–79, viii.

19. Thordarson DB, Greene N, Shepherd L, et al. Facilitating edema resolution with a foot pump after calcaneus fracture. J Orthop Trauma 1999;13(1):43–6.

20. Rammelt S, Amlang M, Sands A, et al. New techniques in the operative treatment of calcaneus fractures. Unfallchirurg 2016;119(3):225–38.

21. Abidi NA, Dhawan S, Gruen GS, et al. Wound-healing risk factors after open reduction and internal fixation of calcaneal fractures. Foot Ankle Int 1998; 19(12):856–61.

22. Buckley RE, Tough S. Displaced intraarticular calcaneal fractures. J Am Acad Orthop Surg 2004;12(3):172–8.

23. Zhang T, Su Y, Chen W, et al. Displaced intra-articular calcaneal fractures treated in a minimally invasive fashion. J Bone Joint Surg Am 2014;96:302–9.

24. Schepers T. The sinus tarsi approach in displaced intra-articular calcaneal fractures: a systematic review. Int Orthop 2011;35(5):697–703.

25. Xia S, Lu Y, Wang H, et al. Open reduction and internal fixation with conventional plate via L-shaped lateral approach versus internal fixation with a percutaneous plate via a sinus tarsi approach for calcaneal fractures: a randomized controlled trail. Int J Surg 2014;12(5):475–80.

26. Kline AJ, Anderson RB, Davis WH, et al. Minimally invasive technique versus an extensile lateral approach for intra-articular calcaneal fractures. Foot Ankle Int 2013;34(6):773–80.

27. Yeo J, Cho H, Lee K. Comparison of two surgical approaches for displaced intra-articular calcaneal fractures: sinus tarsi versus extensile lateral approach. BMC Musculoskelet Disord 2015;16:63.

28. Weber M, Lehmann O, Sägesser D, et al. Limited open reduction and internal fixation of displaced intra-articular fractures of the calcaneum. J Bone Joint Surg Br 2008;90(12):1608–16.

29. Mehta S, Mirza A, Dunbar R, et al. A staged treatment plan for the management of type II and type IIIA open calcaneus fractures. J Orthop Trauma 2009;24(3):142–7.

30. Berry GK, Stevens DG, Kreder HJ, et al. Open fractures of the calcaneus: a review of treatment and outcome. J Orthop Trauma 2004;18:202–6.

31. Thornton SJ, Cheleuitte D, Ptaszek AJ, et al. Treatment of open intraarticular calcaneal fractures: evaluation of a treatment protocol based on wound location and size. Foot Ankle Int 2006;27:317–23.

32. Zhang T, Yan Y, Xie X, et al. Minimally invasive sinus tarsi approach with cannulated screw fixation combined with vacuum-assisted closure for treatment of severe open calcaneal fractures with medial wounds. J Foot Ankle Surg 2016;55:112–6.

Managing Complications of Calcaneus Fractures

Michael P. Clare, MD[a],*, William S. Crawford, MD[b]

KEYWORDS

- Calcaneus fracture • Complications • Wound dehiscence • Malunion

KEY POINTS

- The treatment of calcaneus fractures includes management of sequela of the injury as well as complications regardless of treatment strategy.
- The goal of operative management is to restore native anatomy in order to maximize function and maximize the life span of the joint.
- Meticulous operative technique and a thorough 3-dimensional knowledge of the involved pathoanatomy are pivotal to minimizing perioperative complications surrounding calcaneus fractures.
- A thorough knowledge of these injury sequela and complications should be part of the orthopedic armamentarium for the treatment of fractures of the calcaneus.

INTRODUCTION

Despite the many advances in orthopedic surgery techniques and implants over the past several decades, the management of fractures of the calcaneus remains one of the most challenging problems in the field. Complications can occur with both operative and nonoperative management. Therefore, management of these complications is as important as operative technique for the management of calcaneus fractures.

Wound Complications

The most common complication associated with operative treatment of calcaneus fractures is delayed wound healing, likely a reflection of the limited surrounding soft tissue envelope and the extent of soft tissue trauma associated with the injury.

Extensile lateral approach

Although a variety of surgical approaches have been used historically, the extensile lateral approach has been the most commonly used approach over the past 30 years.[1]

The authors have nothing to disclose.
[a] Foot and Ankle Fellowship, Florida Orthopaedic Institute, 13020 Telecom Parkway North, Tampa, FL 33637, USA; [b] Texas Foot and Ankle Orthopaedics, 800 5th Avenue, #500, Fort Worth, TX 76104, USA
* Corresponding author.
E-mail address: mpclaremd@gmail.com

The incidence of delayed wound healing has been significantly decreased by delaying treatment of calcaneus fractures until the initial postinjury swelling has sufficiently resolved, as indicated by a return of skin wrinkles overlying the calcaneus.[2] Patience is certainly required on the part of both the patient and the surgeon, as this may require up to 3 weeks following injury.

Despite this, the incidence of postsurgical wound breakdown can still occur in up to 25% of patients, usually at the apex of the lateral extensile incision.[3–10] Preoperative risk factors that predispose to wound breakdown include smoking, diabetes, open fractures, high body mass index, and closure of the incision in a single layer.[5,11] Although initial closure may approximate the tissues well, wound dehiscence can still occur up to 4 weeks out from surgery.

Sinus tarsi approach

The sinus tarsi approach has become increasingly popular in recent years. Advantages include much earlier time to fixation, often within 2 to 3 days of injury, and theoretically less wound healing difficulties. Use of this approach requires a thorough 3-dimensional understanding of the pathoanatomy of calcaneal fractures, as this approach affords, by definition, less exposure of the fracture site. Although early reports are encouraging, there are no long-term studies assessing the wound complication rate relative to the malunion rate.[12–14]

Treatment of delayed wound healing

In the event of wound breakdown, all range-of-motion exercises should be stopped and a prophylactic empirical course of oral antibiotics should be started. Treatment should include either a short leg cast with a window (**Fig. 1**) over the wound to allow for wound care with damp-to-dry dressing changes (or other granulation tissue-promoting wound therapy) or placement of a pneumatic fracture boot with daily whirlpool treatments.

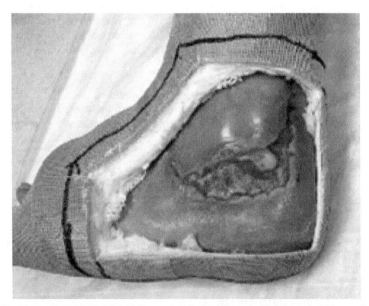

Fig. 1. Postoperative wound breakdown treated with a short leg cast with a window to allow for damp-to-dry dressings.

These methods are generally successful if the wound breakdown is partial thickness. As soon as the wound is healed, range-of-motion exercises are resumed. Recalcitrant wounds may benefit from negative-pressure wound therapy to accelerate formation of granulation tissue. Alternatively, negative-pressure wound therapy may be initiated with the postoperative dressing as a preventative measure.[15] If these methods are not successful, a fasciocutaneous flap may be necessary for wound coverage.[8]

In the case that gross purulence is encountered, hospitalization with serial operative debridements is required. It is important to obtain intraoperative cultures to identify the offending organism and to guide culture-specific antimicrobial treatment. When this presents, it is generally in the early postoperative period; most patients have an osteitis from the adjacent wound, rather than frank osteomyelitis.[16] Regardless, these patients are generally treated with culture-specific intravenous antibiotics for 6 weeks.

If the wound is relatively superficial, hardware should be maintained, at least until fracture union or a minimum of 6 months. Once the wound is determined to be clean after serial debridements, wound closure is performed, either primarily in a delayed fashion or secondarily with the aid of negative-pressure wound therapy. If the wound is too large to accomplish the aforementioned treatments, a free-tissue transfer is performed into the defect.

Osteomyelitis
Despite the aforementioned treatments, the incidence of osteomyelitis following surgical management of calcaneus fractures is 1% to 4% of closed fractures[3,7,9,17] and up to 19% in open fractures.[3,18–20]

In the case of diffuse osteomyelitis, all implants must be removed, necrotic bone debrided, and an antibiotic-impregnated spacer should be placed. Serial debridements and antibiotic spacer exchange is indicated until the wound is determined to be clean. Patients should then complete a 6-week course of culture-specific intravenous antibiotics. Following this treatment, after a 1- to 2-week antibiotic holiday, patients are readmitted to the hospital for surgical reconstruction.

If the wound is clean, and intraoperative gram stain is negative, a subtalar fusion is performed with a large structural iliac crest autograft, based on the remaining calcaneal bone stock. In exceptional cases, if infection persists or is not adequately treated with the aforementioned methods, below-knee amputation is required.

Peroneal Tenosynovitis and Stenosis
Peroneal tenosynovitis and stenosis are generally seen after nonsurgical treatment of calcaneus fractures, because of the expanded lateral wall of the calcaneus, which subluxates the peroneal tendons, causing them to impinge on the tip of the fibula or causing frank dislocation over the fibula.

Peroneal tenosynovitis and stenosis are relatively uncommon following operative treatment, particularly with use of the extensile lateral approach.[1,21] Soft tissue adhesions and implant prominence, however, can contribute to peroneal tendon symptoms following surgical management.

Treatment of peroneal tenosynovitis/stenosis
The initial management of peroneal tenosynovitis and stenosis following calcaneus fractures consists of nonoperative treatment with a combination of temporary immobilization, nonsteroidal antiinflammatory medications, and physical therapy for manual mobilization, stretching, and eversion strengthening. If nonoperative management fails, surgical treatment consists of peroneal tenolysis with possible concurrent

implant removal if applicable. If peroneal symptoms coexist with a malunion, concurrent treatment of the peroneal tendons and the malunion is appropriate (see *Malunion* section).

Peroneal Dislocation

Peroneal tendon dislocation after calcaneus fracture typically occurs in the setting of a joint-depression–type fracture due to the concomitant lateral wall expansion and loss of calcaneal height. The more lateral the intra-articular fracture line, the greater likelihood of superior peroneal retinaculum (SPR) injury. The diagnosis can be made clinically (**Fig. 2**) or radiographically with a fibular fleck sign but is often subtle.

Intraoperatively, the integrity of the SPR should be assessed before wound closure. A Freer elevator is introduced into the peroneal sheath and slid proximally to the retrofibular area. The elevator is levered anteriorly; with an incompetent SPR, the elevator will slide anterior to the posterolateral rim of the fibula; with an intact SPR, the elevator will be met with a firm end point.

Treatment of peroneal dislocation

Dislocating peroneal tendons should be repaired at the time of surgery by tacking the periosteal sleeve to the posterolateral corner of the fibula in order to close the soft tissue defect over the fibula to maintain peroneal tendon location.[22–26]

The calcaneal incision is closed first so as to restore tension of the soft tissue envelope. A small, separate incision is made along the posterolateral rim of the fibula. The peroneal sheath is incised, and the peroneal tendons are assessed for intrasubstance tears. The so-called false pouch[22] is identified, and suture anchors are placed along the

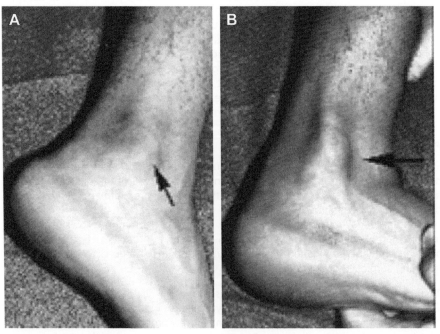

Fig. 2. (*A*) Clinical photograph after calcaneus fracture with foot in plantar flexion-inversion with located peroneal tendons (*arrow*). (*B*) The foot is taken into dorsiflexion-eversion, demonstrating dislocation of the peroneal tendons (*arrow*).

posterolateral rim. The sutures are passed into the detached SPR and periosteal sleeve as anteriorly as possible and tied in horizontal mattress fashion, thereby restoring the posterolateral checkrein (**Fig. 3**). The peroneal sheath is closed in routine fashion.

Posttraumatic Arthritis

Intra-articular incongruity of the posterior facet can result in rapid deterioration of the joint surface, leading to severe pain and disability.[10,27,28] Subtalar arthrosis may still develop despite anatomic reduction due to direct chondrocyte damage at the time of injury.[2,29] Posttraumatic arthrosis can also develop at the calcaneocuboid joint, due to the secondary fracture line projecting anteriorly, which creates the anterolateral fragment and often exits in the calcaneocuboid joint (**Fig. 4**).

Treatment of posttraumatic arthritis

If posttraumatic arthritis is present clinically and radiographically, it can be confirmed by diagnostic/therapeutic injection of the subtalar or calcaneocuboid joint. Initial nonsurgical management consists of temporary immobilization, nonsteroidal antiinflammatory medication, and/or shoe wear modifications with a lace-up ankle brace or a University of California Berkeley Laboratory orthosis. If symptoms persist despite these modalities, surgical treatment is warranted.

In the setting of anatomic or near-anatomic alignment, treatment of end-stage subtalar arthritis consists of an in situ subtalar arthrodesis with large cannulated lag screws (**Fig. 5**). Previous calcaneal implants typically have to be removed in order to provide space for the lag screws.

Treatment of posttraumatic calcaneocuboid arthritis includes exostectomy versus arthrodesis, depending on the extent of calcaneocuboid joint involvement. Typically the arthritic change is limited to the lateral one-quarter to one-third of the joint surface, such that exostectomy alone will suffice.

Calcaneal Malunion

Calcaneal malunions typically result from displaced intra-articular fractures that were treated nonsurgically, often related to a lack of familiarity or comfort with operative techniques or fear of potential operative complications.[30,31] Resulting sequela of such treatment include posttraumatic arthritis due to residual joint displacement;

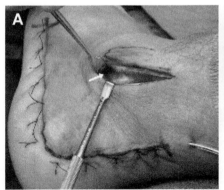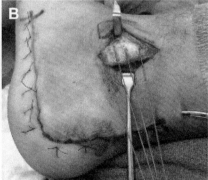

Fig. 3. (*A*) Intraoperative photograph demonstrating SPR avulsed from the fibula, allowing the peroneal tendons to dislocate anteriorly over the fibula. Note the false pouch from incompetence of the posterolateral checkrein (*white arrow*). (*B*) The SPR has been repaired with suture anchors. The peroneal sheath is then closed over the peroneal tendons, keeping them located.

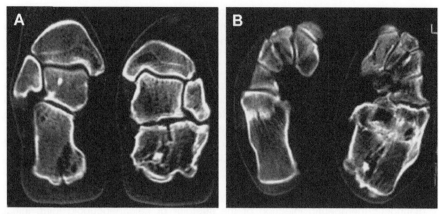

Fig. 4. (*A*). Coronal computed tomography (CT) scan demonstrating posttraumatic subtalar arthrosis. (*B*) Axial CT scan of the same patient demonstrating posttraumatic calcaneocuboid arthrosis.

subfibular impingement due to lateral wall expansion; peroneal tendon impingement, stenosis, or dislocation due to lateral wall expansion; anterior ankle impingement with loss of dorsiflexion due to a loss in calcaneal height resulting in relative dorsiflexion of the talus; hindfoot varus of valgus malalignment resulting in alteration of gait and foot biomechanics; and/or posterior tibial or sural neuritis.[27,32–42]

Malunion can also occur after surgical treatment. Poeze and colleagues[43] showed that there is an inverse relationship between postoperative subtalar arthrosis and institutional fracture volume, suggesting the real presence of a learning curve with operative treatment of these injuries.

Classification of calcaneal malunions
The Stephens and Sanders classification (**Fig. 6**) and treatment algorithm for calcaneal malunions has been shown to be prognostic for the treatment of this condition with long-term follow-up.[44,45] Under this system, a type I includes those with a large lateral

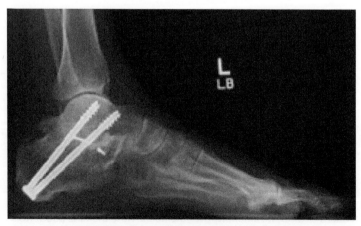

Fig. 5. Postoperative radiograph of an in situ subtalar arthrodesis following posttraumatic arthritis after minimally displaced intra-articular calcaneus fracture.

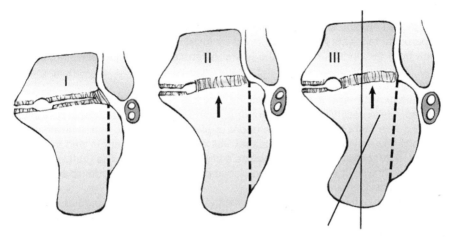

Fig. 6. Stephens and Sanders classification for calcaneal malunion. Note the lateral wall exostosis (*dashed line*), and post-traumatic subtalar arthrosis (*black arrow*).

exostosis with or without far-lateral subtalar arthrosis; a type II includes those with a large lateral exostosis with extensive subtalar arthrosis without hindfoot malalignment; a type III includes those with a large lateral exostosis and extensive subtalar arthrosis in the setting of varus or valgus hindfoot malalignment.

Treatment of calcaneal malunions
Treatment of all 3 malunion types is performed through a lateral extensile approach. Type I malunions are treated with lateral wall exostectomy (including the lateral-most portion of the subtalar joint if far-lateral subtalar arthrosis is present) with peroneal tenosynovectomy. Type II malunions are treated with lateral wall exostectomy, peroneal tenolysis, and bone-block subtalar arthrodesis, using the resected exostosis as structural bone graft to increase calcaneal height and increase talar declination. Type III malunions are treated the same as type II malunions with the addition of a calcaneal osteotomy to correct varus or valgus malalignment.

Despite the good results of the aforementioned treatment algorithm for those initially treated with nonoperative management after calcaneus fracture, patient outcomes are still significantly lower than those patients treated originally by open reduction internal fixation (ORIF) who subsequently developed posttraumatic subtalar arthrosis.[44,46] This finding suggests that initial ORIF allows restoration of calcaneal height, length, and overall morphology, which is beneficial to patients, even if posttraumatic arthritis develops over time.

Surgical technique for the treatment of calcaneal malunion
Patients are placed in a lateral decubitus position, and a standard lateral extensile approach to the calcaneus is performed. Using a sagittal saw, a lateral exostectomy is performed from posterior to anterior, while angling the blade in the coronal plane such that more bone is excised dorsally to decompress the subfibular area and thereby preserve more bone plantarly. The distal fibula and talofibular joint should be protected, and the exostectomy is continued distally to the calcaneocuboid joint. The exostectomy can include the far-lateral portion of the posterior facet articular surface where involved and can also include the far-lateral portion of the calcaneocuboid

articular surface where involved. The exostectomy is completed with an osteotome and removed en bloc for later use as structural autograft (where indicated).

A peroneal tenolysis is then performed by incising the 2 to 3 cm of the peroneal sheath from the undersurface of the lateral extensile flap. A Freer elevator is introduced within the peroneal sheath and advanced proximally to the retro-fibular groove and distally to the cuboid tunnel.

In patients with type II or III malunions, any remaining subtalar joint cartilage is debrided, while preserving the subchondral bone. The subchondral bone is perforated using 2.5-mm drill bit. A laminar spreader is placed posteriorly within the posterior facet, and the previously resected lateral wall expansion fragment is wedged within the posterior facet of the subtalar joint as a structural autograft. The graft is oriented within the joint with the thickest portion placed posteromedially, in order to avoid hindfoot varus malalignment.

The subtalar joint is then positioned in neutral to slight valgus and stabilized using 2 large cannulated, partially threaded lag screws in diverging fashion. In patients with type III malunions, a calcaneal osteotomy is performed before final screw placement. In patients with a varus malunion, a Dwyer closing-wedge osteotomy is performed. In patients with a valgus malunion, a medializing calcaneal osteotomy is performed. If desired, a third cannulated lag screw can be placed from the anterior process of the calcaneus to the talar neck and head (**Fig. 7**).

Routine layered closure is performed over a drain, from the ends of the incision toward the apex to adequately distribute skin tension. In patients with a type I malunion, weight bearing and range-of-motion exercises are initiated once the lateral extensile incision is healed. In patients with a type II or II malunion, weight bearing is not permitted for 10 to 12 weeks, at which point radiographic union should be confirmed.

Ankle Pain

Ankle pain following calcaneus fracture can be multifactorial, which can be due to anterior ankle impingement due to a relative increase in talar dorsiflexion due to a loss in calcaneal height. It can also be due to projected inversion-eversion forces across the ankle joint due to loss of subtalar range of motion.

Initial nonoperative management includes temporary boot immobilization, nonsteroidal antiinflammatory medication, or the use of a lace-up ankle brace. In the event of recalcitrant pain, arthroscopic debridement of intra-articular adhesions or chronic capsular scarring is preferred.

Heel Pad Pain

During the impact of initial injury, there can direct damage to the soft tissues of the heel pad itself. This tissue is composed of a unique architecture of soft tissue septations. Because of that unique architecture, there is no suitable tissue transfer technique to replicate this architecture. There does not seem to be any benefit for operative management of this complication.[47,48] Aside from a gel-type heel pad shoe insert, there remains no effective treatment to date for this complication.

Heel Exostoses

Painful plantar heel exostoses can develop after fractures of the calcaneus. Initial treatment of nonoperative management with a gel-type heel pad shoe insert is the mainstay. If nonoperative management fails, surgical resection of the plantar exostoses can be performed[35]; but a plantar incision should be avoided, so as to avoid painful scarring.

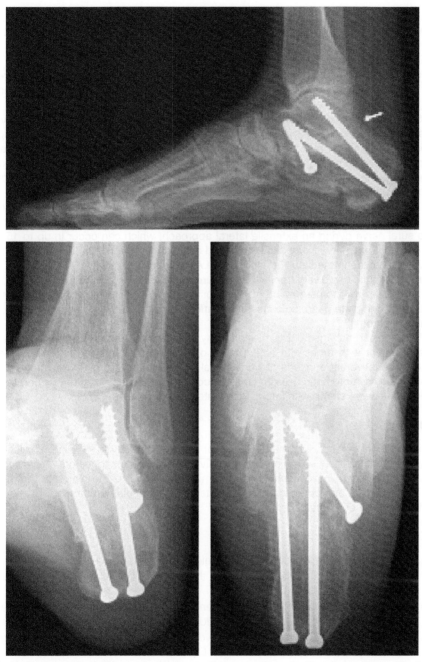

Fig. 7. Postoperative radiographs demonstrating correction of a type II calcaneal malunion using 3 large cannulated lag screws. Note the excised lateral wall exostosis used as a auto-graft bone block (*white arrow*).

Cutaneous Nerve Injury/Nerve Entrapment

Neurologic symptoms following fracture of the calcaneus can occur with either operative or nonoperative management.

The most common neurologic complication following nonsurgical management is nerve entrapment. The most commonly involved nerve is the posterior tibial nerve, as this can become entrapped from soft tissue scarring, fracture fragment malunion, or exostosis.[9,49,50]

Symptoms include medial heel pain and paresthesias in the posterior tibial nerve distribution. Often, these symptoms are worse at night or with standing or walking. Clinical examination may demonstrate a positive Tinel sign over the tarsal tunnel. Diagnosis can be confirmed with electrodiagnostic testing or a local anesthetic injection in the tarsal tunnel. With a confirmed diagnosis, surgical nerve decompression may be indicated.

The most common neurologic complication following operative treatment of fractures of the calcaneus is iatrogenic injury to a sensory cutaneous nerve, particularly the sural nerve during an extensile lateral approach, which can occur in up to 15% of cases.[9] Sural nerve injury can be avoided if the vertical limb of the extensile lateral incision is made immediately anterior to the Achilles tendon.

Injuries to the nerve vary from traction neuropraxia to nerve laceration. With traction neuropraxia, symptoms may be transient or permanent. Patients may experience a partial or complete neurologic loss in the affected neurologic distribution, or even a painful neuroma.

Nonsurgical management is the mainstay of treatment, including pharmacologic management with drugs like amitriptyline or gabapentin, physical therapy, and/or accommodative shoe inserts. If nonsurgical modalities fail, surgical treatment of a persistently symptomatic neuroma may be considered, including neurolysis or resection of the nerve stump with implantation into muscle or bone.

SUMMARY

Complications surrounding the treatment of calcaneus fractures remain a challenge for orthopedic surgeons. The goal of operative management is to restore native anatomy in order to maximize function and maximize the life span of the joint. Management of injury sequela and complications is pivotal for the complete treatment of patients with a fracture of the calcaneus.

REFERENCES

1. Gould N. Lateral approach to the os calcis. Foot Ankle 1984;4:218–20.
2. Sanders R. Intra-articular fractures of the calcaneus: present state of the art. J Orthop Trauma 1992;6:252–65.
3. Benirschke SK, Kramer PA. Wound healing complications in closed and open calcaneal fractures. J Orthop Trauma 2004;18:1–6.
4. Benirschke SK, Sangeorzan BJ. Extensive intra-articular fractures of the foot. Surgical management of calcaneal fractures. Clin Orthop Relat Res 1993;(292):128–34.
5. Folk JW, Starr AJ, Early JS. Early wound complications of operative treatment of calcaneus fractures: analysis of 190 fractures. J Orthop Trauma 1999;13:369–72.
6. Harty M. Anatomic considerations in injuries of the calcaneus. Orthop Clin North Am 1973;4:179–83.
7. Howard JL, Buckley R, McCormack R, et al. Complications following management of displaced intra-articular calcaneal fractures: a prospective randomized

trial comparing open reduction internal fixation with nonoperative management. J Orthop Trauma 2003;17:241–9.

8. Levin LS, Nunley JA. The management of soft-tissue problems associated with calcaneal fractures. Clin Orthop Relat Res 1993;(290):151–6.

9. Lim EV, Leung JP. Complications of intraarticular calcaneal fractures. Clin Orthop 2001;(391):7–16.

10. Sanders R, Fortin P, DiPasquale T, et al. Operative treatment in 120 displaced in-traarticular calcaneal fractures. Results using a prognostic computed tomography scan classification. Clin Orthop Relat Res 1993;(290):87–95.

11. Abidi NA, Dhawan S, Gruen GS, et al. Wound-healing risk factors after open reduction and internal fixation of calcaneal fractures. Foot Ankle Int 1998;19:856–61.

12. Kline AJ, Anderson RB, Davis WH, et al. Minimally invasive technique versus an extensile lateral approach for intra-articular calcaneal fractures. Foot Ankle Int 2013;34(6):773–80.

13. Kikuchi C, Charlton TP, Thordarson DB. Limited sinus tarsi approach for intra-articular calcaneus fractures. Foot Ankle Int 2013;34(12):1689–94.

14. Zhang T, Su Y, Chen W, et al. Displaced intra-articular calcaneal fractures treated in a minimally invasive fashion: longitudinal approach versus sinus tarsi approach. J Bone Joint Surg Am 2014;96(4):302–9.

15. Stannard JP, Volgas DA, McGwin G III, et al. Incisional negative pressure wound therapy after high-risk lower extremity fractures. J Orthop Trauma 2012;26:37–42.

16. Cierny G. Classification and treatment of chonic osteomyelitis. In: Evarts CM, editor. Surgery of the musculoskeletal system. New York: Churchill Livingstone; 1989. p. 10–35.

17. Harvey EJ, Grujic L, Early JS, et al. Morbidity associated with ORIF of intra-articular calcaneus fractures using a lateral approach. Foot Ankle Int 2001;22:868–73.

18. Aldridge JM III, Easley M, Nunley JA. Open calcaneal fractures: results of operative treatment. J Orthop Trauma 2004;18:7–11.

19. Berry GK, Stevens DG, Kreder HJ, et al. Open fractures of the calcaneus: a review of treatment and outcome. J Orthop Trauma 2004;18:202–6.

20. Heier KA, Infante AF, Walling AK, et al. Open fractures of the calcaneus: soft-tissue injury determined outcome. J Bone Joint Surg Am 2003;85-A:2276–82.

21. Tufescu TV, Buckley R. Age, gender, work capability, and worker's compensation in patients with displaced intraarticular calcaneal fractures. J Orthop Trauma 2001;15:275–9.

22. Das De S, Balasubramanium P. A repair operation for recurrent dislocation of peroneal tendons. J Bone Joint Surg Br 1985;67:585–7.

23. Mason RB, Henderson JP. Traumatic peroneal tendon instability. Am J Sports Med 1996;24:652–8.

24. Slatis P, Santavirta S, Sandelin J. Surgical treatment of chronic dislocation of the peroneal tendons. Br J Sports Med 1988;22:16–8.

25. Sobel M, Geppert MJ, Warren RF. Chronic ankle instability as a cause of peroneal tendon injury. Clin Orthop Relat Res 1993;(296):187–91.

26. Steinbock G, Pinsger M. Treatment of peroneal tendon dislocation by transposition under the calcaneofibular ligament. Foot Ankle Int 1994;15:107–11.

27. Myerson M, Quill GE Jr. Late complications of fractures of the calcaneus. J Bone Joint Surg Am 1993;75:331–41.

28. Paley D, Hall H. Intra-articular fractures of the calcaneus. A critical analysis of results and prognostic factors. J Bone Joint Surg Am 1993;75:342–54.

29. Borelli J Jr, Torzilli PA, Grigiene R, et al. Effect of impact load on articular cartilage: Development of an intra-articular fracture model. J Orthop Trauma 1997;11: 319–26.
30. Lindsay WRN, Dewar FP. Fractures of the os calcis. Am J Surg 1958;95:555–76.
31. Pozo JL, Kirwan OE, Jackson AM. The long term results of conservative management of severely displaced fractures of the calcaneus. J Bone Joint Surg Br 1984; 66B:386–90.
32. Isbister JF. Calcaneo-fibular abutment following crush fracture of the calcaneus. J Bone Joint Surg Br 1974;56:274–8.
33. Braly WG, Bishop JO, Tullos HS. Lateral decompression for malunited os calcis fractures. Foot Ankle 1985;6(2):90–6.
34. Carr JB, Hansen ST, Benirske SK. Subtalar distraction bone block fusion for late complications of os calcis fractures. Foot Ankle 1988;9:81–6.
35. Cotton FJ. Old os calcis fractures. Ann Surg 1921;74:294–303.
36. Cotton FJ, Henderson FF. Results of fractures of the os calcis. Am J Orthop Surg 1916;14:290.
37. Gallis WE. Subastragalar arthrodesis in fractures of the os calcis. J Bone Joint Surg Am 1943;XXV:731–6.
38. Kalamchi A, Evans JG. Posterior subtalar fusion. A preliminary report on a modified Gallie's procedure. J Bone Joint Surg Br 1977;59:287–9.
39. Magnuson PB. An operation for relief of disability in old fractures of the os calcis. JAMA 1923;80:1511–3.
40. Miller WE. Pain and impairment considerations following treatment of disruptive os calcis fractures. Clin Orthop Relat Res 1983;177:82–6.
41. Romash MM. Reconstructive osteotomy of the calcaneus with subtalar arthrodesis for malunited calcaneal fractures. Clin Orthop Relat Res 1993;(290):157–67.
42. Sanders R, Fortin P, Walling A. Subtalar arthrodesis following calcaneal fracture. Orthop Trans 1991;15:656.
43. Poeze M, Verbruggen JP, Brink PR. The relationship between the outcome of operatively treated calcaneal fractures and institutional fracture load. A systematic review of the literature. J Bone Joint Surg Am 2008;90:1013–21.
44. Clare MP, Lee WE III, Sanders RW. Intermediate to long-term results of a treatment protocol for calcaneal fracture malunions. J Bone Joint Surg Am 2005;87: 963–73.
45. Stephens HM, Sanders R. Calcaneal malunions: results of a prognostic computed tomography classification system. Foot Ankle Int 1996;17:395–401.
46. Radnay CS, Clare MP, Sanders RW. Subtalar fusion after displaced intra-articular calcaneal fractures: does initial operative treatment matter? J Bone Joint Surg Am 2009;91:541–6.
47. Bernard L, Odegard JK. Conservative approach in the treatment of fractures of the calcaneus. J Bone Joint Surg Am 1955;37-A:1231–6.
48. Lance EM, Carey EJ Jr, Wade PA. Fractures of the os calcis: treatment by early immobilization. Clin Orthop Relat Res 1963;30:76–90.
49. Kitaoka HB, Schaap EJ, Chao EY, et al. Displaced intra-articular fractures of the calcaneus treated non-operatively. Clinical results and analysis of motion and ground-reaction and temporal forces. J Bone Joint Surg Am 1994;76A:1531–40.
50. Myerson MS, Berger BI. Nonunion of a fracture of the sustentaculum tali causing a tarsal tunnel syndrome: a case report. Foot Ankle Int 1995;16:740–2.

Gastrocnemius or Achilles Lengthening at Time of Trauma Fixation

Stephen K. Benirschke, MD[a], Patricia Ann Kramer, PhD[b],*

KEYWORDS

- Gastrocnemius recession • Strayer procedure • Gastrocnemius equinus

KEY POINTS

- Patients with traumatic foot injuries should be evaluated for the presence of gastrocnemius equinus.
- Even when a surgical technique is perfect and anatomic reconstruction of the fracture is obtained, the outcome can be poor if the gastrocnemius equinus is not addressed.
- Gastrocnemius lengthening should be done at the time the injury is initially surgically treated.
- Maintenance of the "stretch" on the calf should be maintained until the gastrocnemius has reattached in a more-proximal position on the soleus.

INTRODUCTION

Patients with traumatic injuries to their feet, particularly the fracture patterns listed in **Table 1**, often have undiagnosed gastrocnemius equinus. Gastrocnemius equinus causes the foot to plantarflex, and in the case of a fall from height or motor vehicle accident, this plantar flexion predisposes the foot to these injuries. In these situations, even with perfect surgical technique and anatomic reconstruction of the injury, the maintenance of the fixation will be problematic and long-term sequelae occur if the underlying condition is not addressed. Problems that occur when the gastrocnemius is not released are as follows:

1. Early osteoarthrosis
2. Failure of fixation
3. Subluxation of affected joints

The authors have nothing to disclose.

[a] Department of Orthopaedics and Sports Medicine, Harborview Medical Center, University of Washington, Box 359798, Seattle, WA 98195-9798, USA; [b] Departments of Anthropology and Orthopaedics and Sports Medicine, University of Washington, Box 313500, Seattle, WA 98195-3100, USA
* Corresponding author.
E-mail address: pakramer@uw.edu

Table 1
Injuries typically associated with gastrocnemius equinus

Type of Initial Injury	At Risk for
Weber B fracture (fracture dislocation only)	Posttraumatic arthrosis
Weber C fracture (syndesmotic injury)	Posttraumatic arthrosis
Pilon fracture (anterior fracture dislocation)	Anterior subluxation
Posteromedial talar body fracture	Varus subluxation
Hawkins 2 talar neck fracture (subtalar dislocation)	Posttraumatic arthrosis
Hawkins 3 fracture	Posttraumatic arthrosis
Tongue-type calcaneal fracture	Posttraumatic arthrosis; failure of implants
Choparts injury (anterior process of calcaneus-navicular body)	Early talonavicular joint degradation
Lisfranc injury	Loosening of screws/medial column instability
Cuboid fracture	Posttraumatic arthrosis
Navicular fracture	Posttraumatic arthrosis
Recurrent sprains	Posttraumatic arthrosis

4. More rapid deterioration of the joint of interest
5. Loosening or failure of fixation

A key point to remember in a patient with gastrocnemius equinus comorbid with a foot injury is that the longer the gastrocnemius release is delayed, the worse the outcome for the foot fracture.

An important question, then, becomes: how is a patient determined to have gastrocnemius equinus, which, therefore, requires lengthening? The following should be considered:

1. If a patient has one of the injuries listed in **Table 1**, suspect gastrocnemius equinus.
2. Look for the telltale radiographic and clinical signs listed in **Box 1**.
3. If possible, examine the contralateral limb. Gastrocnemius equinus on one side almost always means equinus on the other.
4. Ask the questions listed in **Box 2**. The more characteristics a patient expresses, the likelier it is that the patient has equinus.

Once the diagnosis of equinus is made, the gastrocnemius should be released (using the technique described in later discussion) because

1. Releasing the gastrocnemius will make obtaining an anatomic reduction of the injury less difficult;
2. Relieving the tension of the gastrocnemius allows the anatomic reduction to be maintained until the bone and soft tissue injuries heal.

If the release is done at the time of definitive surgery, the patient is not subjected to two surgical procedures and the attendant rehabilitation periods. The recovery from the traumatic injury is not impeded when the release is done at the time of definitive fixation. Delay in releasing the gastrocnemius risks the failure of the fixation and reduction. Finally, if gastrocnemius is present in both limbs, the questions arise: should the equinus in the contralateral limb be addressed and, if so, when?

Box 1
Clinical and radiographic examinations

Clinical examination:

Are the patient's feet planus?

Does the patient have bunions?

Is the navicular dorsally prominent?

Are circulation issues present, ie, is venous insufficiency present?

Radiographic findings:

Anteroposterior view:
   Lateralization of hallucal sesamoids
   Hallux valgus and/or MTP1 arthrosis
   Hypertrophic second ray
   Dorsolateral peritalar subluxation
   Stress fractures of metatarsals 2 to 5
   Lesser toe deformities
   Arthrosis of talonavicular and/or naviculocuneiform and/or tarsometatarsal joints

Lateral view:
   Sag at talonavicular and/or naviculocuneiform and/or tarsometatarsal joints
   Pes planus (talar pitch/calcaneal pitch/Schrades line)
   Closing of sinus tarsi
   Spur on calcaneus (plantar fasciitis)
   Calcification of Achilles tendon
   Spur on/increased diameter of talar neck
   Arthrosis of or spur on talonavicular and/or naviculocuneiform and/or tarsometatarsal joints
   Arthrosis of or spur on metatarsophalangeal joints
   Claw toes
   Anterior spur on distal tibia
   Fowler angle >75°

SURGICAL TECHNIQUE/PROCEDURE

- The following is an adaptation of the technique described by Benirschke and Kramer.[1] The procedure proceeds in 5 main steps that are outlined in later discussion.
- The order should not be changed, and short cuts are not advised.

Box 2
Questions for patient

Do you have foot pain when you stand for longer than a few minutes?

Do your calves hurt if you stand for more than a few minutes?

Have you ever sprained your ankle?

If so, how often? And what was the circumstance?

Do you consider yourself to be flexible?

Do you wear or have you ever worn an arch support?

Do your feet or calves limit what you can do?

Do you choose your shoes based on comfort? What type of shoes is most comfortable?

Do you know of anyone else in your family with any of these issues?

- The senior authors' Sofield retractors were modified to eliminate the angulation at the terminal end and to narrow the blade. The removal of the angulation prevents traumatic injury to the soleus fascia, while the narrowing (to 1.5 cm) improves visualization.

PATIENT POSITIONING AND SURGICAL APPROACH

- The patient is positioned supine with the leg elevated, the heel resting on a triangular pad, and the knee extended (**Fig. 1**).
- The area where the gastrocnemius recession will occur should be visible to the seated surgeon, who accesses the medial surface of affected calf across the contralateral limb.
- A 3- to 5-cm incision is made on the medial surface approximately 2 cm distal to the insertion of the muscle belly of the medial head of the gastrocnemius muscle.[2] If the insertion point is not apparent, it can be approximated as the midway point between the fibular head and lateral malleolus transferred to the medial surface of the calf.[3]
- In the sagittal plane, the incision should be located approximately one thumb's breadth posterior to the posterior border of the tibia.
- Adequate hemostasis throughout the procedure is necessary, so a tourniquet should not be used for this procedure.

SURGICAL PROCEDURE

- After the skin incision is made, an auxiliary venous plexus is usually encountered and will need to be cauterized (**Fig. 2**).
- The tributaries of the great saphenous vein may be identified (during the initial skin incision) and should be retracted and/or ligated.
- The saphenous nerve should lie anterior to the operative field.

Step 1—Identification of the "V"

- Using the skin incision as a guide, the superficial posterior compartment fascia is incised, which exposes the areolar tissue and paratenon surrounding the gastrocnemius-soleus complex.
- The auxiliary venous plexus beneath the superficial posterior compartment is the only structure that could produce substantial bleeding during the procedure. The plexus should be identified and cauterized as necessary.

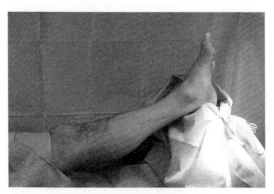

Fig. 1. Positioning of leg. Note line of incision marked in black.

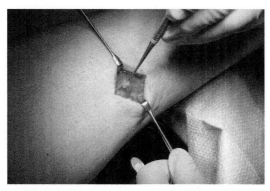

Fig. 2. Perfusing vessel (a branch of the posterior tibial artery) identified. The vessel will need to be cauterized. Note that this is an approximate marker of the gastrocnemius-soleus interval.

- Freeing the areolar tissue and paratenon from the fascia exposes the interval between the gastrocnemius and soleus musculature.
- Beginning proximally and anterior to the medial head of the gastrocnemius (the muscle belly of which is usually distal to that of the lateral head), the gastrocnemius tendon is freed from the soleus beyond the muscular extent of the medial head.
- When the medial head is free, attention is directed to the lateral head. Release of the lateral border of the gastrocnemius tendon will reveal the lateral areolar tissue surrounding the gastrocnemius-soleus complex and, subsequently, the fatty tissue of the lateral subcutaneous layer.
- Careful dissection results in an open interval of approximately 2 to 3 cm, referred to as the "V."
- Dissection of the gastrocnemius from the soleus should continue beyond the muscle belly of the medial head. Both medial and lateral heads of the gastrocnemius should be separated from the underlying fascia of the soleus.
- To minimize the potential for adhesions, do not damage the soleus muscle fascia during this part of the procedure. The goal of this step is to obtain an interval between the gastrocnemius heads and the soleus that is smooth and will allow smooth retraction of the gastrocnemius once it has been transected.
- Some patients may not have a readily identifiable interval between the gastrocnemius and soleus, due to prior injury or other inherent issues. In these cases, slowly dissect through the areolar tissue until the muscle bellies are visible. Once the interval is identified, usually by beginning more proximally, the dissection proceeds as detailed above. It is imperative that both heads of the gastrocnemius are freed from adjacent tissues.

Step 2—Resection of the Plantaris

- Once the interval is freed, the plantaris tendon is identified on the anteromedial surface of the gastrocnemius tendon (**Fig. 3**). Although this muscle is vestigial, it has been retained in most people.
- Approximately 5 cm of the plantaris tendon is resected to prevent possible adhesion formation (**Fig. 4**).

Step 3—Dissection

- With the anterior interval freed and the plantaris resected, the posterior paratenon and areolar tissue are carefully freed from the gastrocnemius tendon. As

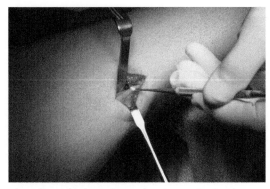

Fig. 3. Plantaris tendon. Note the bent Freer elevator under tendon.

with the anterior separation, dissection proceeds from proximal to distal and from medial to lateral.

- As the dissection approaches the lateral edge, identify and protect the sural nerve and venae comitantes, which typically lie within this lateral areolar tissue.
- Once the sural nerve has been identified, it should be gently teased off the gastrocnemius fascia and retracted posteriorly with a retractor.

Step 4—Recession

- Once the posterior soft tissues are free of the gastrocnemius tendon and the neurovascular structures are protected with the retractor, the scalpel with a number 15 blade on a number 7 handle can be inserted into the base of the V, where the gastrocnemius tendon coalesces with that of the soleus.
- With the blade always held away from the sural nerve, the gastrocnemius tendon is transected (**Fig. 5**).
- At this point, the gastrocnemius muscle belly retracts proximally 3 to 5 cm and the foot moves into a neutral position.
- Active dorsiflexion of the foot/ankle should be avoided, in order to minimize the risk of stretching the sural nerve.

Step 5—Closure

- Closure of the superficial posterior compartment fascia re-establishes the containment of the superficial posterior compartment (**Fig. 6**).

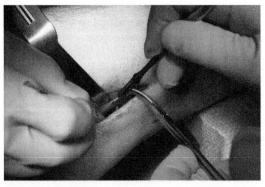

Fig. 4. Recession of plantaris tendon.

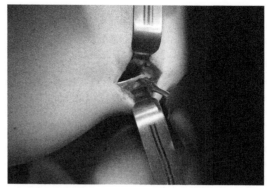

Fig. 5. Initiating recession of dissected gastrocnemius tendon.

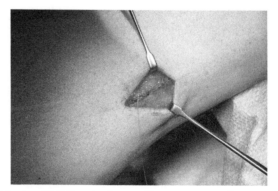

Fig. 6. Closure of fascia with 3-0 undyed monofilament Monocryl on a RB-1 tapered needle.

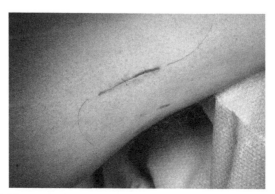

Fig. 7. Closure of skin.

- Closure also minimizes adhesions that prevent movement between the gastrocnemius and the soleus.
- A running, subcuticular 3-0 Prolene suture is used to close the skin (**Fig. 7**).

Postoperative care

The foundational principle of postoperative care is that if allowed, the gastrocnemius reattaches with the ankle in a plantarflexed position. If this is allowed to happen, the gastrocnemius will not have been lengthened. After recession surgery, therefore, the keys to success include the following:

- Immobilization of the ankle in approximately 3° to 5° of dorsiflexion. Neutral ankle positioning will not stretch the gastrocnemius sufficiently to lengthen it.
- Keep the knee extended as much as tolerable for the first 2 weeks.
- Cast if necessary and use wheelchair to maintain the extended knee position.

SUMMARY

Patients with traumatic foot injuries should be evaluated for the presence of gastrocnemius equinus. Even when surgical technique is perfect and anatomic reconstruction of the fracture is obtained, the outcome can be poor if gastrocnemius equinus is not addressed. Gastrocnemius lengthening should be done at the time the injury is definitely treated. The "stretch" on the calf should be maintained until the gastrocnemius has reattached in a more-proximal position on the soleus.

REFERENCES

1. Benirschke SK, Kramer PA. High energy acute Lisfranc fractures and dislocations. Techniques in Foot and Ankle Surgery 2010;9:82–91.
2. Pinney SJ, Sangeorzan BJ, Hansen ST Jr. Surgical anatomy of the gastrocnemius recession (Strayer procedure). Foot Ankle Int 2004;25:247–50.
3. DiGiovanni CW, Kuo R, Tejwani N, et al. Isolated gastrocnemius tightness. J Bone Joint Surg Am 2002;84-A:962–70.

Posterior Malleolar Fractures

Changing Concepts and Recent Developments

Jan Bartoníček, MD[a,b,*], Stefan Rammelt, MD, PhD[c], Michal Tuček, MD[a]

KEYWORDS

- Ankle fractures • Trimalleolar fractures • Posterior malleolus • Classification
- Posterior approaches

KEY POINTS

- Injuries to the posterior malleolus (PM) have a prognostic impact for patients with ankle fracture-dislocations.
- The three-dimensional outline of the fragments as seen on CT, involvement of the fibular notch of the distal tibia (incisura), and the presence of depressed intercalary joint fragments seem to be of greater therapeutic relevance than the size of the fragment and the amount of the fractured articular surface alone.
- Although extraincisural fractures (type 1 according to Bartoníček and Rammelt) can be treated nonoperatively, operative treatment of type 2 to 4 fractures aims at reconstruction of the posterior tibial plafond, the fibular notch, and the integrity of the posterior tibiofibular syndesmosis.
- The individual choice of approaches depends on the fracture pattern of the PM and associated injuries to the medial and lateral malleolus.
- Direct open reduction and fixation of PM fragments via posterolateral and posteromedial approaches is biomechanically more stable than indirect reduction and anteroposterior screw fixation.

INTRODUCTION

Fractures of posterior rim of the distal tibia have been the subject of continuing interest for more than 200 years and are one of the most controversial issues in the treatment

The authors have nothing to disclose.
[a] Department of Orthopaedics, First Faculty of Medicine, Central Military Hospital Prague, Charles University, U Vojenské Nemocnice 1200, Prague 6 169 02, Czech Republic; [b] Department of Anatomy, First Faculty of Medicine, Charles University Prague, U Nemocnice 3, Prague 2 120 00, Czech Republic; [c] University Center of Orthopaedics and Traumatology, University Hospital Carl Gustav Carus Dresden, Fetscherstrasse 74, Dresden 01307, Germany
* Corresponding author. Department of Anatomy, First Faculty of Medicine, Charles University Prague, U Nemocnice 3, Prague 2 120 00, Czech Republic.
E-mail address: bartonicek.jan@seznam.cz

of ankle injuries.[1–8] They have also been referred to as posterior malleolar fractures or posterior pilon fractures. Despite a continuously growing number of studies, no consensus has been reached yet as for classification and treatment of these injuries. The more generous use of computed tomography (CT) scanning in the diagnosis of trimalleolar ankle fractures over the recent decade has brought a deeper understanding of the fracture patterns and a changed perception of the issues related to them.[9–15]

Earle,[16] in 1828, was probably the first to describe a fracture of the posterior rim of the distal tibia in an ankle fracture dislocation. In the huge body of German literature on that subject, this fragment is commonly referred to as Volkmannsches Dreieck (Volkmann triangle).[17–19] However, the original description and figures published in 1875 show that Volkmann presented an avulsion of the anterolateral part of the distal tibia in the sagittal plane instead.[19,20] The term Volkmann triangle was probably introduced by Ludloff[21] in 1926 and by Felsenreich[22] in 1931.

The posterior tibial rim fragment was studied radiologically by Chaput[23] in 1907 and later by Destot[24] who introduced the term "malléole postérieure" (posterior malleolus [PM]) in 1911. In 1915, Cotton[25] described a new type of ankle fracture, which was later named after him. It was a bimalleolar fracture in combination with a fracture of PM. However, this type of fracture had been described by Adams[26] in 1836. In 1932, Henderson[27] introduced the term trimalleolar fracture.

The first reports on fixation of the posterior rim of the distal tibia via a posterior approach appear in the 1920s, published by Lounsbury and Metz[28] and Leveuf.[29] In 1940, Nelson and Jensen[30] classified fractures of PM of the distal tibia as classical, affecting more than one-third of the articular surface, and minimal, involving less than one third. For the classical type they recommended screw fixation from the posteromedial approach and introduced the "one-third rule" still used by many surgeons until today.

ANATOMIC AND BIOMECHANICAL ASPECTS

The distal tibia or the tibial pilon ends in a concave articular surface and serves to transmit axial compression forces.[8,31] The medial malleolus is not part of the tibial pilon; rather, it controls movement and position of the talus. Because of the tibial slope, the posterior articular rim of the distal tibia projects more distally than the anterior rim (**Fig. 1**). The medial part of PM is separated from the medial malleolus by the malleolar groove containing the posterior tibial tendon. The lateral half of PM is formed by a marked bony prominence, the posterior tubercle of the distal tibia that also forms the posterior part of the fibular notch (incisura fibularis tibiae).

The posterior tubercle of the distal tibia also serves as the origin of the strong superior, obliquely oriented fibers of the trapezoidally shaped posterior tibiofibular ligament.[31] Its inferior, more horizontally oriented fibers originate from the rim of the articular surface of the distal tibia, medial to the posterior tubercle. The superior and inferior fibers of the ligament converge distally toward the posterior fibula, where they insert at the circumference of the malleolar fossa (**Fig. 2**).

A variable reinforcement of the posterior joint capsule, the intermalleolar ligament, arises from the distal tip of the fibula and inserts into the angle formed by PM and the medial malleolus.[31]

Given these anatomic facts, it seems logical that PM contributes significantly to stability and load transfer within the ankle. However, results from the few available biomechanical studies on cadaveric specimens are inconclusive at best.[32–39]

Harper[32] found that resection of up to 50% of the posterior articular surface of the distal tibia had no measurable effect on ankle stability. Vrahas and colleagues[35] came

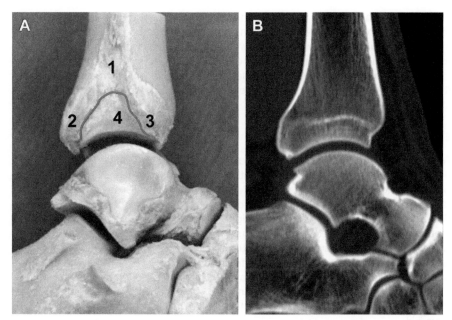

Fig. 1. Anatomy of posterior malleolus. (*A*) Lateral aspect of right distal tibia. 1, interosseous tibiofibular ligament; 2, posterior tibiofibular ligament; 3, anterior tibiofibular ligament; 4, superior recessus of ankle joint cavity (*red line*). (*B*) CT scan in sagittal plane.

to the conclusion that removal of PM did not lead to significant changes in tibiotalar peak contact stresses. Hartford and colleagues[36] revealed that reduction of the articular surface by 25%, 33%, and 50% resulted in a progressive reduction of the tibiotalar contact area by 4%, 13%, and 22%, respectively. Papachristou and colleagues[37] demonstrated that with a normal range of motion, the posterior quarter of the articular surface of the distal tibia bears almost no load, provided the medial and lateral structures are intact or fixed. Fitzpatrick and colleagues[38] found that a fragment of PM carrying 50% of the articular surface got displaced anteriorly in the region

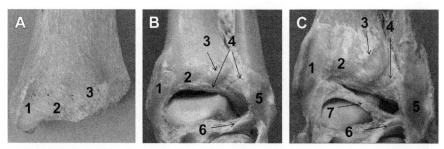

Fig. 2. Anatomy of posterior aspect of ankle joint. (*A*) Posterior aspect of right distal tibia. (*B*) Posterior aspect of right ankle joint. (*C*) Posterior aspect of right ankle joint with intermalleolar ligament. 1, malleolar groove; 2, posterior rim of distal tibia; 3, posterior tibial tubercle; 4, posterior tibiofibular ligament; 5, peroneal groove; 6, posterior talofibular ligament; 7, intermalleolar ligament.

of maximum load, if there was a 2-mm step-off or gap. Gardner and colleagues[39] found that in pronation-external rotation stage 4 fractures on cadaveric specimens, stability of the tibiofibular syndesmosis was restored better by fixation of the posterior fragment than with a standard syndesmotic screw.

Thus, it seems that not the total articular surface involved in PM fractures but rather the involvement of the posterior tubercle and the fibular notch is a relevant factor for stability.

EVALUATION AND CLASSIFICATION

A fracture of PM occurs in about 46% of Weber type B or C ankle fracture-dislocations.[40] The initial radiographic examination of the injured ankle includes true antero-posterior, mortise, and lateral views. PM fractures are usually obvious in the lateral radiograph. In addition, they may be detected indirectly in the anteroposterior projection by the so-called "flake fragment sign" or "spur sign," a double contour of the medial malleolus in case of a PM fracture involving the medial malleolus (**Fig. 3**).[41] An atypical, vertical course of the fracture line of medial malleolus in Weber type B and C fractures may also indicate a PM fracture with medial extension. The true anatomy of the fragment, its medial propagation, and depressed intermediate fragments may be diagnosed only by CT scanning.[10–15,42,43] Most instructive is a three-dimensional (3D) inferior view of the tibiofibular mortise after subtraction of the talus.[8,13]

First classifications of PM fractures were proposed a few years after the introduction of x-rays to the clinical practice.[23,30,44] Overall, the historical classifications do not differ much from more recent radiologic classifications.

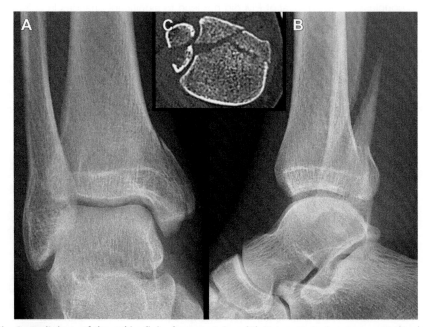

Fig. 3. Radiology of the ankle: flake fragment sign. (*A*) Anteroposterior view, note the double contour of the medial malleolus (flake fragment sign or spur sign). (*B*) Lateral view. (*C*) CT transversal scan demonstrating two-part type fracture of posterior malleolus.

AO Radiologic Classification

This classification published in 1987[45] identified three types of PM fractures with regard to the amount of articular surface involved: (1) extra-articular fracture, (2) small fragment of the articular surface, and (3) large fragment of the articular surface.

Haraguchi Two-Dimensional Computed Tomography Classification

This first CT-based classification of 2006 was developed based on the analysis of axial CT scans of 57 patients.[11] These authors distinguished three types:

- Type I: posterolateral oblique fracture as the most common variant (67%). The fracture involves a triangular fragment separated from the posterolateral part of the distal tibia.
- Type II: medial extension fracture (19%) affects the posterior part of the medial malleolus and may be formed by one or two fragments.
- Type III: small-shell fracture (14%) involves small fragments of the PM cortex.

However, the authors, used only transverse sections, without two-dimensional (2D) or 3D CT reconstructions that would show the exact outline of the PM fragment.

Bartoníček and Rammelt Three-Dimensional Computed Tomography Classification

These authors, in 2015, analyzed 141 consecutive CT scans of individuals with an ankle fracture or fracture-dislocation of types Weber B or Weber C with fracture of PM.[13] The fragments were analyzed in the transverse, sagittal, and frontal planes; a 3D CT reconstruction was performed in 91 patients. The fractures of PM were classified into four basic types having constant pathoanatomic features, with special reference to involvement of the fibular notch (**Fig. 4**). The anatomic features of these types are summarized in **Table 1**.

Type 1: extraincisural fragment

This type was recorded in 11 (8%) patients with a mean age of 53 years. In three cases only the posterior tibial tubercle was avulsed, in five cases the fragment was formed by the posterior tubercle and the medial posterior rim, and in three cases the fracture involved only the medial posterior rim (**Fig. 5**). The average transverse area of the fragment comprised 9% of the cross-sectional area of the tibial pilon. A Weber type B fibular fracture was observed seven times and Weber type C fracture four times (three low fractures and one high fracture).

Type 2: posterolateral fragment

This type was the most frequent, occurring in 74 (52%) patients, with a mean age of 50 years. In 43 cases the fragment was formed by the posterior tubercle only. In 20 cases the fragment consisted of the posterior tubercle and the medial posterior rim, and in one case the fracture line extended to the malleolar groove. By contrast, in 11 cases the fragment was small and carried only the lateral portion of the posterior tubercle. One-quarter to one-third of the fibular notch was affected in 48 cases, less than a quarter in 24 cases, and half of the notch in two cases (**Fig. 6**). Transverse and sagittal CT scans showed a depressed intercalary joint fragment in 25 cases (**Fig. 7**). The average transverse area of the fragment comprised 14% of the cross-sectional area of the tibial pilon. A Weber type B fibular fracture was recorded 53 times and Weber type C fracture 21 times (12 low, three midshaft, and six high fractures).

Type 3: posteromedial, two-part fragment

This type was identified in 39 (28%) patients, with a mean age of 44 years. A flake-fragment sign (double contour of the medial malleolus) was seen in the anteroposterior

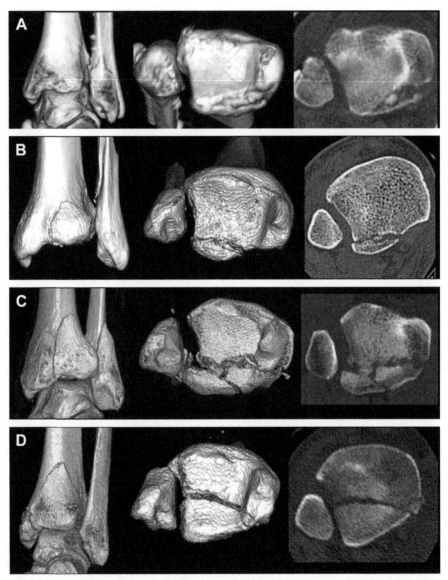

Fig. 4. Bartoníček and Rammelt classification of fractures of posterior malleolus. (*A*) Extra-incisural fragment with an intact fibular notch. (*B*) Intraincisural posterolateral fragment. (*C*) Intraincisural two-part fragment involving the medial malleolus. (*D*) Intraincisural large triangular fragment.

view in 11 cases. All fragments consisted of two triangular portions of different size and involved the medial malleolus. The fracture line extended into the posterior colliculus in 10 cases, into the intercollicular groove in 28 cases, and into the malleolar groove in one case. One-quarter to one-third of the fibular notch was affected in 25 cases, less than one-quarter in nine cases, and one-half of the notch in five cases (**Fig. 8**). The average transverse area of the fragment comprised 24% of the cross-sectional area of the tibial

Table 1
Anatomic features of PM fractures according to the Bartoníček and Rammelt classification

Type	Common Feature	Frequency (%)	Male: Female	Talus Subluxation (%)	Transverse Area (%)	Fragment Height (mm)	Fragment Depth (mm)
1	Extraincisural	8	8:3	36	9	11.2	8.1
2	Posterolateral	52	41:33	39	14	17.9	8.7
3	Two-part	28	13:26	59	24	29.1	12.7
4	Large triangular	9	1:12	85	29	37.4	18.1

pilon. A Weber type B fibular fracture was observed 31 times, and a Weber type C fracture eight times (six low and two high fractures).

Type 4: large, posterolateral triangular fragment

This type occurred in 13 (9%) patients with a mean age of 59 years. The solid posterior tibial fragment (without depressed intercalary interfragment in all cases) displayed a triangular geometry. The fragment involved the posterior tubercle and the medial posterior rim in nine cases, the malleolar groove in two cases, and the posterior colliculus in two cases (**Fig. 9**). One-half of the fibular notch was affected in all 13 cases. The average transverse area of the fragment comprised 29% of the cross-sectional area of the tibial pilon. A Weber type B fibular fracture of was recorded 11 times, and a low Weber type C fracture twice.

Type 5: irregular osteoporotic fracture

In four (3%) women with a mean age of 70 years, it was impossible to classify the posterior malleolar fracture using the previously mentioned criteria, despite 3D CT

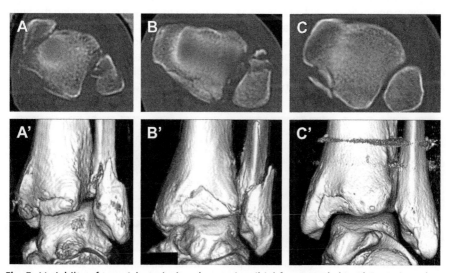

Fig. 5. Variabilty of type 1 (extraincisural posterior tibial fragments). (*A, A'*) Posterior tubercle avulsion. (*B, B'*) Posterior tubercle and posterior rim avulsion. (*C, C'*) Posteromedial corner avulsion, probably by pull of the intermalleolar ligament.

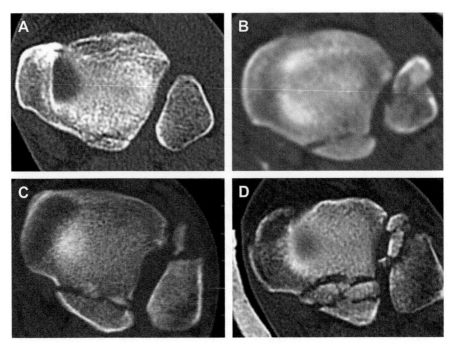

Fig. 6. Variabilty of type 2 (intraincisural posterolateral fragment). (*A*) Small undisplaced fragment. (*B*) Small displaced fragment. (*C*) Typical, most frequent fragment. (*D*) Large, displaced fragment with interfragments.

reconstruction. The reason was a considerable comminution of fragments, most likely caused by osteoporosis.

The course of fracture lines as detailed in this classification correlates with the findings of Magnus and colleagues[14] who used a CT mapping technique summarizing the findings of 45 patients with PM fractures. The lines showed a continuous spectrum of posterolateral and posteromedial fragments. Similar to the studies of Weber[46] and Magnus and colleagues,[14] a high percentage of fractures with depressed intercalary fragments was seen. In contrast to the Müller/AO[45] and Heim[17] classifications, Bartoníček and coworkers[13] did not observe any extra-articular PM fragments. Analysis of the

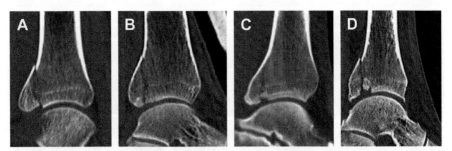

Fig. 7. Variabilty of type 2 (intraincisural posterolateral fragment) on CT scans in sagittal plane. (*A*) Displaced single fragment. (*B*) Minimally displaced fragment with interfragment. (*C*) Undisplaced fragment with impacted interfragment. (*D*) Displaced fragment with impacted interfragment.

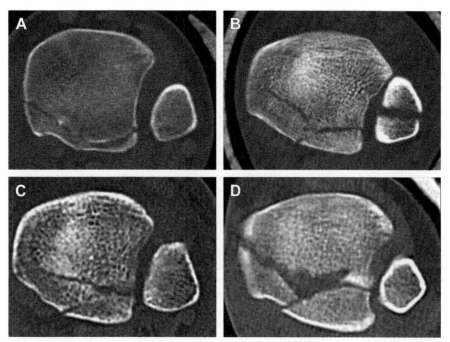

Fig. 8. (*A–D*) Variabilty of type 3 (intraincisural two-part fragment involving the medial malleolus) from the viewpoint of the size of fragments and involvement of fibular notch on CT scans.

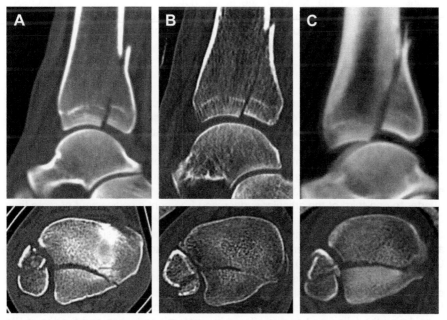

Fig. 9. Variabilty of type 4 (intraincisural large posterolateral triangular fragment). (*A*) Involvement of posterior tubercle and rim. (*B*) Involvement of malleolar groove. (*C*) Involvement of posterior colliculus of medial malleolus.

sagittal CT scans revealed that all fragments, including the extraincisural ones (type 1), carried a part of the articular surface of the distal tibia. The number of cases with subluxation or dislocation of the talus, the cross-sectional area of the fragment, the height of the fragment, and the extent of involvement of the fibular notch increased throughout the classification groups.[13] This indicated that the types proposed by Bartoníček and Rammelt indeed represent a scale of increasing injury severity.

Posterior Malleolar Versus Posterior Pilon Fractures

The question how to distinguish between a fracture of the posterior tibial rim in ankle fracture-dislocations and posterior fractures of the tibial pilon caused by compressive forces has not yet been satisfactorily resolved. It is difficult to explain the mechanism of these injuries solely on the basis of the Lauge-Hansen classification.[47] PM fractures most likely result from a combination of tensile, compression, and shear forces. Smaller fragments, as seen in Bartoníček and Rammelt types 1 and 2, are most likely produced by ligamentous and capsular avulsions in rotational injuries. Larger and multifragmentary fractures as seen in types 3 and 4 are predominately caused by compression forces, because these fragments usually carry a larger part of the articular surface. Therefore, trimaleollar ankle fractures with types 3 and 4 PM fragments already represent a transition to posterior fractures of the tibial pilon.

Thus, the dividing line between ankle fractures with PM fragments and partial pilon fractures is a matter of convention. Haraguchi and colleagues[11] used the transmalleolar line, although they included two cases where the posterior fragment carried the whole medial malleolus. Switaj and colleagues[48] and Klammer and colleagues[49] termed the medial extension type of a fracture of the posterior rim (Haraguchi type II, Bartoníček and Rammelt type 3) a posterior pilon fracture. Weber[46] considers this type as a part of trimalleolar ankle fractures. Bartoníček and coworkers[13] set the line connecting the center of the fibular notch and the intercollicular groove as the conventional criterion. If the posterior fragment carries the anterior colliculus of the medial malleolus or more than 50% of the fibular notch, the injury was classified as a partial fracture of the tibial pilon.

INDICATIONS TO SURGERY

The first authors to perform surgical fixation of PM fractures back in the 1920s and 1930s saw the indication to operative treatment because of ankle instability.[7,21,28–30] Later, the AO/Association for the Study of Internal Fixation (ASIF) group coined the principles of restoration of the articular surface of the tibial pilon as a basic prerequisite for good long-term treatment results.[50–53] Thus, for a long period the decisive factor for indication to surgery was the size of the articular surface carried by the PM fragment and its displacement.[30,50,51,53] The critical size was considered to be one-quarter to one-third of the articular surface and fragment displacement of more than 2 mm on the lateral radiograph. However, recent studies using CT have challenged these criteria because it is impossible to determine the exact size of the fragment and articular surface involvement merely by a lateral radiograph[42,43] and even in 2D CT scans compared with 3D CT scans.[15]

Over the last 10 years more attention has been paid to the importance of restoration of the fibular notch and stability of the tibiofibular syndesmosis through fixation of PM fractures.[39,54] The indications to operative treatment have become more aggressive considering the following benefits offered by anatomic reduction and fixation of PM fractures[8]: restoration of the congruence of the articular surface of the tibial pilon and thus posterior ankle stability; restoration of the competence of the posterior tibiofibular ligament and thus syndesmotic stability; and restoration of the integrity of the fibular notch facilitating reduction of the distal fibula, particularly in high fibular fractures (Weber type C including Maisonneuve fractures).

Using the classification of PM fractures by Bartoníček and coworkers[13] based on 3D CT scanning, the following treatment recommendations may be proposed:

- Type 1 (extraincisural): nonoperative treatment of the PM fracture.
- Type 2 (posterolateral): generous indication to anatomic reduction and fixation of the PM fracture, particularly in the presence of an impacted intercalary fragment and high fibular fractures (Weber type C), to reconstruct the fibular notch to alleviate anatomic reduction of the distal fibula and restoring syndesmotic stability.
- Type 3 (two-part): open reduction and internal fixation of displaced fragments to restore tibiotalar joint congruity and stability, integrity of the fibular notch, syndesmostic stability, and congruity of the medial malleolus with medial propagation of the fracture
- Type 4 (large triangular): open reduction and internal fixation to restore the articular surface and ankle stability.

Apart from the type of PM fracture, the choice of treatment depends on the overall pattern of injury to the ankle, that is, the type of fibular fracture (Danis-Weber B or low C types vs high C Maisonneuve type) and the type of injuries to the medial structures (bicollicular fracture of medial malleolus, rupture of deltoid ligament, or combined lesion [fracture of the anterior colliculus and rupture of the tibiotalar part of the deltoid ligament]).[55]

SURGICAL APPROACHES AND OPEN REDUCTION INTERNAL FIXATION TECHNIQUE

Internal fixation of PM fractures may be performed by direct and indirect techniques.[56–63] The choice of approaches depends on the type of the PM fracture and the overall malleolar fracture pattern.[8]

- In most Bartoníček and Rammelt type 2 to 4 fractures, the posterolateral approach allows simultaneous direct reduction of the PM fragments and the distal fibular fracture. Any impacted intercalary fragments hampering indirect reduction should be approached from posterior.
- Displaced bony avulsions of the anterior tibiofibular syndesmosis (Chaput or Wagstaffe fragments) should be anatomically reduced via a small additional anterolateral approach.
- In Bartoníček and Rammelt type 3 fractures with posterolateral and posteromedial fragments, reduction and fixation of the posterolateral fragment is best achieved via a posterolateral approach. If the posteromedial fragment cannot be visualized and fixed adequately via the same approach, it should be addressed via a separate medial approach extended posteromedially that allows simultaneous reduction and fixation of the medial malleolus, if fractured. Alternatively, a single posteromedial approach is used.
- Single, large Bartoníček and Rammelt type 4 fractures without impacted joint fragments are best reduced via a posterolateral approach and fixed by buttress plate and/or screws.

Indirect Reduction and Anterior-to-Posterior Fixation

This approach has been widely popularized in classical textbooks including the AO Manual.[50,51,53] It is most suitable for single, large triangular fragments (Bartoníček and Rammelt type 4). Typically, the posterior fragment is reduced after internal fixation of the medial and lateral malleoli.

- In the authors' preference, reduction of the posterior tibial fragment is performed first, because hardware in the medial and lateral malleoli overlaps with the line of the tibial plafond thus rendering the control of joint reduction difficult, if not impossible.[8]
- The posterior fragment is reduced by dorsiflexion of the ankle, percutaneous manipulation with a K-wire, or sharp elevator, introduced behind the fibula. Bone forceps may be placed between the anterolateral and posterolateral tubercle of the tibia to achieve anatomic reduction.
- The fragment is held temporarily by a K-wire introduced anteroposteriorly. A small incision is made over the anterolateral aspect of the distal tibia. Care is taken not to injure the extensor tendons and the anterior neurovascular bundle.
- Definitive fixation is achieved by cancellous compression screws introduced parallel to the joint surface. The threads must be completely within the posterior fragment to obtain a lag effect. The smaller the fragments, the more difficult it is to obtain solid fixation and compression. If the threads of a standard screw exceed the joint line it is necessary to cut the screw thread short.[51,53] However, in many cases these short threads do not provide adequate fixation. Therefore, fragments with a diameter of less than 15 mm should be fixed directly from posterior.

Transfibular Reduction According to Weber

- In long, oblique Weber type B fractures of the distal fibula beginning at the joint level of the tibial plafond, the fracture line can be opened by external rotating the distal fragment and displacing it distally, such as with a gently introduced laminar spreader.[60,61,63] This visually exposes the fibular notch as far as PM.
- Subsequently, the PM fragment is reduced under direct visual control with a pointed reduction clamp introduced between the anterior and posterior tubercle of the tibia.
- The fragment is fixed temporarily by a K-wire and definitely by anterior-to-posterior screw fixation.
- With short and irregular fibular fractures, adequate visual control of the tibial plafond may be difficult to obtain. This technique is not useful in the presence of a multifragmentary or high (Weber type C) fibular fracture.

Direct Reduction and Fixation from the Posterolateral Approach

With this approach fractures of the posterior tibial rim and the distal fibula are reduced and fixed via the same incision. It is especially useful with relatively small PM fragments and in the presence of intercalary fragments that cannot be reduced indirectly.[5,60,61]

- The patient is placed in a prone or semiprone position. The incision runs longitudinally along the posterior rim of the distal fibula until the apex of the lateral malleolus, where it turns slightly anteriorly. To obtain better visualization of the posterior tibia, the incision is placed halfway between the distal fibula and the Achilles tendon as a classical posterolateral (Gallie) approach.
- The sural nerve is identified in the subcutaneous tissue and gently held away laterally. The peroneal fascia is dissected longitudinally in the same interval and the peroneal tendons are retracted anterolaterally. Subsequently, a longitudinal incision through the deep fascia of the flexor hallucis longus muscle is made.

- The distal flexor hallucis longus muscle belly and tendon is retracted medially thus protecting the deep posterior neurovascular bundle and exposing the complete posterior aspect of the distal tibia. The posterolateral fragment is gently mobilized and hinged on the posterior tibiofibular ligament, which is left intact. After debriding the fracture surfaces, the fragment is reduced using the metaphyseal fracture line as a reference and temporarily fixed by posteroanterior K-wires.
- Intercalary fragments of sufficient size and cartilage quality are reduced toward the tibial plafond using the talus as a template and fixed with lost K-wires or resorbable pins. Comminuted osteochondral or chondral fragments not amenable to fixation are resected. Reduction of the joint surface is controlled with a lateral image intensifier view.
- Definite internal fixation may be performed using 3.5-mm lag screws with a washer and/or a buttress plate, preferably T-shaped, from the small fragment set. The choice of implants depends on the size and bone quality of the PM fragment. Biomechanical studies revealed a higher strength of posterior plates compared with anteroposterior and posteroanterior screws.[64,65] In osteoporotic bone, plating is preferred.
- During screw insertion, the concave shape of the articular surface of the distal tibia in the lateral view must be respected to avoid intra-articular penetration or perforation of the fibular notch. For maximum stability the distal screws should be inserted close to the articular surface and purchase the anterior cortex of the tibia (**Fig. 10**).
- Internal fixation of PM is followed by internal fixation of the fractured distal fibula via the same approach with posterior antiglide plating.[61]

Direct Reduction and Fixation from the Posteromedial Approach

This approach provides access to the posterior tibial rim and the medial malleolus.[49,56] It is especially useful in certain Bartoníček and Rammelt type 3 PM fractures with a posteromedial fragment involving the medial malleolus.[8]

- The patient is placed in a supine position. The longitudinal incision runs along the posterior border of the distal tibia to the apex of the medial malleolus, where it slightly turns anteriorly.
- The crural fascia is incised and the tendons of the tibialis posterior and flexor digitorum longus muscles are mobilized and retracted anteriorly. Care is taken not to injure the posteromedial neurovascular bundle.
- The fractures of the posterior tibial fragment and of the medial malleolus are identified. Reduction and fixation is performed in analogy to the posterolateral fragments. Horizontal medial malleolar fracture are typically fixed with obliquely placed compression screws. Multifragmentary fractures are fixed with either a cerclage technique or a medial plate. Fractures of the posterior tibial rim extending into the medial malleolus in the frontal plane are fixed with posterior-to-anterior screws. When inserting the screws, irritation of the flexor tendons has to be avoided.

In the authors' practice, direct reduction and fixation from posterior is preferred over indirect reduction and anterior-to-posterior fixation because it allows a more accurate and stable fixation of PM fractures and removal or reduction of impacted or displaced osteochondral interfragments. Most of the PM fracture patterns can be addressed through a posterolateral approach; however, the optimal approach is chosen on a case-by-case basis in view of the exact fracture anatomy on CT examination (**Fig. 11**).

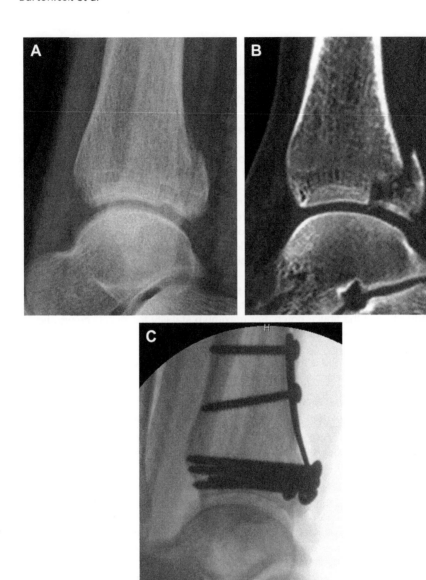

Fig. 10. Reduction and fixation of posterior tibial fragment (type 3) from posterolateral approach. (*A*) Preoperative lateral radiograph. (*B*) Preoperative sagittal CT scan. (*C*) Intraoperative lateral radiograph after direct reduction and fixation by screws and buttress plate.

POSTOPERATIVE CARE

Aftertreatment is tailored individually to the overall injury pattern, type of fixation, bone quality, soft tissue conditions, and patient compliance. Active, compliant patients are treated in a boot or walker with partial weight-bearing of 15 to 20 kg for 6 weeks. Older, noncompliant patients are offloaded in a wheelchair and a below-knee cast. In cases of poor bone quality (osteoporosis, poorly controlled diabetes with neuropathy) longer offloading times are needed up to 12 weeks. Gradual increase of weight-bearing is

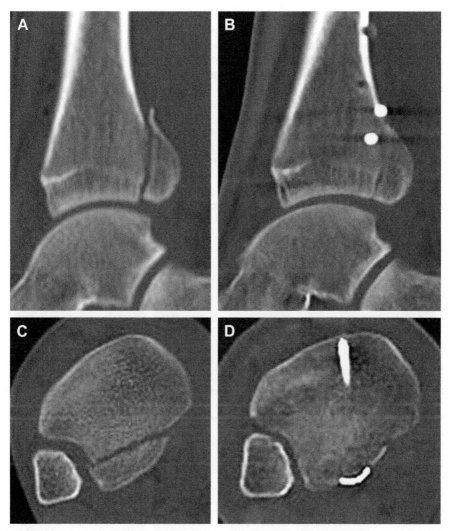

Fig. 11. Postoperative CT control of reduction of fractured posterior malleolus, type 2. (*A, C*) Sagittal and transverse CT scans before surgery. (*B, D*) Sagittal and transverse CT scans after direct reduction and direct fixation from posterolateral approach. Note the perfect reduction of distal fibula into fibular notch after anatomic reduction of posterior fragment. (*From* Bartoníček J, Rammelt S, Tuček M, et al. Posterior malleolar fractures of the ankle. Eur J Trauma Emerg Surg 2015;41:597; with permission.)

allowed after radiographic evidence of bony consolidation. An active physical therapy protocol including range of motion exercises, muscle balancing, and proprioceptive and gait training aims at functional rehabilitation.

COMPLICATIONS AND THEIR MANAGEMENT
Malalignment

An early report documented problems with obtaining anatomic fixation via a posterior approach in 5 of 30 patients and related this to the lack of experience in such patient's position or placement of the plate too far proximal.[66] Still, the quality of reduction was superior to percutaneous anteroposterior screw fixation done by the same authors, which yielded anatomic reduction in 8 of 30 patients only. More recent studies consistently reported a high rate of anatomic reduction and favorable results with posterolateral plating of PM fractures.[67,68] In any case of doubt, a postoperative CT scan should be obtained and repeat reduction is indicated for relevant malalignment of the articular surface of tibial plafond or the malreduction of fractured fibula, which results in syndesmotic malalignment.

Symptomatic malunions or nonunions of PM fragments may be treated by joint-preserving osteotomies and secondary anatomic fixation if no or only mild posttraumatic arthritis is present.[69,70] Ankle fusion with realignment remains a salvage option in patients with severe osteoarthritis at the time of presentation.

Posttraumatic arthritis can result from direct cartilage damage at the time of injury and residual malalignment of PM fractures (**Fig. 12**). The fact that there is a higher incidence and severity of posttraumatic arthritis with the presence and increasing size of a

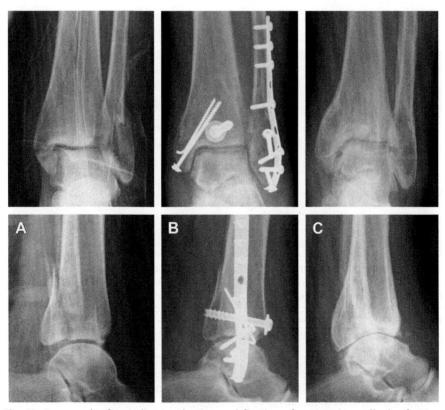

Fig. 12. Poor result after indirect reduction and fixation of a posterior malleolus fracture (type 4). (*A*) A 42-year-old man, trimalleolar fracture. (*B*) Indirect incomplete reduction and anterior-to-posterior fixation of posterior malleolus. (*C*) Malunion and severe posttraumatic osteoarthritis 2 years after surgery. (*From* Bartoníček J, Rammelt S, Tuček M, et al. Posterior malleolar fractures of the ankle. Eur J Trauma Emerg Surg 2015;41:598; with permission.)

posterior tibial fragment probably reflects the overall severity of injury compared with isolated fibular fractures and bimalleolar fractures.[18,71–73]

RESULTS

It is well established that the mere presence of a small posterior fragment has a negative effect on the clinical outcome of ankle fractures.[64,72–75] Both the clinical results and the degree of posttraumatic arthritis are reported to correspond to the size of the posterior tibial fragment.[64,72,73] However, the size of the PM fragment was judged on plain radiographs, which does not allow adequate assessment.[76]

The results of comparative studies are inconsistent. Although some studies did not reveal statistically significant differences in the results after nonoperative versus operative treatments of PM fractures with fragments carrying up to 25% of the articular surface,[18,48,64] others have found that for larger PM fragments, the results of open reduction and internal fixation are better compared with nonoperative treatment.[30,73] The evidence from the existing studies is limited because of a retrospective design, assessment of fractures and reduction based on radiographs only, lack of uniform treatment of PM fractures and associated injuries, and the predominant use of indirect reduction techniques without adequate control.

Several reports on malunited posterior malleolar fractures documented poor results of nonanatomic reduction and internal fixation of PM fractures requiring operative correction.[69,70,77] In a prospective study, Heim and coworkers[18] found a tendency toward deterioration 7 years after the injury in patients with a PM fragment involving more than one-third of the articular surface despite anatomic reduction and stable internal fixation. Langenhuijsen and colleagues[77] found that not the size but rather the accuracy of reduction obtained affected outcome even in small fragments containing only 10% of the joint surface. Miller and colleagues[54] found in a clinical study that with PM reconstruction the distal fibula is reduced more accurately into the restored fibular notch. O'Connor and colleagues[62] saw superior clinical outcomes after posterior buttress plating versus anteroposterior screw fixation for PM fracture fixation. With increasing awareness of these issues and the regular use of CT scanning to assess the 3D geometry of PM fractures, an increasing number of authors recommend internal fixation of any displaced PM involving the fibular notch regardless of its size because it recreates the notch for fibular reduction and substantially contributes to syndesmotic stability.[8,39,54,62,67,68]

SUMMARY

Injuries to the PM have gained increased attention over the last decade. The mere presence of a posterior fragment leads to significantly poorer outcomes in ankle fracture-dislocations. Adequate diagnosis, classification, and treatment require preoperative CT examination, preferably with 3D reconstructions. The 3D outline of the fragments, involvement of the fibular notch of the distal tibia (incisura), and the presence of depressed intercalary fragments seem to be of greater therapeutic relevance than the size of the fragment and the amount of the fractured articular surface alone. Operative treatment aims at reconstruction of the posterior tibial plafond, the fibular notch (thus facilitating tibiofibular reduction), and the integrity of the posterior inferior tibiofibular syndesmosis. The individual choice of approaches depends on the fracture pattern of PM and all associated lateral and medial malleolar fractures. Direct open reduction and fixation of PM fragments via posterolateral and posteromedial approaches is biomechanically more stable than indirect reduction and anteroposterior screw fixation.

ACKNOWLEDGMENTS

This study was supported by grant of AZV ČR (Agentura pro zdravotnický výzkum České republiky) 16-28458A: Trimalleolar ankle fractures - CT diagnostics of fractures of posterior tibial rim, their CT classification and operative treatment.

REFERENCES

1. Lauge N. Fractures of the ankle. Arch Surg 1948;56:259–317.
2. van den Bekerom MPJ, Haverkamp D, Kloen P. Biomechanical and clinical evaluation of posterior malleolar fractures. A systematic review of the literature. J Trauma 2009;66:279–84.
3. Gardner MJ, Streubel PN, McCormick JJ, et al. Surgeon practices regarding operative treatment of posterior malleolus fractures. Foot Ankle Int 2011;32: 385–93.
4. Streubel PN, McCormick JJ, Gardner MJ. The posterior malleolus: should it be fixed and why? Curr Orthop Pract 2011;22:17–24.
5. Heim D. Der posterior Malleolus bzw. Das Volkmann-Dreieck. Unfallchirurg 2013; 116:781–8.
6. Irwin TA, Lien J, Kadakia AR. Posterior malleolus fracture. J Am Acad Orthop Surg 2013;21:32–40.
7. Bartoníček J, Kostlivý K. The history of fractures of the posterior lip of the tibia in fracture-dislocations of the ankle [in Czech]. Ortopedie 2014;8:132–6.
8. Bartoníček J, Rammelt S, Tuček M, et al. Posterior malleolar fractures of the ankle. Eur J Trauma Emerg Surg 2015;41:587–600.
9. Friedburg H, Hendrich V, Wimmer B, et al. Computertomographie bei komplexen Sprunggelenksfrakturen. Radiologie 1983;23:421–5.
10. Magid D, Michelson JD, Ney DR, et al. Adult ankle fractures: comparison of plain films and interactive two- and three dimensional CT scans. AJR Am J Roentgenol 1990;154:1017–23.
11. Haraguchi N, Haruyama H, Toga H, et al. Pathoanatomy of posterior malleolar fractures of the ankle. J Bone Joint Surg 2006;88-A:1085–92.
12. Yao L, Zhang W, Yang G, et al. Morphologic characteristics of the posterior malleolar fragment: a 3-D computer tomography based study. Arch Orthop Trauma Surg 2014;134:389–94.
13. Bartoníček J, Rammelt S, Kostlivý K, et al. Anatomy and classification of the posterior tibial fragment in ankle fractures. Arch Orthop Trauma Surg 2015;135: 506–16.
14. Magnus L, Meijer DT, Stufkens SA, et al. Posterior malleolar fracture patterns. J Orthop Trauma 2015;29:428–35.
15. Meijer DT, de Muinck Keizer RJO, Doornberg JN, et al. Diagnostic accuracy of 2-dimensional computed tomography for articular involvement and fracture pattern of posterior malleolar fractures. Foot Ankle Int 2016;37:75–82.
16. Earle H. Simple, succeeded by compound dislocation forwards, of the inferior extremity of the tibia, with fracture of its posterior edge, comminuted fracture of the fibula, amputation of the leg, and death. Lancet 1828–29;II/6:346–8.
17. Heim U. Indikation und Technik der Stabilisierung des hinteren Kantendreiecks nach Volkmann bei Malleolarfrakturen. Unfallheilkunde 1982;85:388–94.
18. Heim D, Niederhauser K, Simbray N. The Volkmann dogma: a retrospective, long-term, single-center study. Eur J Trauma Emerg Surg 2010;36:515–9.
19. Bartoníček J. Avulsed posterior edge of tibia: Earle's or Volkmann's triangle? J Bone Joint Surg 2004;86-B:746–50.

20. Volkmann R. Beiträge zur Chirurgie anschliessend an einen Bericht über die Thätigkeit der Chirurgischen Universitätsklinik zu Halle im Jahre 1873. Leipzig (Germany): Breitkopf und Härtel; 1875. p. 104–9.

21. Ludloff K. Zur Frage der Knöchelbrüche mit Heraussprengung eines hinteren Volkmann'schen Dreiecks. Zentralbl Chir 1926;53:390–1.

22. Felsenreich F. Untersuchung über die Pathologie des sogenannten Volkmann-schen Dreiecks neben Richtlinien moderner Behandlung schwerer Luxationsfrakturen des oberen Sprunggelenkes. Arch Orthop Unfallchir 1931;29:491–529.

23. Chaput V. Les fractures malléolaires du cou-de-pieds et les accidents du travail. Paris: Masson; 1907.

24. Destot E. Traumatisme du pied et rayons X. Paris: Masson; 1911.

25. Cotton FJ. A new type of ankle fracture. Am J Med Assoc 1915;64:318–21.

26. Adams R. Ankle Joint, abnormal conditions. In: Todd RB, editor. The cyclopaedia of anatomy and physiology of man, vol. II. London: Longman; 1835–1836. p. 154–64.

27. Henderson MS. Trimalleolar fractures of the ankle. Surg Clin North Am 1932;12: 867–72.

28. Lounsbury BF, Metz AR. Lipping fracture of lower articular end of tibia. Arch Surg 1922;5:678–90.

29. Leveuf J. Traitment des fractures et luxations des membres. Paris: Masson; 1925.

30. Nelson MC, Jensen NK. The treatment of trimalleolar fractures of the ankle. Surg Gynec Obst 1940;71:509–14.

31. Bartoníček J. Anatomy of the tibiofibular syndesmosis and its clinical relevance. Surg Radiol Anat 2003;25:379–86.

32. Harper MC. Talar shift. The stabilizing role of the medial, lateral, and posterior ankle structures. Clin Orthop Relat Res 1990;257:177–83.

33. Macko VW, Matthews IS, Zwirkoski P, et al. The joint-contact area of the ankle. The contribution of posterior malleolus. J Bone Joint Surg 1991;73-A:347–51.

34. Raasch WG, Larkin JJ, Draganich LF. Assessment of the posterior malleolus as a restraint to posterior subluxation of the ankle. J Bone Joint Surg 1992;74-A: 1201–6.

35. Vrahas M, Fu F, Veenis B. Intraarticular contact stresses with simulated ankle malunions. J Orthop Trauma 1994;8:159–66.

36. Hartford JM, Gorczyca JT, McNamara JL, et al. Tibiotalar contact area. Contribution of posterior malleolus and deltoid ligament. Clin Orthop Relat Res 1995;20: 182–7.

37. Papachristou G, Efstathopoulos N, Levidiotis C, et al. Early weightbearing after posterior malleolus: an experimental and prospective clinical study. J Foot Ankle Surg 2003;42:99–104.

38. Fitzpatrick DC, Otto JK, McKinley TO, et al. Kinematic and contact stress analysis of posterior malleolus fractures of the ankle. J Orthop Trauma 2004;18:271–8.

39. Gardner MJ, Brodsky A, Briggs SM, et al. Fixation of posterior malleolar fractures provides greater syndesmotic stability. Clin Orthop Relat Res 2006;447:165–71.

40. Jehlička D, Bartoníček J, Svatoš F, et al. Fracture-dislocations of the ankle in adults. Part I: Epidemiological evaluation of one-year group of patients. Acta Chir Orthop Tramatol Čech 2002;69:243–7 [in Czech].

41. Hinds RM, Garner MR, Lazaro LE, et al. Ankle fracture spur sign is pathognomic for a variant ankle fracture. Foot Ankle Int 2015;36:159–64.

42. Ferries JS, DeCoster TA, Firoozbakhsh KK, et al. Plain radiographic interpretation in trimalleolar ankle fractures poorly assesses posterior fragment size. J Orthop Trauma 1994;8:328–31.

43. Büchler L, Tannast M, Bonel HM, et al. Reliability of radiologic assessment of the fracture anatomy at the posterior tibial plafond in malleolar fractures. J Orthop Trauma 2009;23:208–12.

44. Ashhurst APC, Bromer RS. Classification and mechanism of fractures of the leg bones involving the ankle. Arch Surg 1922;4:51–129.

45. Müller ME, Nazarian S, Koch P, et al. The comprehensive classification of long bones. Berlin: Springer; 1987.

46. Weber M. Trimalleolar fractures with impaction of the posteromedial tibial plafond: Implications for talar stability. Foot Ankle Int 2004;25:716–27.

47. Lauge-Hansen N. Fractures of the ankle. Part 2. Combined experimental-surgical and experimental-roentgenologic investigations. Arch Surg 1950;60:957–87.

48. Switaj PJ, Weatherford B, Fuchs D, et al. Evaluation of posterior malleolar fractures and the posterior pilon in operatively treated ankle fractures. Foot Ankle Int 2014;35:886–95.

49. Klammer G, Kadakia AR, Joos DA, et al. Posterior pilon fractures: a retrospective case series and proposed classification system. Foot Ankle Int 2013;34:189–99.

50. Weber BG. Die Verletzungen des oberen Sprunggelenkes. Bern (Switzerland): Huber; 1966.

51. Müller ME, Allgöwer M, Schneider R, et al, editors. Manual der Osteosynthese. 3. Aufl. Berlin: Springer; 1991. p. 595–612.

52. Zenker H, Nerlich M. Prognostic aspects in operated ankle fractures. Arch Orthop Trauma Surg 1982;100:237–41.

53. Heim U. Trimalleoar fractures: late results after fixation of the posterior fragment. Orthopedics 1989;12:1053–9.

54. Miller AN, Carroll EA, Parker RJ, et al. Posterior malleolar stabilization of syndesmotic injuries is equivalent to screw fixation. Clin Orthop Relat Res 2010;468: 1129–35.

55. Pankovich AM, Shivaram MS. Anatomical basis of variability in injuries of the medial malleolus and the deltoid ligament. II. Clinical studies. Acta Orthop Scand 1979;50:223–36.

56. Bois AJ, Dust W. Posterior fracture dislocation of the ankle: technique and clinical experience using a posteromedial surgical approach. J Orthop Trauma 2008;22: 629–36.

57. Karachalios T, Roidis N, Karoutis D, et al. Trimalleolar fracture with a double fragment of the posterior malleolus: a case report and modified operative approach to internal fixation. Foot Ankle Int 2001;22:144–9.

58. Amorosa LF, Brown GD, Greisberg J. A surgical approach to posterior pilon fractures. J Orthop Trauma 2010;24:188–93.

59. Rammelt S, Zwipp H. Ankle fractures. In: Bentley G, editor. European instructional course lectures 12. Berlin: Springer; 2012. p. 205–19.

60. Rammelt S, Heim D, Hofbauer LC, et al. Problems and controversies in the treatment of ankle fractures. Unfallchirurg 2011;114:847–60.

61. Rammelt S, Zwipp H, Mittlmeier T. Operative treatment of pronation fracture-dislocations of the ankle. Oper Orthop Traumatol 2013;25:273–93 [in German].

62. O'Connor TJ, Mueller B, Ly TV, et al. A to P" screw vs posterolateral plate for posterior malleolus fixation in trimalleolar ankle fractures. J Orthop Trauma 2015;29: e151–6.

63. Kim MB, Lee YH, Kim JH, et al. Lateral transmalleolar approach and miniscrews fixation for displaced posterolateral fragments of posterior malleolus fractures in adults: a consecutive study. J Orthop Trauma 2015;29:105–11.

64. DeVries JS, Wijgman AJ, Sierevelt IN, et al. Long term results of ankle fractures with a posterior malleolar fragment. J Foot Ankle Surg 2005;44:211–7.
65. Li YD, Liu SM, Jia JS, et al. Choice of internal fixation methods for posterior malleolus fracture in both biomechanics and clinical application. Beijing Da Xue Xue Bao 2011;43:718–23.
66. Huber M, Stutz PM, Gerber C. Open reduction and internal fixation of the posterior malleolus with a posterior antiglide plate using a posterolateral approach- a preliminary report. Foot Ankle Surg 1996;2:95–103.
67. Abdelgawad AA, Kadous A, Kanlic E. Posterolateral approach for treatment of posterior malleolus fracture of the ankle. J Foot Ankle Surg 2011;50:607–11.
68. Forberger J, Sabandal PV, Dietrich M, et al. Posterolateral approach to the displaced posterior malleolus: functional outcome and local morbidity. Foot Ankle Int 2009;30:309–14.
69. Weber M, Ganz R. Malunion following trimalleolar fracture with posterolateral subluxation of the talus: reconstruction including the posterior malleolus. Foot Ankle Int 2003;24:338–44.
70. Rammelt S, Zwipp H. Intra-articular osteotomy for correction of malunions and nonunions of the tibial pilon. Foot Ankle Clin 2016;21:63–76.
71. Leed HC, Ehrlich MG. Instability of the distal tibiofibular syndesmosis after bimalleolar and trimalleolar ankle fractures. J Bone Joint Surg 1984;66-A:490–503.
72. Lindsjø U. Operative treatment of ankle fracture-dislocations. A follow-up study of 306/321 consecutive cases. Clin Orthop Relat Res 1985;199:28–38.
73. Jaskulka RA, Ittner G, Schedl R. Fractures of the posterior tibial margin: their role in the prognosis of malleolar fractures. J Trauma 1989;29:1565–70.
74. McKinley TO, Rudert MJ, Koos DC, et al. Incongruity versus instability in the etiology of posttraumatic arthritis. Clin Orthop Relat Res 2004;423:44–51.
75. Tejwani NC, Pahk B, Egol AE. Effect of posterior malleolus fracture on outcome after unstable ankle fracture. J Trauma 2010;69:666–9.
76. Evers J, Barz L, Wähnert D, et al. Size matters: the influence of posterior fragment on patient outcomes in trimalleolar ankle fractures. Injury 2015;46(Suppl 4): S109–13.
77. Langenhuijsen JF, Heetveld MJ, Ultee JM, et al. Results of ankle fractures with involvement of the posterior tibial margin. J Trauma 2002;53:55–60.

Primary Arthrodesis for Tibial Pilon Fractures

Bryant Ho, MD[a], John Ketz, MD[b],*

KEYWORDS

- Pilon fracture • Distal tibia fracture • Primary fusion • Ankle arthrodesis
- Ankle fusion

KEY POINTS

- Primary arthrodesis for pilon fractures can potentially accelerate recovery, decrease complications, and decrease pain compared with open reduction internal fixation in certain scenarios.
- Indications for primary ankle arthrodesis include 43.B and 43.C fractures that are nonreconstructible, in patients with delay in treatment or multiple medical comorbidities, or in patients with peripheral neuropathy.
- Initial reduction of the posterior malleolus and fibula can decrease the difficulty of staged ankle arthrodesis.
- In patients with peripheral neuropathy, increase fixation by adding independent lag screws to an anterior or posterior plate. Alternatively, consider a tibiotalocalcaneal arthrodesis with an intramedullary nail.

INTRODUCTION

Pilon fractures are intra-articular fractures of the distal tibia that typically result from high-energy injuries. This can result in fractures with significant displacement, articular comminution, and extensive surrounding soft tissue injuries. Treatment strategies have evolved due to improved understanding on the management of the surrounding soft tissue. Staged treatment involves initial establishment of gross length and alignment with an external fixator with or without fixation of the fibula, followed by definitive fixation once the soft tissue envelope has improved. Although these techniques have improved complication rates, Sirkin and colleagues[1] reported a 17% superficial wound complication rate and 3.4% deep wound complication rate with staged treatment. Deep infections prolong treatment, often requiring multiple operative procedures and extended immobilization, and can increase the risk of ankle arthritis that requires eventual arthrodesis (**Fig. 1**).

The authors have nothing to disclose.
[a] Hinsdale Orthopaedics, 550 W Odgen Ave, Hinsdale, IL, USA; [b] Department of Orthopaedics, University of Rochester Medical Center, 601 Elmwood Avenue, Box 665, Rochester, NY 14642, USA
* Corresponding author.
E-mail address: John_Ketz@urmc.rochester.edu

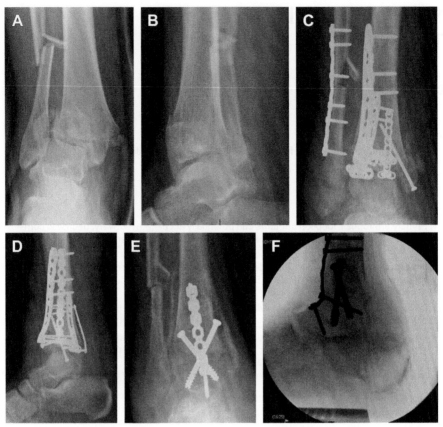

Fig. 1. (*A, B*) Initial anteroposterior (AP) and lateral radiographs of a 30-year-old man who fell from a ladder and sustained a high-energy intra-articular pilon fracture. The patient was treated by another surgeon with initial fixation of the posterior malleolus and fibula with external fixation followed by staged definitive treatment through an anterior approach (*C, D*). The patient developed an infected nonunion 2 months postoperatively that required removal of his hardware, antibiotics, 3 debridements, and 7 total months in an external fixator. He was treated with an ankle arthrodesis 7 months after his initial injury (*E, F*).

Pilon fractures are very difficult to manage for a variety of reasons. Although postoperative complications have improved with staged treatment, outcomes after operative treatment are modest. At average 3.2-year follow-up, Pollak and colleagues[2] reported ankle stiffness in 35% of patients, and persistent pain in 33%. Harris and colleagues[3] found posttraumatic arthritis in 39% of patients with Orthopaedic Trauma Association (OTA) 43.B or 43.C fractures at average 26-month follow-up. Improved clinical results have been associated with the quality of articular reduction.[4,5] However, evaluation of computed tomography (CT) scans demonstrates that malreduction after operative treatment can be as high as 70%.[6]

Primary ankle arthrodesis has been proposed as an alternative treatment for high-energy pilon fractures with complex articular comminution that have a low chance of adequate reduction.[7–10] Potential advantages include accelerated recovery, decreased complications including wound infections, and improved functional outcome and pain. Although previously reported literature has limited primary arthrodesis to nonreconstructible pilon fractures, there are other possible indications for high-energy 43.C-type fractures. These include delayed definitive treatment from soft tissue injuries or infection, patient factors, medical comorbidities, and peripheral neuropathy.

EVALUATION AND WORKUP

Initial evaluation consisting of a thorough history and physical examination is crucial in determining treatment options. Comorbidities that can increase complications with operative intervention should be evaluated, such as diabetes, hypertension, chronic alcohol abuse, schizophrenia, and peripheral neuropathy.[11–13] Other possible potential comorbidities that have been associated with complications in ankle fractures include American Society of Anesthesiologists (ASA) class, age older than 60, pulmonary disease, body mass index greater than 40, and wound-compromising medications such as corticosteroids.[14–17]

The mechanism of injury is also important in that lower-energy injury patterns can be treated acutely and have shown to yield good results with open reduction internal fixation (ORIF).[18] High-energy fractures with metaphyseal and diaphyseal comminution are associated with surrounding soft tissue trauma and have higher reported complication rates with lower functional outcome scores.[3]

Physical examination consists of evaluation of the soft tissues and vascular status of the ankle. The location of soft tissue injuries should be noted for preoperative planning of surgical incisions. Patients with open injuries, significant soft tissue swelling, or fracture blisters should be treated in a staged fashion (see **Fig. 4**F). Sensory examination in patients with suspicion for neuropathy, such as patients with diabetes, should include 5.07-g Semmes-Weinstein monofilament testing over the plantar foot to evaluate protective sensation.

Plain radiographs of the ankle and tibia and fibula should be obtained, as they provide significant information on injury pattern and status of the fibula. In high-energy fracture patterns, a CT scan should be obtained if provisional fixation of the fibula or tibia is being considered by the treating surgeon. Images from the CT provide detailed information about the articular surface, displacement, shortening, and rotation. If provisional treatment consists of external fixation alone, a CT is best reserved following stabilization in preparation for staged treatment. Tornetta and Gorup[19] showed that a CT scan to be useful, as it can change surgical planning based on fracture pattern. Pilon fractures are classified by the Arbeitsgemeinschaft für Osteosynthesefragen (AO)/OTA system, with subgroups B3, C2, and C3 having increasing metaphyseal and articular comminution, which often make anatomic reduction difficult. In these patterns, primary arthrodesis can be considered as a treatment option.

Initial treatment for staged fixation usually consists of external fixation. It is important to reestablish length and alignment in the coronal and sagittal planes. This can be done in isolation or with fixation of the fibula and/or limited fixation of the tibia. This aids in restoration of length and alignment of the fracture. The authors recommend against initial fixation of the tibia or fibula if the surgeon is not going to be definitively managing the fracture. For pilon fractures with a displaced posterior malleolus with amenable posterior soft tissues, initial treatment may include fixation of the fibula and posterior malleolus through a posterolateral approach in the prone position followed by placement of an external fixator. This staged method was reported by Ketz and Sanders[20] for treating high-energy C2 and C3 fractures with improved anatomic reduction (**Fig. 2**).

The affected extremity should be closely monitored, with definitive treatment scheduled once the soft tissue envelope has recovered. Once swelling has decreased

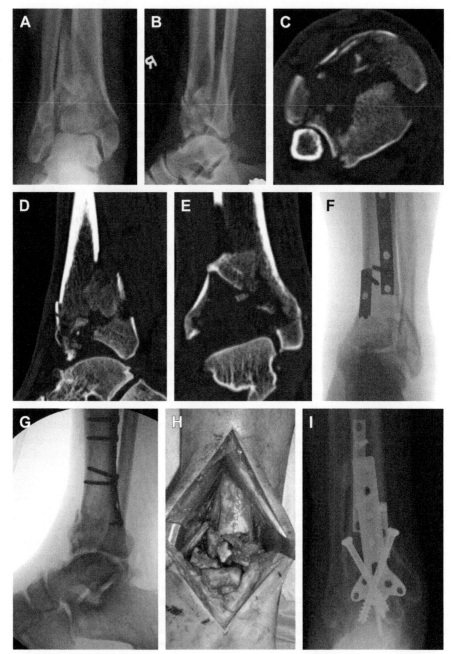

Fig. 2. (*A, B*) Initial AP and lateral radiographs of a 43-year-old man who sustained a pilon fracture from a soccer injury that was treatment at an outside institution with external fixation. (*C–E*) Axial, sagittal, and coronal CT views demonstrate a posterior malleolus fragment with extensive anterior articular comminution. He was treated 2 weeks after injury with posterior fixation and placed in an external fixator (*F, G*). He was treated definitively 6 weeks after injury with an ankle arthrodesis through an anterior approach (*H*). Radiographs at 12 months demonstrate fusion (*I, J*). The patient returned fully to duty as a manual laborer. (*From* Ketz J, Sanders R. Pilon Fractures. Mann's surgery of the foot and ankle. 9th edition. Philadelphia: Elsevier Health Sciences; 2013. p. 1995; with permission.)

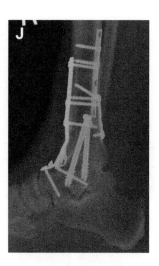

Fig. 2. (*continued*).

sufficiently, patients will demonstrate the wrinkle sign, in which the ankle around the skin will demonstrate wrinkling without manipulation. Other signs of soft tissue recovery include epithelialization of fracture blisters, and complete healing of initial open wounds. This process typically takes 1 to 2 weeks, although severe high-energy injuries can take up to 6 weeks. During this time, several factors may lead the surgeon toward primary arthrodesis versus ORIF.

INDICATIONS FOR PRIMARY ANKLE ARTHRODESIS
Nonreconstructible Pilon Fractures

AO/OTA 43.C2 and C3 and even some B3 fractures with extensive articular comminution are candidates for primary ankle arthrodesis (**Fig. 3**). Fractures with significant comminution or small articular fragments make anatomic reduction extremely difficult. Without anatomic reduction, there can be rapid progression of radiographic and potentially symptomatic arthritis. In a younger, more active population, the main reconstructive option is arthrodesis. Also, areas of comminution can develop aseptic avascular necrosis, which can lead to collapse and nonunion. During surgery, the articular surface of the joint may have cartilage delamination or injury that may lead to rapid arthrosis. If this is suspected, primary arthrodesis should be discussed with the patient before the procedure.

Delayed Definitive Treatment

There are multiple reasons that can delay definitive treatment. High-energy pilon injuries are often polytraumas with other injuries, or unstable hemodynamics that may postpone definitive ORIF beyond 3 to 4 weeks. After that time, mobilization of the fragments can be difficult, limiting reduction. The cartilage layer also can be destabilized and may delaminate with manipulation. Open fractures with traumatic wounds can limit surgical incisions that may be needed for reduction purposes. Fracture blisters and abrasions also can produce the same effect. Open fractures with acute infections may similarly postpone definitive treatment and require intravenous antibiotics before placement of indwelling hardware (**Fig. 4**).

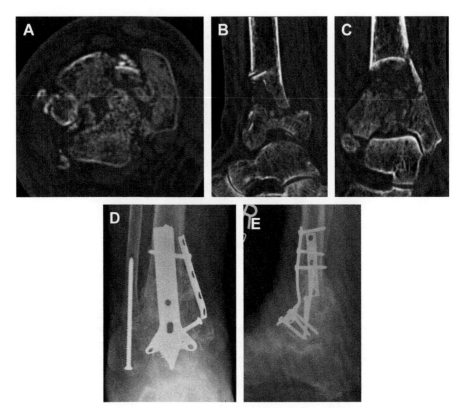

Fig. 3. (*A–C*) Axial, sagittal, and coronal CT views of a 70-year-old woman with extensive metaphyseal and articular comminution of the distal tibia. Three-month radiographs show consolidation and she was ambulating in an ankle brace without pain (*D, E*).

Multiple Medical Comorbidities

Patients with medical comorbidities have increased complications and reoperation rates after operative treatment of pilon fractures.[11–13] In a retrospective cohort of 95 pilon fractures (43C) treated in a staged fashion, White and colleagues[13] reported reoperation rates of 50% in patients with diabetes or schizophrenia, and 40% in patients with alcohol abuse, compared with 6% for entire cohort. Primary arthrodesis for these patients allows for increased time for the soft tissues to recover. It also allows more time for medical optimization, such as improved glucose control. Poor glucose control has been found to be associated with increased complications in ankle arthrodesis.[21] Additionally, ankle arthrodesis can be done through a posterior approach, avoiding the tenuous anterior skin.

Patient Factors

A small select population of patients may not tolerate or adhere to an extended 8-week to 12-week course of non–weight bearing. These include comorbidities, such as obesity or altered mental status, and patient factors, such as limited mobility or living alone. In these patients, staged definitive treatment with a tibiotalocalcaneal (TTC) arthrodesis using an intramedullary nail is an option that allows for earlier weight bearing with a load-sharing implant (**Fig. 5**); however, this comes at the cost of

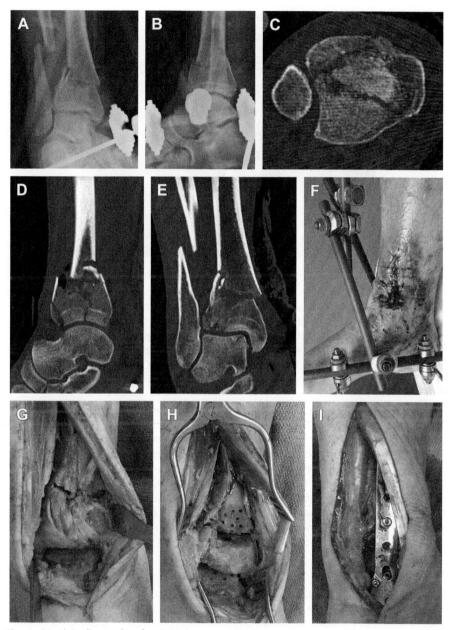

Fig. 4. (*A, B*) Radiographs after initial external fixation in a 60-year-old man with an open pilon fracture. Axial, sagittal, and coronal CT views demonstrate minimal comminution (*C–E*). He had severe initial soft tissue injury (*F*). He was treated with staged primary arthrodesis after infection with osteomyelitis delayed his treatment for 3 months. Intraoperative images of an anterior approach demonstrate exposure of the fracture (*G*) followed by joint preparation with drilling of the articular surface as well as the anterior distal metaphysis (*H*). An ankle arthrodesis plate was used (*I*) in addition to an independent lag screw. Final radiographs at 4 months demonstrate consolidation (*J, K*).

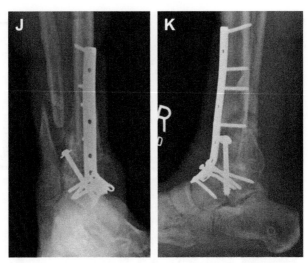

Fig. 4. (*continued*).

subtalar motion. Hsu and Szatkowski[22] reported on a patient with a history of seizures, stroke, hypertension, smoking, and cocaine abuse who had a 43.C pilon fracture treated with staged TTC arthrodesis. Despite immediately weight bearing against medical advice, she achieved fusion and was satisfied at final 17-month follow-up with an American Orthopaedic Foot and Ankle Society (AOFAS) score of 79.

Peripheral Neuropathy

Staged primary arthrodesis in these patients allows for more rigid fixation, an advantage in these patients that lack protective sensation. This can lead to noncompliance of weight bearing. In higher energy patterns, ORIF may create failures and wounds due to early weight bearing. Arthrodesis does not require maintained articular reduction and may be beneficial in this patient population. As a general principle, additional hardware should be used to prevent failure. This can be accomplished by anterior or posterior plating supplemented by independent lag screws. In scenarios in which there is significant metaphyseal comminution, additional fully threaded large lag screws can be used. Consideration also can be given to hindfoot intramedullary nailing, as the implant is stronger, although it sacrifices the subtalar joint.

SURGICAL TECHNIQUE
Initial Treatment

Initial treatment consists of reestablishing length and alignment with an external fixator. For fractures without a displaced posterior malleolar fracture, a standard external fixator is placed in the supine position with fixation of the fibula through a posterior or posterolateral approach. If the patient has a 43.C pilon fracture that includes the posterior malleolus, our preferred treatment is with initial fixation of the posterior malleolus and fibula.

- The patient is positioned in the prone position with a proximal thigh tourniquet.
- A posterolateral incision is made midway between the lateral border of the Achilles and the posterior border of the fibula.
- The sural nerve is protected during superficial dissection.

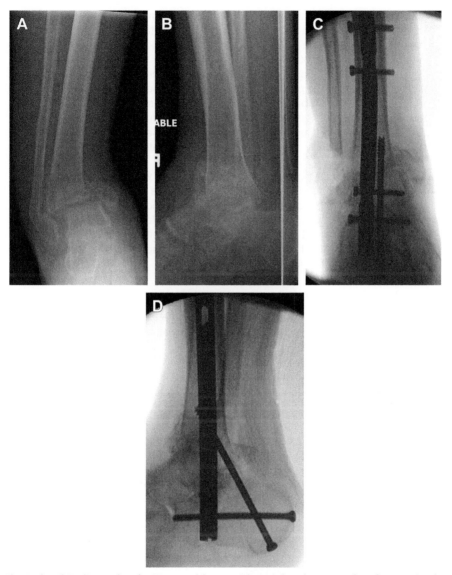

Fig. 5. (*A, B*) Radiographs of a 65-year-old man with peripheral neuropathy who sustained a pilon fracture with extensive articular comminution. (*C, D*) Intraoperative radiographs after tibiotalocalcaneal arthrodesis with an intramedullary nail supplemented with an independent lag screw.

- The peroneal fascia is incised and the peroneal tendons are reflected medially to expose the fibula. For simple fractures, the fibula is reduced with clamps and a lag screw is placed with a neutralization plate if there is no comminution. There is often significant comminution of the fibula that requires bridge fixation. In these instances, contralateral ankle films are obtained preoperatively to help judge fibular length and rotation. Anatomic reduction of the fibula is critical to reduction of the posterior malleolus fragments.

- The peroneal tendons are reflected laterally and the flexor hallucis longus tendon is reflected medially to expose to the posterior distal tibia. Dissection is maintained superficial to the periosteum and posterior ankle capsule to avoid damage to the posterior tibiofibular ligament.
- In patients without posterior metaphyseal comminution, there is typically a cortical read along the proximal fracture fragment that helps reduce the fracture. A 3.5-mm one-third tubular plate is applied in buttress mode with fixation only in the proximal fragment (see **Fig. 2**F–G). If the distal fragments are smaller or unstable, mini-fragment locking fixation can be used. Care should be taken to make sure that any distally placed screw does not interfere with future anterior reduction.
- After reduction of the posterior malleolus and fibula, we place an external fixator. The knee is flexed to 90° and two 5.0-mm half pins are placed proximal to the fracture site and our planned definitive anterior or posterior arthrodesis plate. A 5.0-mm centrally threaded transcalcaneal pin is placed. A 4.0-mm half pin is placed in the proximal first metatarsal shaft. A Delta frame construct is used with a first metatarsal pin for added stability and to prevent equinus with extended external fixation treatment.

Ankle Arthrodesis with Open Reduction Internal Fixation

After external fixation, a CT scan is obtained to characterize the fracture. The patient is followed in the clinic weekly until the soft tissues have recovered, as evidenced by healing of open wounds, the appearance of a wrinkle sign, and reepithelialization of fracture blisters. If the patient meets indications for ankle arthrodesis, the patient is counseled on associated increased adjacent arthritis and gait changes.

- An anterior approach is performed in the supine position. Alternatively, a direct posterior or a previously used posterolateral approach in the prone position can be performed for patients with tenuous anterior soft tissues.
- For the anterior approach, a midline incision is used. Dissection is carried out through the interval between the anterior tibial tendon and the extensor hallucis longus tendon. Dissection is carried down to bone just lateral to the anterior tibial tendon while persevering the more lateral neurovascular bundle. The anterior tibial tendon sheath is preserved. Subperiosteal dissection is extended medially and laterally to expose the fracture fragments and the entire ankle joint.
- Fracture fragments are debrided of fibrous tissue and callous (see **Fig. 4**F). Larger articular fragments are reduced and stabilized with either Kirschner (K)-wire or screw fixation. Small comminuted articular fragments are removed and all remaining cartilage is debrided.
- All cartilage is then removed from the talus.
- A 2.0-mm drill is used to drill holes spaced approximately 2 to 3 mm apart in the talus as well as the anterior metaphysis of the tibia (see **Fig. 4**G).
- Metaphyseal defects as well as the tibiotalar joint are packed with autologous or allograft bone graft. The authors' preference is autograft from the iliac crest. If more volume is needed, we mix autograft with demineralized bone matrix.
- Proper care is taken to position the ankle. Varus and valgus alignment is corrected first. Then proper rotation of the talus is confirmed. The ankle is placed in neutral dorsiflexion and large K-wires are passed across the fracture and ankle sequentially. Position is then confirmed with fluoroscopy.
- If allowed by the fracture, 1 to 3 large cannulated lag screws are placed across the fracture and ankle joint. If there is significant comminution or bone loss, fully

threaded screws are used. An anterior plate is then placed and screws are placed into the talus and tibia sequentially. In patients with peripheral neuropathy, supplemental fixation is applied, if the fracture pattern allows.

- The wound is closed in a layered fashion, with careful closure of the superior extensor retinaculum to ensure soft tissue coverage over the anterior plate. The patient is then placed into a short-leg splint.

Postoperative Protocol

- The patient is placed in a short-leg splint with no weight bearing.
- At 2 to 3 weeks, the sutures are removed if the wounds have healed, and the patient is placed in a short-leg cast with continued non–weight bearing.
- At 8 weeks, the patient is placed in a walking boot with the initiation of progressive weight bearing if there is evidence of consolidation across the fusion site.
- At 12 weeks, the patient is transitioned to full weight bearing with an ankle brace, which is weaned at 16 weeks.

ANKLE ARTHRODESIS WITH EXTERNAL FIXATION

Scenarios exist in which ORIF with fusion is not possible. The patient's soft tissues may not be able to tolerate large or multiple incisions about the ankle. There may be an early, acute infection from an open injury or ORIF that requires hardware removal, irrigation and debridement, and intravenous antibiotics. In these cases, a ring external fixator can be a useful tool. It allows for stabilization of the fracture. Through previous wounds, small limited incisions, or arthroscopically, the cartilage surfaces can be denuded.[23] Alignment can be stabilized with the fixation and the fracture can be compressed or lengthened with the fixator (**Fig. 6**). Depending on the fracture stability, earlier weight bearing can be initiated. Foot bypass frames also can be applied to allow weight bearing in patients who cannot tolerate non–weight-bearing precautions. These patients need to be followed closely for complications, such as pin tract infections, deep infections, or pin loosening.

ANKLE ARTHRODESIS WITH INTRAMEDULLARY NAILING

Intramedullary nailing also can be used for pilon fractures (see **Fig. 5**). Hindfoot nailing provides a strong implant that theoretically can allow for earlier weight bearing. The cartilage surfaces can be prepared using limited incisions, or arthroscopically.[24,25] However, it is difficult to correct fractures with significant displacement or malalignment with intramedullary nailing.

Intramedullary nailing sacrifices subtalar joint motion, which can accelerate transverse tarsal joint motion. Although tibiotalar arthrodesis rates range from 91% to 97%, tibiotalocalcaneal arthrodesis rates with an intramedullary nail range from 80% to 93% due to the additional fusion site.[23,26–28] This method is reserved for low-demand patients, patients with socioeconomic factors that preclude extended non–weight bearing, or neuropathic patients.

RESULTS

Although there are few studies on staged ankle arthrodesis for high-energy pilon fractures, the results have been good. In the largest study, Zelle and colleagues[10] reported on 17 patients with nonreconstructible pilon fractures who were treated through a posterior Achilles splitting approach with a 95-degree blade plate. All patients had iliac crest autograft and 14 patients had additional allograft. All patients achieved eventual union

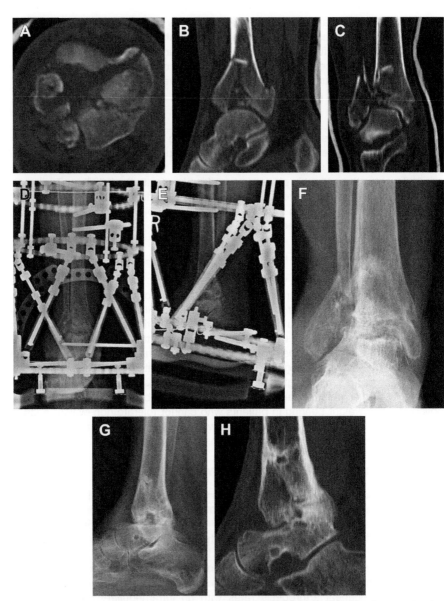

Fig. 6. (*A–C*) Axial, sagittal, and coronal CT views of a 72-year-old woman who sustained an open pilon fracture. (*D, E*) She was treated with primary arthrodesis with a ringed fixator due to delay in treatment from delayed healing and infection of her anterior open wound (*D, E*). Radiographs and sagittal CT view at 7 months demonstrate fusion and she was ambulating in an ankle foot orthosis without pain (*F–H*).

at an average of 132 days. One patient had a nonunion that required a circular frame with fusion at 435 days. At average follow-up of 7.2 years, all patients were ambulating without assistance. Average Short Form (SF)-36 physical component summary scores were 31.2 and SF-36 mental component summary scores were 51.6. There was one superficial infection that resolved with antibiotics and no deep infections.

Bozic and colleagues[8] reported on 14 nonreconstructible pilon fractures treated with staged arthrodesis similarly through a posterior Achilles splitting approach with a 90-degree blade plate and iliac crest autograft. Union was achieved in all cases at an average of 15 weeks. There was one case of deep infection requiring implant removal and intravenous antibiotics.

Beaman and Gellman[7] retrospectively reviewed 63 patients with high-energy pilon fractures, of whom 11 were treated with staged primary fusion due to articular loss greater than 50%. All but 2 patients were treated through an anterior approach. Fixation consisted of anterior ankle arthrodesis plates, ringed fixators, or a combination or both. All fusions eventually united at an average of 4.4 months with an average AOFAS score of 83 at average 14-month follow-up. One patient had an initial nonunion that required a revision procedure. One patient had a superficial wound dehiscence that required a split-thickness skin graft and 1 patient reviewed a revision of fixation for a rotational deformity.

Niikura and colleagues[29] reported on 2 patients with nonreconstructible pilon fractures treated with ankle arthrodesis using an antegrade tibial nail. Both patients achieved union, remained pain free, and ambulated without assistance at final follow-up at 1 and 2 years, respectively.

LIMITATIONS OF ARTHRODESIS

If staged definitive treatment with primary ankle arthrodesis is selected, preoperative discussion with patients should address the potential disadvantages. Ankle arthrodesis increases the risk of arthritis to the adjacent joints in the hindfoot and midfoot.[30] Coester and colleagues[30] reported increased arthritis of the ipsilateral subtalar, talonavicular, calcaneocuboid, naviculocuneiform, tarsometatarsal, and first metatarsophalangeal joints at average 22-year follow-up after ankle arthrodesis for posttraumatic arthritis. Although radiographic rates of adjacent arthritis are high, a systemic review of the literature found an average of only 24% of patients were symptomatic.[31] Reoperation rates for adjacent arthritis are much lower at 2%, most commonly at the subtalar joint (1%). Ankle arthrodesis also leads to decreased walking speed. Thomas and colleagues[32] compared gait in 26 patients after ankle arthrodesis when compared with age-matched controls. They reported decreased gait velocity (1.06 compared with 1.29 m/s), decreased cadence, and decreased stride length in patients with ankle arthrodesis compared with age-matched controls.

SUMMARY

Staged primary ankle arthrodesis is a viable option for high-energy pilon fractures that are nonreconstructible, in patients with delay in treatment or multiple medical comorbidities, or in patients with peripheral neuropathy. Small retrospective series demonstrate high union and low wound complication rates, although further studies are needed to determine the long-term results. Ankle arthrodesis offers decreased complication rates while eliminating the potential of posttraumatic ankle arthritis pain.

REFERENCES

1. Sirkin M, Sanders R, DiPasquale T, et al. A staged protocol for soft tissue management in the treatment of complex pilon fractures. J Orthop Trauma 2004; 18(8 Suppl):S32–8.
2. Pollak AN, McCarthy ML, Bess RS, et al. Outcomes after treatment of high-energy tibial plafond fractures. J Bone Joint Surg Am 2003;85-A(10):1893–900.

3. Harris AM, Patterson BM, Sontich JK, et al. Results and outcomes after operative treatment of high-energy tibial plafond fractures. Foot Ankle Int 2006;27(4):256–65.

4. Korkmaz A, Ciftdemir M, Ozcan M, et al. The analysis of the variables, affecting outcome in surgically treated tibia pilon fractured patients. Injury 2013;44(10): 1270–4.

5. Teeny SM, Wiss DA. Open reduction and internal fixation of tibial plafond fractures. Variables contributing to poor results and complications. Clin Orthop Relat Res 1993;(292):108–17.

6. Knight J, Lauren N, Nickisch F, R B. Plain radiographs versus CT after open reduction internal fixation of tibial pilon fractures: what are we missing. American Academy of Orthopaedic Surgeons Annual Meeting. San Francisco (CA), March, 2012.

7. Beaman DN, Gellman R. Fracture reduction and primary ankle arthrodesis: a reliable approach for severely comminuted tibial pilon fracture. Clin Orthop Relat Res 2014;472(12):3823–34.

8. Bozic V, Thordarson DB, Hertz J. Ankle fusion for definitive management of non-reconstructable pilon fractures. Foot Ankle Int 2008;29(9):914–8.

9. Morgan SJ, Thordarson DB, Shepherd LE. Salvage of tibial pilon fractures using fusion of the ankle with a 90 degrees cannulated blade-plate: a preliminary report. Foot Ankle Int 1999;20(6):375–8.

10. Zelle BA, Gruen GS, McMillen RL, et al. Primary arthrodesis of the tibiotalar joint in severely comminuted high-energy pilon fractures. J Bone Joint Surg Am 2014; 96(11):e91.

11. Kline AJ, Gruen GS, Pape HC, et al. Early complications following the operative treatment of pilon fractures with and without diabetes. Foot Ankle Int 2009;30(11): 1042–7.

12. Molina CS, Stinner DJ, Fras AR, et al. Risk factors of deep infection in operatively treated pilon fractures (AO/OTA: 43). J Orthop 2015;12(Suppl 1):S7–13.

13. White TO, Guy P, Cooke CJ, et al. The results of early primary open reduction and internal fixation for treatment of OTA 43.C-type tibial pilon fractures: a cohort study. J Orthop Trauma 2010;24(12):757–63.

14. Basques BA, Miller CP, Golinvaux NS, et al. Morbidity and readmission after open reduction and internal fixation of ankle fractures are associated with preoperative patient characteristics. Clin Orthop Relat Res 2015;473(3):1133–9.

15. Belmont PJ Jr, Davey S, Rensing N, et al. Patient-based and surgical risk factors for 30-day postoperative complications and mortality after ankle fracture fixation. J Orthop Trauma 2015;29(12):e476–82.

16. Miller AG, Margules A, Raikin SM. Risk factors for wound complications after ankle fracture surgery. J Bone Joint Surg Am 2012;94(22):2047–52.

17. Ovaska MT, Madanat R, Makinen TJ. Predictors of postoperative wound necrosis following primary wound closure of open ankle fractures. Foot Ankle Int 2016; 37(4):401–6.

18. Chen SH, Wu PH, Lee YS. Long-term results of pilon fractures. Arch Orthop Trauma Surg 2007;127(1):55–60.

19. Tornetta P 3rd, Gorup J. Axial computed tomography of pilon fractures. Clin Orthop Relat Res 1996;(323):273–6.

20. Ketz J, Sanders R. Staged posterior tibial plating for the treatment of Orthopaedic Trauma Association 43C2 and 43C3 tibial pilon fractures. J Orthop Trauma 2012; 26(6):341–7.

21. Myers TG, Lowery NJ, Frykberg RG, et al. Ankle and hindfoot fusions: comparison of outcomes in patients with and without diabetes. Foot Ankle Int 2012;33(1):20–8.

22. Hsu AR, Szatkowski JP. Early tibiotalocalcaneal arthrodesis intramedullary nail for treatment of a complex tibial pilon fracture (AO/OTA 43-C). Foot Ankle Spec 2015;8(3):220–5.
23. Townshend D, Di Silvestro M, Krause F, et al. Arthroscopic versus open ankle arthrodesis: a multicenter comparative case series. J Bone Joint Surg Am 2013;95(2):98–102.
24. Carranza-Bencano A, Tejero S, Del Castillo-Blanco G, et al. Minimal incision surgery for tibiotalocalcaneal arthrodesis. Foot Ankle Int 2014;35(3):272–84.
25. Malekpour L, Rahali S, Duparc F, et al. Anatomic feasibility study of posterior arthroscopic tibiotalar arthrodesis. Foot Ankle Int 2015;36(10):1229–34.
26. Abicht BP, Roukis TS. Incidence of nonunion after isolated arthroscopic ankle arthrodesis. Arthroscopy 2013;29(5):949–54.
27. Pellegrini MJ, Schiff AP, Adams SB Jr, et al. Outcomes of tibiotalocalcaneal arthrodesis through a posterior Achilles tendon-splitting approach. Foot Ankle Int 2016;37(3):312–9.
28. Thomas AE, Guyver PM, Taylor JM, et al. Tibiotalocalcaneal arthrodesis with a compressive retrograde nail: a retrospective study of 59 nails. Foot Ankle Surg 2015;21(3):202–5.
29. Niikura T, Miwa M, Sakai Y, et al. Ankle arthrodesis using antegrade intramedullary nail for salvage of nonreconstructable tibial pilon fractures. Orthopedics 2009;32(8). http://dx.doi.org/10.3928/01477447-20090624-26.
30. Coester LM, Saltzman CL, Leupold J, et al. Long-term results following ankle arthrodesis for post-traumatic arthritis. J Bone Joint Surg Am 2001;83-A(2): 219–28.
31. Ling JS, Smyth NA, Fraser EJ, et al. Investigating the relationship between ankle arthrodesis and adjacent-joint arthritis in the hindfoot. A systematic review. J Bone Joint Surg Am 2015;97(9):e43.
32. Thomas R, Daniels TR, Parker K. Gait analysis and functional outcomes following ankle arthrodesis for isolated ankle arthritis. J Bone Joint Surg Am 2006;88(3): 526–35.

Chopart Injuries
When to Fix and When to Fuse?

Stefan Rammelt, MD, PhD[a],*, Tim Schepers, MD, PhD[b]

KEYWORDS

- Midtarsal joint • Cuboid • Navicular • Anterior calcaneal process • Talar head
- Fracture • Internal fixation • Corrective fusion

KEY POINTS

- Fractures and dislocations at the midtarsal (Chopart) joints have a relatively low incidence but a highly variable clinical presentation and care must be taken to address all bony and ligamentous components of the injury.
- Surgical treatment aims at joint reconstruction and axial alignment with restoration of the normal relationship of the lateral and medial foot columns while type of internal fixation depends on the individual fracture pattern, including Kirschner wires, resorbable pins, screws, and plates.
- In cases of severe soft tissue trauma, internal fixation is supplemented by tibiometatarsal external fixation until soft tissue consolidation.
- Primary fusion of the talonavicular or calcaneocuboid joint should be reserved for rare cases of severe destruction of the articular surface because of the pivotal role of these joints for global foot function.
- The best predictor for acceptable results after midtarsal and tarsometatarsal dislocations is primary anatomic reduction and adequate internal fixation, whereas inadequate joint reduction and/or stabilization almost invariably leads to painful malunions or nonunions, residual instability, and deformity.

INTRODUCTION

The midtarsal joint is crucial for foot function. Among clinicians it bears the name of the French surgeon François Chopart (1732–1795) of whom just 1 exarticulation at the midtarsal joint has been reported.[1] Fractures and fracture-dislocations at the Chopart joint are among the most frequently overlooked and underestimated injuries. It is held that these are either missed completely or not adequately diagnosed in about 30% to 40% of cases[2–4] mainly because of their relatively low incidence, the variability of the clinical presentation, the high prevalence of accompanying injuries, lack of knowledge

The authors have nothing to disclose.
[a] Foot & Ankle Section, University Center for Orthopaedics and Traumatology, University Hospital Carl-Gustav Carus, Fetscherstrasse 74, Dresden 01307, Germany; [b] Trauma Unit, Academic Medical Center, Meibergdreef 9, PO Box 22660, Amsterdam 1100 DD, The Netherlands
* Corresponding author.
E-mail address: strammelt@hotmail.com

of subtle clinical radiographic signs, and underestimation of the ligamentous component of the injury.[5]

The Chopart joint consists of the talonavicular joint at the medial column, which is pivotal for the 3-dimensional movement between the forefoot and midfoot, and the calcaneocuboid joint, which provides essential elasticity to the lateral foot column. Both joints closely interact with each other and the subtalar joint within the triple joint complex. Consequently, malfunction of 1 joint will negatively affect the 2 other joints, thus substantially impeding global foot function.[6,7] Both the talonavicular and calcaneocuboid joints are stabilized by strong plantar and dorsal ligaments with the central bifurcate ligament acting as a pivot of the Chopart joint as a whole.[8] Intrinsic and extrinsic foot muscles provide additional dynamic support to the longitudinal foot arch that has its highest point at the level of the talonavicular joint.

In their classic study from 1975, Main and Jowett[2] analyzed the mechanism of midtarsal joint injuries in 71 cases and discussed the problems that almost invariably arise from inadequate treatment, which, at that time, was typically closed reduction and cast immobilization. The investigators stated that longitudinal forces (axial load) on the foot were responsible for about 40% of the injuries. The individual fracture pattern depended on the position of the foot (ie, plantarflexion or dorsiflexion) during the impact. Medial forces with forefoot adduction resulted in fractures of the tarsal navicular or talar head. Main and Jowett[2] further observed lateral forces (forefoot abduction) leading to fractures of the anterior calcaneal process and the cuboid. Rotational forces produced swivel dislocations as subtypes of these injuries. Rarely, plantar forces resulted in plantar dislocation of the midfoot and forefoot with bony avulsions. Finally, crush injuries with irregular fracture patterns and compound soft tissue wounds resulted from heavy objects falling on the foot. In a biomechanical study, high pressures at the Chopart joint and subsequent fractures at the midfoot could be reproduced with plantar impact.[9]

When considering the proposed injury mechanisms at the Chopart joint, compression fractures at the medial or lateral side are most likely combined with distraction forces at the opposite side (**Fig. 1**), regularly leading to either ligamentous injuries, bony avulsions, or fractures.[10,11] Consequently, about half of the patients with injuries at the Chopart joint have fractures of 2 or more bony components.[4] When assessing acute injuries, ligamentous injuries, avulsions, or fractures of the opposite side must be ruled out before diagnosing isolated navicular or cuboidal fractures. Pure dislocations with isolated ligamentous injuries of both the medial and lateral side are exceedingly rare and bony injuries must be ruled out with the generous use of computed tomography (CT) scanning.[12] In their classic paper from 1953, Hermel and Gershon-Cohen[13] observed that what they termed nutcracker fractures of the cuboid were rarely isolated because of the considerable forces that were required to produce them.

ASSESSMENT
Clinical Examination

Patients with injuries at the Chopart joints display a wide range of clinical symptoms ranging from localized pain that is exaggerated by weightbearing, to severe swelling and hematoma over the midfoot, to compound soft tissue wounds. In cases of severe dislocations, there is a marked deformity with pale skin over prominent bone fragments that will rapidly lead to blistering and skin necrosis if left unreduced. In more subtle injuries, there is pain on palpation over the midfoot, and eversion and inversion of the foot is painful and restricted. A pathognomonic sign of relevant injuries of

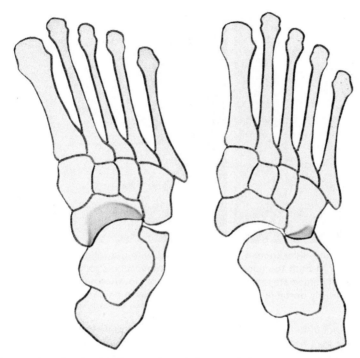

Fig. 1. Proposed mechanism leading to Chopart fracture dislocations according to Main and Jowett.[2] Forced adduction of the forefoot against the hindfoot leads to medial stress and forced abduction of the forefoot leads to lateral stress at the midtarsal joint. This may be combined with longitudinal forces (axial load). Compression fractures at the medial or lateral side are most likely combined with distraction forces at the opposite side. Consequently, there should be a high index of suspicion for ligamentous injuries, bony avulsions, or accompanying fractures. (*From* Rammelt S, Grass R, Schikore H, et al. [Injuries of the Chopart joint.] Unfallchirurg 2002;105:371–83 [Article in German]; with permission.)

Chopart joint is the presence of a plantar ecchymosis that indicates the rupture of the strong plantar ligaments at the midtarsal joint.[14]

Open wounds are dressed sterile at the site of the accident and are inspected again in the operating room at the time of lavage and debridement. Because a sizable number of Chopart joint injuries result from high-energy trauma, care must be taken not to overlook closed injuries in multiple injuries or polytraumatized patients.[15,16]

Radiographic Examination

Standard radiographs with suspected Chopart joint injuries include dorsoplantar (anteroposterior), lateral, and 45°oblique projections.[17] For obtaining the dorsoplantar view, the tube is tilted caudally 30° to minimize overprojection of adjacent bones. In the lateral view, the Chopart joint has a harmonic double wave appearance, hence the name cyma line from the Greek word κυμα for wave. If this line is disrupted, incongruity at the Chopart joint must be suspected (**Fig. 2A**).

If relevant instability at the Chopart joint must be ruled out in the presence or absence of bony avulsions,[11] stress radiographs with forced abduction and adduction are carried out under sufficient local anesthesia.[4,17] If a bony injury at the Chopart joint is seen or suspected on plain radiographs, CT scanning should be used generously to

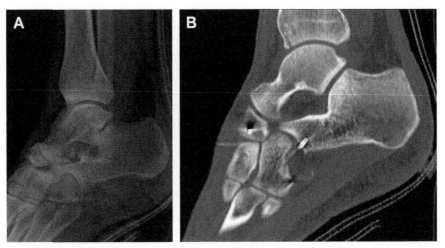

Fig. 2. (A) Fracture-dislocation at the Chopart joint with disruption of the cyma line and a double contour in both the talonavicular and calcaneocuboid joints. (B) Emergency treatment consists of immediate reduction of the marked dislocation and Kirschner wire transfixation of the grossly unstable talonavicular and calcaneocuboid joints.

reveal the exact fracture anatomy and to allow for adequate treatment planning.[10] Severe Chopart joint fracture-dislocations that occur without a relevant trauma should raise the suspicion of a Sanders and Frykberg type 3 Charcot neuroarthropathy.[15]

Classification

Besides the generic classification of Main and Jowett[2] with respect to the supposed mechanism of injury, fractures and dislocations at the Chopart joint can be classified with respect to the affected anatomic structures according to Zwipp[17] (**Fig. 3**):

1. Transligamentous
2. Transtalar

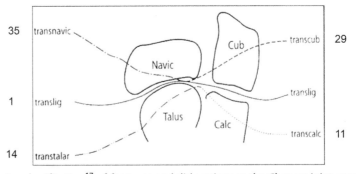

Fig. 3. Zwipp classification[17] of fractures and dislocations at the Chopart joint according to the affected anatomic structures. The numbers represent the total number of individual injuries of each type in the study by Rammelt and colleagues[4] with a total of 61 subjects. Almost 50% had injuries of 2 or more bones at the Chopart joint. Calc, Calcaneus; Cub, Cuboid; Navic, Navicular; transcalc, transcalcanear; transcub, transcuboidal; translig, transligamentous; transnav, transnavicular. (*From* Rammelt S, Grass R, Schikore H, et al. [Injuries of the Chopart joint.] Unfallchirurg 2002;105:371–83 [Article in German]; with permission.)

3. Transcalcaneal
4. Transnavicular
5. Transcuboidal
6. Combinations of 2 to 5.

Purely transligamentous dislocations are rare because of the strong ligamentous support at the talonavicular and calcaneocuboid joints.[4,18,19] Instead, bony avulsions on 1 or more bones at the Chopart joint are seen. The distal bones (ie, navicular and cuboid) are fractured more than twice as often as the proximal bones (ie, talar head and anterior calcaneal process).[4] Combined injuries with more than 1 fractured bony component make up almost half of all Chopart joint injuries and every combination of bony injuries may be observed, including fractures of all 4 bones.[20]

INDICATIONS TO SURGERY

Midfoot sprains, including stable ligamentous ruptures or bony avulsions around the Chopart joint, are treated nonoperatively with full weightbearing in an orthosis that limits eversion and inversion of the foot for 6 weeks. Undisplaced tarsal fractures, as verified by CT scanning, are treated in a below-knee cast or stable boot in a neutral position of the foot and ankle with partial weightbearing on the affected leg of 15 to 20 kg for 6 weeks. The cast or boot is then removed and gradual increase of weight-bearing as tolerated is allowed, provided that radiographic union has occurred.

All displaced fractures and fracture-dislocations at the midtarsal joint should be treated by anatomic reduction and stable internal fixation. Contraindications to a formal open reduction include contaminated or infected soft tissues, advanced peripheral vascular disease, chronic venous insufficiency with skin ulceration, poor patient compliance (substance abuse), diabetic neuro-osteoarthropathy (Charcot foot), manifest immunodeficiency, and a critical overall condition of the patient that does not allow meticulous reconstruction of midtarsal joint injuries.

Gross dislocations and fracture-dislocations must be reduced as early as possible under sufficient analgesia to prevent further damage to the soft tissues (**Fig. 2**B). Frequently, closed reduction will be impossible because of locked dislocations or interposed capsuloligamentous and bony debris. In these cases, repeated attempts on closed reduction will only further compromise soft tissue and open reduction is mandatory. If definite internal fixation is not feasible at the time of initial treatment (eg, in polytraumatized patients or because of the lack of experience with these particular injuries), an approximate reduction may be achieved with direct, limited incisions and preliminary fixation achieved with Kirschner (K) wires supplemented by tibiometatarsal external fixation. Anatomic reduction and definite internal fixation via standard approaches is then performed after soft tissue consolidation, improvement of the patient's overall condition, and detailed preoperative planning, including CT scanning.

In open fractures and fracture-dislocations, primary treatment consists of emergent reduction of gross dislocations, copious irrigation, and generous debridement of contaminated and avital tissue. Open reduction and internal fixation is carried out, possibly by extending the existing open wound. If a primary definite internal fixation is not feasible, an approximate reduction and temporary internal and external fixation is carried out. In the presence of a manifest foot compartment syndrome, a single or double longitudinal dorsal dermatofasciotomy, including the extensor retinaculum, is carried out emergently.[21,22] Alternatively, a medial fasciotomy (modified Henry approach) may be performed. In cases with compound wounds, early definite internal fixation combined with free tissue transfer aims at functional rehabilitation even in cases of complex foot trauma.[23]

Primary fusion of the talonavicular or calcaneocuboid joint should be reserved for rare cases of severe destruction of the articular surface because of the pivotal role of these joints for global foot function.[6,15] In particular, a fusion of the talonavicular joint significantly limits motion in the calcaneocuboid (by 81%–92%) and subtalar (by 62%–86%) joints.[6,7]

OPERATIVE TECHNIQUE
Patient Placement and Preparation

The patient is placed in a supine position with a tourniquet at the thigh. The lower leg is draped free and mobile, so that both the medial and lateral aspect of the Chopart joint can be easily approached. A wedge is placed under the ipsilateral hip to allow better access to the lateral side. In cases of severe compression fracture, the iliac crest is also draped free to allow for harvesting of autologous bone graft if necessary. Alternatively, bone graft may be obtained from the proximal or distal tibial metaphysis.

Internal Fixation of Talar Head Fractures

The talar head is accessed through a curved anteromedial incision starting below the medial malleolus and extending to the navicular tuberosity. The superficial fascia is opened and the tibialis posterior tendon held away plantarly with a soft strap. The joint capsule is opened and the medial plantar aspect of the talonavicular and subtalar joints exposed. If the fracture extends far laterally, an additional anterolateral approach distal and medial to the sinus tarsi is needed.[15]

The talar head fragments are gently reduced and fixed according to the individual fracture pattern. Options include resorbable pins (**Fig. 4**) for small chondral or osteochondral fragments, lost K-wires, 3.5 mm and 2.7 mm screws for simple fracture patterns with relatively large fragments, small curved 2.7 mm interlocking plates bridging the talar head to the talar neck and body with comminuted and compression fractures, supplemented by additional bone grafting in the case of resulting defects.[4] If, for stability reasons, screws are introduced near or through the joint surface, the heads must be countersunk. Alternatively, headless screws may be used. To avoid shortening of the talar head, interfragmentary compression is not desirable.

Internal Fixation of Navicular Fractures

Most navicular fractures can be accessed through a longitudinal dorsomedial or dorsomedian incision centered over the talonavicular joint, depending on the site of the fracture as assessed before surgery with CT scanning (**Fig. 5A**). During subcutaneous dissection, care is taken not to injure the intermediate dorsal cutaneous nerve arising from the superficial peroneal nerve. The central portion of the tarsal navicular is accessed in the interval between the tibialis anterior and extensor hallucis longus tendons. Fractures that are located at the lateral aspect are accessed between the extensor hallucis longus and extensor digitorum longus tendons.[15] In both instances, the dorsalis pedis artery and deep peroneal nerve are gently mobilized and held away laterally together with the extensor digitorum longus tendon. A mini-distractor placed between the talar neck and the first cuneiform is most useful to restore the length of the medial column of the foot and to expose the central and plantar aspects of the spherical joint surface (**Fig. 5B**).

The joint and the fracture edges are cleared from clots and loose fragments. The main fragments are identified and carefully mobilized with sharp elevators, K-wires, and fracture-picks. Reduction is carried out stepwise starting with the relatively constant plantar fragments and then from lateral to medial.[24] The fragments are held

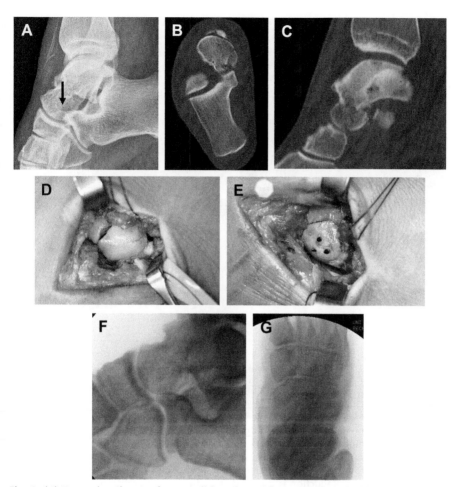

Fig. 4. (*A*) Transtalar Chopart fracture-dislocation with a suspicious double contour in the talar head (*arrow*) on plain radiographs with the patient still in the pneumatic splint. (*B–C*) CT scanning reveals a talar head fracture with multiple fragmentation and displacement at the medial aspect of the talonavicular and subtalar joints. (*D*) Intraoperative aspect of the displaced medial talar head fragment. (*E–G*) Treatment consists of open reduction via a medial approach, removal of intra-articular debris and fixation of the talar head with resorbable pins that are introduced through the cartilage and perpendicular to the main fracture lines. This restores both the medial aspect of the talonavicular joint and the anteromedial facet of the subtalar joint.

temporarily with K-wires introduced preferably at the margins close to the cortical bone (**Fig. 5**C, D). Defects resulting from central compression are filled with autologous bone graft from the medial malleolus or the iliac crest, depending on the defect size. The navicular tuberosity fragment is reduced to the reconstructed navicular body with a clamp and fixed with compression screws via a stab incision directly over the tuberosity. Internal fixation is achieved with 3.5 and 2.7 mm screws in simple fracture patterns and 2.7 mm anatomically shaped interlocking plates in cases of more complex fractures.[24–26] K-wires that are important for stabilization are cut flush to the cortex or buried beneath the cortex and left in place as lost K-wires.[15]

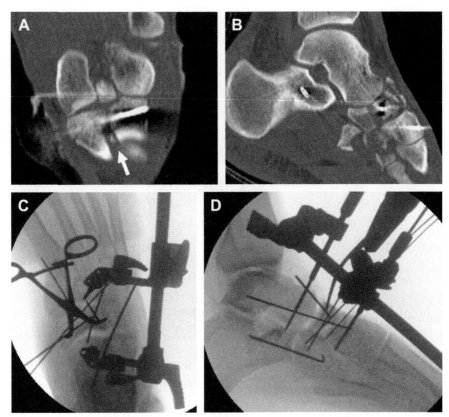

Fig. 5. (*A, B*) Open reduction of the multiply fragmented navicular (*arrow* in A and sagittal cut in B showing multiple joint fragments) in a transnavicular and transcuboidal Chopart fracture-dislocation after primary transfixation (same patient as in **Fig. 2**). (*C, D*) A mini-distractor is used to restore length of the medial foot column and to allow evaluation of the whole joint facet. Reduction is achieved stepwise from lateral to medial and plantar to dorsal with temporary K-wire fixation.

Internal Fixation of Cuboid Fractures

The cuboid is accessed via an oblique anterolateral approach starting at the upper aspect of the anterior calcaneal process and extending to the fourth tarsometatarsal joint. The incision is carried out above and parallel to the peroneal tendons on a line between the tip of the fibula and the fourth metatarsal base. Care is taken not to injure the sural nerve that is running subcutaneously parallel to the peroneal tendons. The tendons are gently mobilized and held away plantarly within their sheaths. The joint is visualized and the cuboid brought out to length using a mini-distractor placed between the anterior calcaneal process and the tuberosity of the fifth metatarsal. The joint and the fracture edges are cleared from clots and debris. The calcaneal joint facet of the cuboid is reduced gently by introducing a sharp elevator or osteotome beneath the joint surface into the compression zone of the cancellous bone, then mobilizing the articular surface together with the subcortical bone, using the uninjured corresponding joint facet of the calcaneus as a template.[4] After the calcaneocuboid joint has been reduced anatomically, the resulting subchondral defect is filled with bone graft from the distal tibia or iliac crest to maintain the correct anatomic length of the cuboid. The cuboid is fixed with an anatomically shaped 2.7 mm plate (**Fig. 6**). The use of locking plates seems useful to avoid secondary settling of these nutcracker fractures[13] and thus shortening of the lateral column of the foot leading to posttraumatic planovalgus foot.[15]

Internal Fixation of Anterior Process Fractures of the Calcaneus

The anterior calcaneal process is visualized via an oblique anterolateral approach starting at the sinus tarsi and extending to the calcaneocuboid joint. The incision is carried out above and parallel to the peroneal tendons. Care is taken not to injure the sural nerve that is running subcutaneously parallel to the peroneal tendons. The tendons are gently mobilized at the inferior retinacula, which must be detached, and held away together plantarly or dorsally with a soft strap. The joint is visualized and the lateral column brought out to length using a mini-distractor placed between the calcaneal body and the cuboid.

The calcaneocuboid joint and the fragments are cleared from clots and debris. The depressed joint fragment of the anterior calcaneal process is reduced gently by introducing a sharp elevator or osteotome beneath the joint surface into the compression zone of the cancellous bone. The joint-bearing fragment is then mobilized toward the articular surface together with the subcortical bone using the uninjured surface of the cuboid as a template (**Fig. 7**). If both calcaneus and cuboid are fractured, reduction starts with the less complex fracture. Multifragmentary fractures are reduced stepwise under direct vision and held temporarily with K-wires. If a relevant subchondral defect remains after reduction of the calcaneocuboid joint surface, it is filled with bone graft

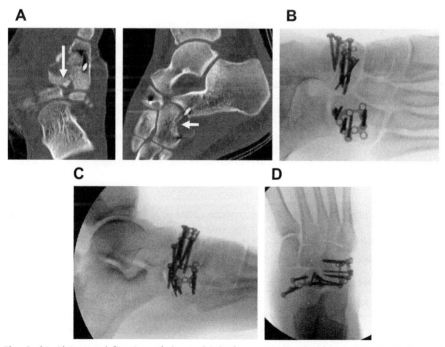

Fig. 6. (*A, B*) Internal fixation of the multiple fragmented cuboid in a transnavicular and transcuboidal Chopart fracture-dislocation (same patient as in **Figs. 2** and **5**). Note the impression and dislocation of the cuboidal joint surface (*white arrows* in A, B). (*C, D*) Both the navicular and cuboid fractures are fixed with small, anatomically shaped interlocking plates and 2.7 mm screws.

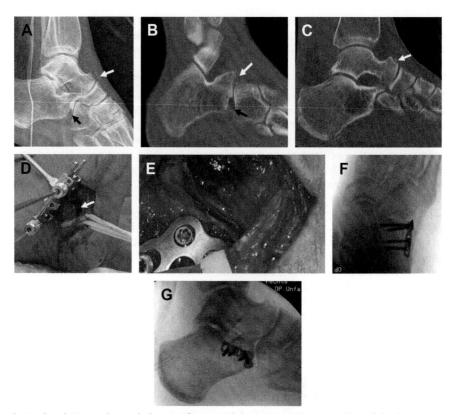

Fig. 7. (*A–C*) Transcalcaneal Chopart fracture-dislocation with impression of the lower part of the calcaneal facet to the calcaneocuboidal joint (*black arrow*). Also note the bony avulsions at the upper margin of the cuboid and the talus at the talonavicular joint (*white arrows*) as a result of the force transgressing the whole Chopart joint. (*D*) Intraoperative aspect of the depressed plantar portion of the joint facet of the anterior calcaneal process to the cuboid. The peroneal tendons are held away with a soft strap. (*E–G*) The depressed joint fragment it elevated, supported with autologous cancellous bone graft taken from the central portion of the calcaneal body via the same approach, and buttressed with a small interlocking L-plate and 2.7 mm screws.

from the distal tibia or iliac crest. The anterior process of the calcaneus is fixed with short T-shaped or L-shaped plates.[27] The use of locking plates seems useful to sustain the length of the lateral column of the foot.[15] Simple fractures of the upper part of the anterior process can be fixed with screws.[4,27]

Combined Injuries

Approximately half of all Chopart joint injuries involve 2 or more bones.[4] Treatment is tailored to the individual fracture pattern according to these principles (see **Figs. 5** and **6**). If bilateral incisions are used, they should run in a parallel manner and approximately 5 cm apart.

Temporary Joint Transfixation

After completion of internal fixation the talonavicular and calcaneocuboid joints are checked for residual instability. In cases of gross joint instability following internal fixation, the affected joint is transfixed temporarily with a 1.8 mm K-wire to allow ligamentous healing and to avoid chronic posttraumatic instability.[4] In severely comminuted fractures, temporary bridge plating of the medial column from the talus to the first metatarsal base has been advocated to ensure solid bony union.[28,29]

Primary Fusion

In the authors' practices, primary talonavicular and/or calcaneocuboid fusion is performed in exceptional cases with subtotal loss of the articular cartilage because these joints are essential for global foot function.[6,15] Fusion should, therefore, be restricted to the affected joint. After reconstruction of the medial and lateral foot column, the affected joint is freed from remaining cartilage and the subchondral bone perforated. Fusion is achieved with screws and/or plates according to the individual anatomy and fracture pattern (**Fig. 8**). An acute fusion may warrant bone grafting to maintain the relative length of the medial and lateral foot columns.

POSTOPERATIVE CARE AND REHABILITATION

Postoperatively, a splint or a split below-knee cast is applied and the affected leg is elevated. The foot may be taken out of the splint for active and passive range-of-motion exercises, except for joints that have been transfixed due to instability. In patients with open fractures or severe soft tissue damage, including compartment syndrome, external fixation is kept in place until soft tissue consolidation and definite wound closure, usually for 5 to 10 days. After wound healing, a below-knee cast is applied for 6 weeks. After that time, any temporary K-wires are removed and range-of-motion exercises are started. Patients are restricted to partial weightbearing of 15 to 20 kg for 6 to 10 weeks, depending on the individual fracture anatomy, the type of fixation, the amount of bone grafting, and overall bone quality.[15]

In the authors' practices, transarticular K-wires are removed 6 weeks after surgery and then weightbearing is increased gradually over the following 2 to 6 weeks, depending on the overall injury pattern. A similar regime is advocated when using bridge plates. Removal of implants is indicated only if there is a direct irritation to the skin or restricted range of motion (**Fig. 9**). In the latter case, it is combined with arthrolysis of the talonavicular and/or calcaneocuboid joints (**Fig. 10**).

COMPLICATIONS AND THEIR MANAGEMENT
Soft Tissue Problems

Infections of the soft tissues are rare after closed Chopart joint injuries. They are seen between zero and 10%, almost exclusively after open injuries or delayed treatment.[3,18] Other complications related to soft tissue, such as wound edge necrosis, peroneal or sural nerve injury, deep venous thrombosis, and compartment syndrome, have been reported anecdotally.[3,4,18] Complex regional pain syndrome has been described exclusively after initially overlooked Chopart injuries.[3]

Avascular Necrosis

Avascular necrosis (AVN) of the navicular has been observed predominately in middle-aged or elderly women.[12,20,26,30] The patients typically complain about persisting or revolving pain on increased weightbearing. AVN is diagnosed with the help of standard radiographs at 4 to 6 months after the injury and characterized by a radiopaque appearance of the navicular. The exact extension of the necrotic zone is best seen on MRI. In analogy to the talus, creeping substitution of the navicular may occur

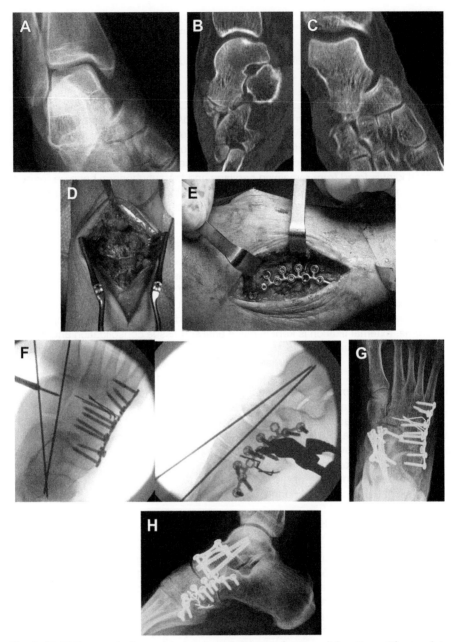

Fig. 8. (*A–D*) Transnavicular and transcuboidal Chopart fracture-dislocation with complete loss of cartilage over the lateral aspect of the navicular and medial aspect of the talar head due to a locked dislocation. (*E–F*) After debridement of the remaining cartilage at the talonavicular joint, axial realignment is achieved with distraction of the lateral foot column, which is stabilised using a temporary bridge plate (removed after 4 months). Primary fusion is carried out with an interlocking plate and additional compression screws across the talonavicular joint. (*G–H*) Radiographs taken at 8 weeks show axial realignment and solid fusion.

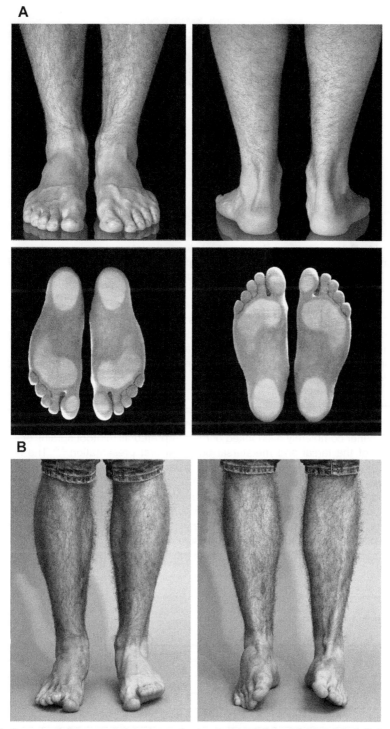

Fig. 9. One-year follow-up of the same patient as in **Figs. 2, 5,** and **6**. He works full time as a construction engineer and has no pain during daily walking and standing (*A*). There is almost full inversion but mild restriction of eversion at the midfoot preventing him from running (*B*).

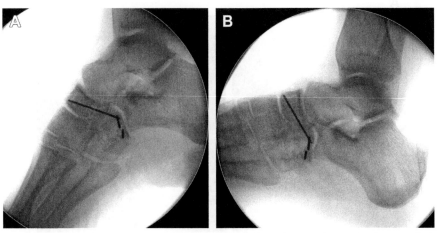

Fig. 10. (*A, B*) Implant removal and arthrolysis of the talonavicular and calcaneocuboid joints may result in considerable functional improvement (same patient as in **Figs. 2, 5, 6,** and **9**). Lost K-wires are left in place when being flush with the cortex or even buried inside the bone.

over several months.[30] Complete AVN leads to collapse of the navicular with subsequent shortening of the medial column and dorsal extrusion of the superior fragment. Treatment consists of necrectomy and talonavicular fusion with tricortical bone grafting. Sometimes the naviculocuneiform joints must be included into the fusion to bridge the defect and achieve adequate stability.

Malunion and Nonunion

It is estimated that between 20% and 40% of fractures and dislocations of the Chopart joint are either completely overlooked or misinterpreted as midfoot sprains or isolated fractures of the tarsal and metatarsal bones at first presentation.[3–5] The resulting 3-dimensional deformity depends on the initial fracture anatomy.[20] Shortening of the medial or lateral foot column leads to horizontal malalignment with forefoot adduction or abduction, respectively. Plantar or dorsal dislocation of the tarsal bones results in a flatfoot or cavus deformity. Rotatory (swivel) dislocations around the talonavicular cuboid or calcaneocuboid joint at the time of the original injury will lead to coronal (frontal) plane malunion with forefoot inversion or eversion.

With respect to possible treatment, malunions of the Chopart joint have been classified into 5 types (**Table 1**).[20]

Table 1 Five types of malunions of the Chopart joint	
Type	**Pathologic condition**
I	Malunion or joint incongruity
II	Nonunion
III	I/II with arthritis at the calcaneocuboid joint
IV	I/II with arthritis at the talonavicular joint
V	Bilateral arthritis and complex deformity

From Rammelt S, Zwipp H, Schneiders W, et al. Anatomical reconstruction after malunited Chopart joint injuries. Eur J Trauma Emerg Surg 2010;36(3):199; with permission.

Corrective osteotomies or resection of fibrous nonunion with secondary anatomic reconstruction and preservation of the talonavicular and calcaneocuboid joints may be considered in selected, compliant patients with type I or II deformity, good bone stock, and cartilage quality at the time of presentation.[5,20] In the authors' experiences, posttraumatic arthritis evolves rapidly in the talonavicular joint, thus limiting the possibility of joint-sparing reconstruction. In most cases, fusion of the affected joints with axial and rotational realignment at the midtarsal joint will be the only feasible salvage option.[31] Because of the close interaction of the joints of the triple joint complex, fusion should be limited to those with symptomatic arthritis in order to preserve a maximum of residual function.[4,6,20]

CLINICAL RESULTS FROM THE LITERATURE

Few studies report the clinical results after operative treatment of Chopart fractures and dislocations. The overall results range from moderate to good with American Orthopaedic Foot & Ankle Society (AOFAS) midfoot scores between 67 and 78.[4,18,26,32–34] There is consensus that early anatomic reduction and stable internal fixation is the single most important prognostic factor in the treatment of Chopart joint injuries.[4,12,19,24,26,30,32–36] Closed reduction, delayed or inadequate fixation, and the presence of concomitant fractures of the lower leg or foot especially with severe soft tissue damage, such as crush injuries, are negative prognostic factors.[2–4,18,26]

There are only anecdotal reports on primary or early fusion of the talonavicular or calcaneocuboid joint for severe initial cartilage destruction.[37,38] Temporary bridge plating has been proposed in severe midfoot injuries but no results were reported.[28,29] Main and Jowett[2] strongly discouraged any early arthrodesis at the Chopart joint but advocated fixation of highly unstable navicular fragments to the stable cuneiforms.

The reported rates of posttraumatic arthritis in the few available studies on open reduction and internal fixation of Chopart fracture-dislocations vary considerably between zero and 95%.[3,4,18] However, radiographic evidence of posttraumatic arthritis does not always correlate with the clinical symptoms and, therefore, the need for a secondary fusion of the talonavicular and/or calcaneocuboid joint. A study using pedobarography after operative treatment of Chopart and Lisfranc fracture dislocations revealed that malunion resulting in shortening of either the medial or lateral foot column had a more severe impact on gait function than the presence of posttraumatic arthritis.[39] The authors are not aware of reported rates of late fusions at the Chopart joint.

In general, posttraumatic fusions at the talonavicular and calcaneocuboid joints are not very well tolerated due to the important role in overall foot function.[40] This is in accordance with the authors' experiences when treating Chopart joint injuries in which patients treated with a primary fusion had significantly worse results than those treated with open reduction internal fixation (Rammelt et al, 2015, unpublished data). It must be remembered, however, that only patients with severe crush injuries and cartilage damage were treated with a primary fusion.

SUMMARY

Fractures and dislocations of the Chopart joints are relatively rare injuries resulting mostly from high-energy trauma. The patients present with a great variety of symptoms ranging from subtle clinical signs, such as a plantar ecchymosis in mostly ligamentous injuries, to complex fracture dislocations with severe soft tissue damage after crush injuries. Careful clinical examination and exact radiographic projections should lead to the correct diagnosis. A high amount of suspicion is required in multiple injuries and polytraumatized patients who make up a considerable part of the patient cohort with midtarsal joint injuries. Urgent reduction of gross dislocations is mandatory to alleviate the strain on the soft tissues and avoid further complications. Open soft tissue injuries require proper debridement and early, stable, soft tissue coverage. CT scanning should be used generously to reveal the true extent of the bony injury and allow for preoperative planning.

The type of internal fixation depends on the individual fracture pattern, including K-wires, resorbable pins, screws, and plates. A wide array of anatomically shaped, interlocking plates is available for the talus, navicular, cuboid, and anterior process of the calcaneus. In cases of severe soft tissue trauma, internal fixation is supplemented by tibiometatarsal external fixation until soft tissue consolidation. With gross instability at the Chopart joint, temporary joint transfixation with K-wires or bridging plates are used to ensure proper ligamentous healing. Primary fusion of the talonavicular or calcaneocuboid joint is restricted to exceptional cases of near-complete loss of cartilage and should be limited to the affected joint.

Several studies have shown that the best predictor for acceptable results after Chopart joint injuries is primary anatomic reduction and adequate internal fixation,[4,18,26,30,34,35] whereas closed reduction and cast immobilization often yields unacceptable results with frequent redislocations and painful malunions.[2,3,5,19,20] In cases of painful malunions, corrective arthrodesis provides significant relief of pain and functional rehabilitation.[31] In selected active and compliant patients with good bone and cartilage quality, a joint-preserving osteotomy may be performed.[5,20]

REFERENCES

1. Wolf JH. Francois Chopart (1743-1795) – inventor of the partial foot amputation at the transtarsal articulation. Operat Orthop Traumatol 2000;4:314–7.
2. Main BJ, Jowett RL. Injuries of the midtarsal joint. J Bone Joint Surg Br 1975;57: 89–97.
3. Kotter A, Wieberneit J, Braun W, et al. The Chopart dislocation. A frequently underestimated injury and its sequelae. A clinical study. Unfallchirurg 1997; 100:737–41 [in German].
4. Rammelt S, Grass R, Schikore H, et al. Injuries of the Chopart joint. Unfallchirurg 2002;105:371–83 [in German].
5. Schneiders W, Rammelt S. Joint-sparing corrections of malunited Chopart joint injuries. Foot Ankle Clin 2016;21:147–60.
6. Astion DJ, Deland JT, Otis JC, et al. Motion of the hindfoot after simulated arthrodesis. J Bone Joint Surg Am 1997;79:241–6.
7. Wülker N, Stukenborg C, Savory KM, et al. Hindfoot motion after isolated and combined arthrodeses: measurements in anatomic specimens. Foot Ankle Int 2000;21:921–7.
8. Manter JT. Movements of the subtalar and transverse tarsal joints. Anat Rec 1941; 80:397–410.
9. Richter M, Wippermann B, Thermann H, et al. Plantar impact causing midfoot fractures result in higher forces in Chopart's joint than in the ankle joint. J Orthop Res 2002;20:222–32.
10. Rammelt S, Grass R, Zwipp H. Nutcracker fractures of the navicular and cuboid. Ther Umsch 2004;61:451–7.
11. Schmitt JW, Werner CM, Ossendorf C, et al. Avulsion fracture of the dorsal talonavicular ligament: a subtle radiographic sign of possible Chopart joint dislocation. Foot Ankle Int 2011 Jul;32(7):722–6.

12. Dhillon MS, Nagi ON. Total dislocations of the navicular: are they ever isolated injuries? J Bone Joint Surg Br 1999;81:881–5.
13. Hermel MB, Gershon-Cohen J. The nutcracker fracture of the cuboid by indirect violence. Radiology 1953;60:850–4.
14. Dewar FP, Evans DC. Occult fracture-subluxation of the midtarsal joint. J Bone Joint Surg Br 1968;50:386–8.
15. Rammelt S. Chopart and Lisfranc joint injuries. In: Bentley G, editor. European surgical orthopaedics and traumatology. The EFORT textbook. Berlin: Springer; 2014. p. 3835–57.
16. Wei CJ, Tsai WC, Tiu CM, et al. Systematic analysis of missed extremity fractures in emergency radiology. Acta Radiol 2006;47:710–7.
17. Zwipp H. Chirurgie des Fusses. Wien (Austria): Springer-Verlag; 1994.
18. Richter M, Thermann H, Huefner T, et al. Chopart joint fracture-dislocation: initial open reduction provides better outcome than closed reduction. Foot Ankle Int 2004;25:340–8.
19. Swords MP, Schramski M, Switzer K, et al. Chopart fractures and dislocations. Foot Ankle Clin 2008;13(4):679–93.
20. Rammelt S, Zwipp H, Schneiders W, et al. Anatomical reconstruction after malunited Chopart joint injuries. Eur J Trauma Emerg Surg 2010;36(3):196–205.
21. Manoli A 2nd. Compartment syndromes of the foot: current concepts. Foot Ankle 1990;10:340–4.
22. Sands AK, Rammelt S, Manoli A. Foot compartment syndrome – a clinical review. FussSprungg 2015;13(1):11–21.
23. Brenner P, Rammelt S, Gavlik JM, et al. Early soft tissue coverage after complex foot trauma. World J Surg 2001;25:603–9.
24. Cronier P, Frin JM, Steiger V, et al. Internal fixation of complex fractures of the tarsal navicular with locking plates. A report of 10 cases. Orthop Traumatol Surg Res 2013;99S:S241–9.
25. Bayley E, Duncan N, Taylor A. The use of locking plates in complex midfoot fractures. Ann R Coll Surg Engl 2012;94:593–6.
26. Evans J, Beingessner DM, Agel J, et al. Minifragment plate fixation of high-energy navicular body fractures. Foot Ankle Int 2011;32:485–92.
27. Sanders RW, Rammelt S. Fractures of the calcaneus. In: Coughlin MJ, Saltzman CR, Anderson JB, editors. Mann's surgery of the foot & ankle. 9th edition. Philadelphia: Elsevier Saunders; 2013. p. 2041–100.
28. Schildhauer TA, Nork SE, Sangeorzan BJ. Temporary bridge plating of the medial column in severe midfoot injuries. J Orthop Trauma 2003;17:513–20.
29. Apostle KL, Younger AS. Technique tip: open reduction internal fixation of comminuted fractures of the navicular with bridge plating to the medial and middle cuneiforms. Foot Ankle Int 2008;29(7):739–41.
30. Sangeorzan BJ, Benirschke SK, Mosca VEA. Displaced intraarticular fractures of the tarsal navicular. J Bone Joint Surg Am 1989;71:1504–10.
31. Rammelt S, Marti RK, Zwipp H. Arthrodesis of the talonavicular joint. Orthopäde 2006;35:428–34 [in German].
32. Holbein O, Bauer G, Kinzl L. Die dislozierte Kuboidfraktur. Klinik und Therapie einer seltenen Fußverletzung. Unfallchirurg 1998;101:214–21.
33. Weber M, Locher S. Reconstruction of the cuboid in compression fractures: short to midterm results in 12 patients. Foot Ankle Int 2002;23:1008–13.
34. van Dorp KB, de Vries MR, van der Elst M, et al. Chopart joint injury: a study of outcome and morbidity. J Foot Ankle Surg 2010;49:541–5.

35. Sangeorzan BJ, Swiontkowski MF. Displaced fractures of the cuboid. J Bone Joint Surg Br 1990;72:376–8.
36. Schmid T, Krause F, Gebel P, et al. Operative treatment of acute fractures of the tarsal navicular body: midterm results with a new classification. Foot Ankle Int 2016;37(5):501–7.
37. Johnstone AJ, Maffulli N. Primary fusion of the talonavicular joint after fracture dislocation of the navicular bone. J Trauma 1998;45(6):1100–2.
38. Kang GC, Rikhraj IS. Salvage arthrodesis for fracture-dislocation of the cuneonavicular and calcaneocuboid joints: a case report. J Orthop Surg (Hong Kong) 2008;16(3):396–9.
39. Mittlmeier T, Krowiorsch R, Brosinger S, et al. Gait function after fracture-dislocation of the midtarsal and/or tarsometatarsal joints. Clin Biomech (Bristol, Avon) 1997;12(3):S16–7.
40. Pinney SJ, Sangeorzan BJ. Fractures of the tarsal bones. Orthop Clin North Am 2001;32(1):21–33.

Treatment of Peripheral Talus Fractures

John R. Shank, MD[a],*, Stephen K. Benirschke, MD[b], Michael P. Swords, DO[c]

KEYWORDS

- Lateral process • Posteromedial talar body • Talar head

KEY POINTS

- Peripheral talus fractures are rare injuries, and careful clinical and radiographic evaluation can lead to prompt diagnosis.
- An attempt at open reduction internal fixation can potentially improve outcome and delay arthrosis.
- Conservative treatment or excision should be reserved for smaller avulsion fractures or severely comminuted fractures that are not amendable to open reduction internal fixation.
- Timely diagnosis and rigid open reduction internal fixation can lead to better results when compared with nonoperative treatment.

INTRODUCTION

Peripheral talus fractures represent a spectrum of injuries, including lateral process talus fractures, posteromedial talar body fractures, and talar head fractures. These injuries are rare and are poorly described in the literature. Initial presentation is often confused with ankle sprains, as initial radiographs may not indicate a fracture.[1–3] Injuries to the peripheral talus can present in an isolated fashion or in combination with talar neck and body fractures and often involve significant portions of articular cartilage.

The optimal treatment of these injuries remains controversial. There is literature to support open reduction internal fixation of peripheral talus fractures, fracture excision, and conservative treatment of minimally displaced fractures.[2,4] Concern exists regarding fracture excision leading to hindfoot instability and altered biomechanics.[5,6]

The authors have nothing to disclose.
^a Colorado Center of Orthopaedic Excellence, 2446 Research Parkway, #200, Colorado Springs, CO 80920, USA; ^b Department of Orthopaedics and Sports Medicine, University of Washington, Box 359798, Seattle, WA 98195-9798, USA; ^c Orthopedic Trauma, Orthopedic Surgery, Michigan Orthopedic Center, Sparrow Hospital, 2815 South Pennsylvania Avenue, #204, Lansing, MI 48190, USA
* Corresponding author.
E-mail address: johnrshank@yahoo.com

Foot Ankle Clin N Am 22 (2017) 181–192
http://dx.doi.org/10.1016/j.fcl.2016.09.012
foot.theclinics.com

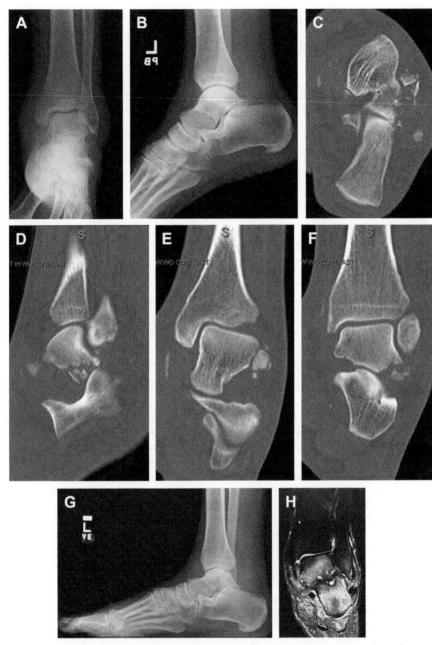

Fig. 1. Patient 1. (A) Injury anteroposterior (AP) radiograph demonstrating lateral process talus fracture. (B) Injury lateral radiograph demonstrating incongruity of the lateral process. (C) Injury axial, (D) sagittal, and coronal (E, F) CT scans. Surgical excision of the lateral process was performed with development of rapid arthrosis of the subtalar joint. The patient was referred with complaints of increasing subtalar pain and stiffness. (G) Weight-bearing lateral radiograph and (H, I) MRI at 6 months postinjury demonstrates severe arthritic changes.

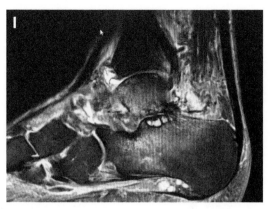

Fig. 1. (*continued*).

There is a similar concern with conservative treatment leading to nonunion and arthrosis. Few long-term studies exist detailing the outcome of peripheral talus injuries. Misdiagnosed and untreated injuries can cause significant pain and functional impairment.[3]

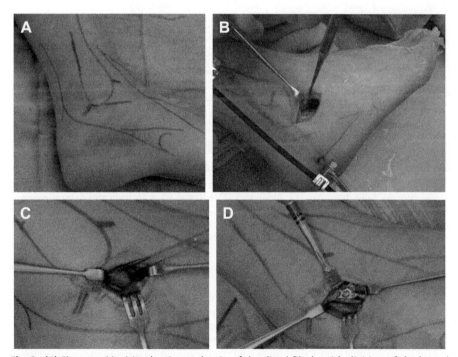

Fig. 2. (*A*) Sinus tarsi incision begins at the tip of the distal fibula with division of the lateral ligamentous complex. (*B*) Intraoperatively placed external fixator placed between the fibula and calcaneus allows for distraction and visualization of the subtalar joint. (*C*) K-wire fixation of the articular surface performed with direct visualization of the articular reduction. (*D*) Plate and screw fixation is used for final fixation.

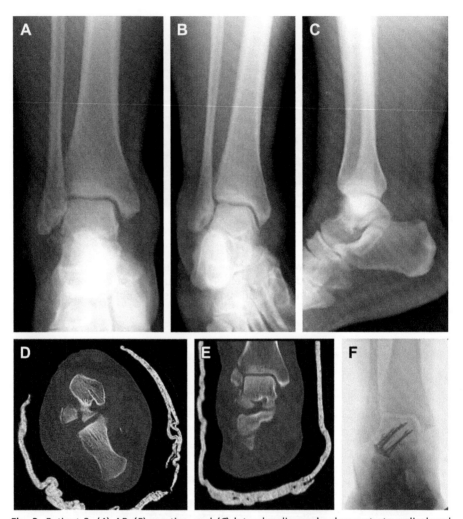

Fig. 3. Patient 2. (A) AP, (B) mortise, and (C) lateral radiographs demonstrate a displaced lateral process talus fracture. (D) Axial and (E) coronal CT scan indicates lateral process displacement. Intraoperative (F) AP, (G) mortise, and (H) lateral fluoroscopy with K-wire, plate and screw fixation of the lateral process. Follow-up (I) AP, (J) mortise, and (K) lateral radiographs indicating anatomic reduction of the lateral process fracture, lateral gutter, and subtalar joint.

Precise identification of peripheral talus fractures is critical. The most common reason these injuries are treated nonoperatively is failure to properly diagnose the fracture, with many injuries missed on initial presentation.[2] A thorough clinical and radiographic evaluation must be used in detecting these fractures, as treatment of missed injuries is associated with a high morbidity. There should be a high index of suspicion of peripheral talus fractures with subtalar dislocations. All subtalar dislocations should be reduced with a postreduction computed tomography (CT) scan obtained.[7]

Judicious use of CT scan is important in defining fracture displacement, comminution, and to assess for intra-articular debris. The advantages of open reduction internal

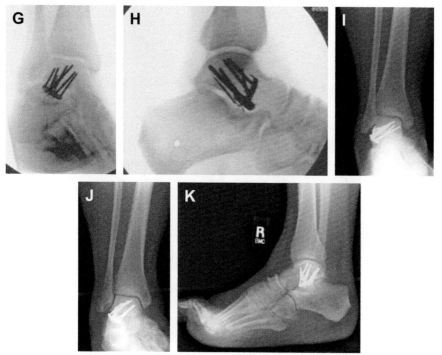

Fig. 3. (*continued*).

fixation include earlier time to fracture union, a lower rate of nonunion, and ability to perform earlier range of motion. Arthrosis can be delayed by debridement of impinging osseous and chondral debris and through precise restoration of articular anatomy. Worse functional outcomes can be seen in association with posttraumatic arthritis and osteonecrosis that progresses to collapse.[8] Late reconstruction, including salvage osteotomy and arthrodesis, can be simplified with initial operative treatment of the peripheral talus. We use multiple patient examples to detail the treatment of peripheral talus fractures.

INDICATIONS

There is controversy in the literature regarding the ideal treatment of peripheral talus injuries and which of these treatments leads to the best long-term outcome. Smaller avulsion-type injuries involving the lateral process, posteromedial talar body, medial tubercle, and talar head can be treated conservatively or excised late if painful. There are data to support improved outcomes with early excision of larger avulsion fractures of the medial tubercle of the posterior process of the talus.[9] Most peripheral talus fractures involve sizable articular components with displacement of the ankle, subtalar, and talonavicular joints. These injuries should be treated with open reduction internal fixation to anatomically restore the articular surfaces of the talus. An attempt to treat severely comminuted injuries with open reduction internal fixation should be performed, as excision of major articular fragments can lead to rapid arthrosis and joint instability. This is demonstrated by patient 1 (whose imaging is

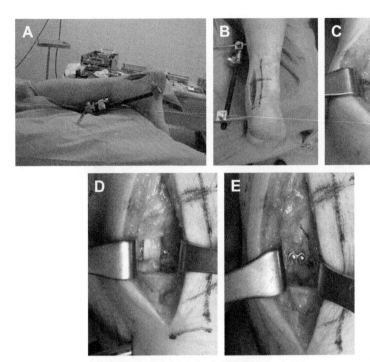

Fig. 4. (*A*) A Prone position is used with (*B*) placement of an intraoperative external fixator with distractor to visualize the (*C*) fracture including both the ankle and subtalar joints. (*D*) Release and retraction of the FHL allows improved visualization of the posteromedial talus (*E*).

shown in **Fig. 1**) Excision or primary arthrodesis should be used as a last-resort primary treatment option.

SURGICAL TECHNIQUE
Preoperative Planning

CT imaging should be critically reviewed in deciding which approach to use. A sinus tarsi incision for the lateral process and posteromedial approach for the posteromedial talar body is used, respectively. The talar head is accessed from a medial utility incision or from the distal extension of the anteromedial approach to the talar neck. An anterolateral approach to the talar head can be used concomitantly.

The anterolateral approach to the talus allows full access to the lateral process of the talus if a more extended approach is needed to treat a talar neck fracture with a lateral process component. A combination of approaches can be used with more complex fractures. A staged approach for a complex talus injury is commonly used for injuries involving the talar neck and posteromedial talar body secondary to prone positioning for the posteromedial talar body.

Equipment

- Tourniquet
- Headlight
- Pointed reduction clamps
- Dental pick

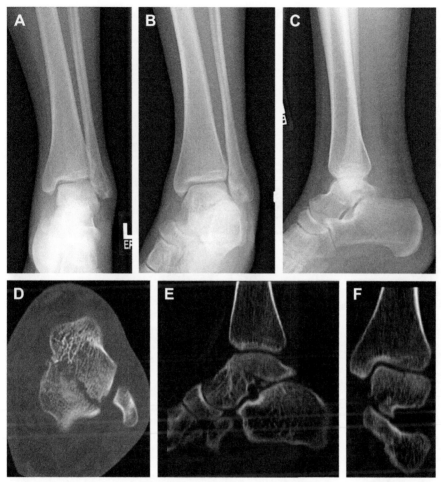

Fig. 5. Patient 3. Injury (*A*) AP, (*B*) mortise, and (*C*) lateral radiographs appear relatively normal with the lateral radiograph demonstrating incongruity of the posteromedial talar body and subtalar joint. (*D*) Axial, (*E*) sagittal, and (*F*) coronal CT scans indicate posteromedial talar body displacement. (*G*) Intraoperative fluoroscopy with K-wire reduction and assessment of the reduction with a freer elevator. (*H*) The plate is slid over and around the K-wires and screw fixation is completed. Final postoperative (*I*) AP, (*J*) mortise, (*K*) lateral, and (*L*) oblique radiographs demonstrate an anatomically reduced ankle and subtalar joint.

- Freer elevator
- Schanz pins (2.5 mm to 4.0 mm)
- External fixator or femoral distractor
- Kirschner (K)-wires

SURGICAL APPROACHES
Sinus Tarsi

Lateral process talus fractures are approached through a sinus tarsi incision (**Fig. 2**). The peroneal tendons, lateral branch of the superficial peroneal nerve, and the sural nerve should be carefully protected throughout the approach. Incision of the lateral

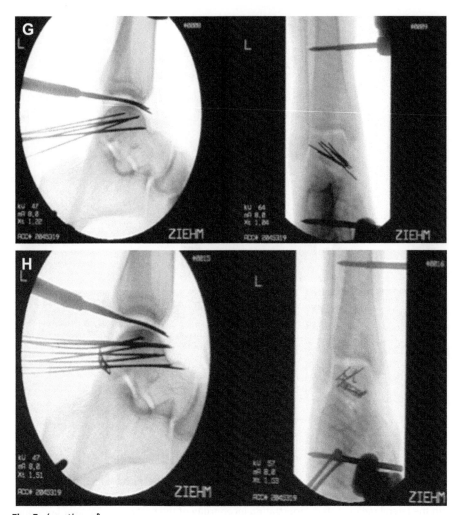

Fig. 5. (*continued*).

joint capsule, including the anterior talofibular ligament, allows for excellent visualization of the lateral process. The lateral ligamentous complex should be carefully repaired at the end of the operative procedure.

An intraoperatively placed external fixator, placed from the fibula to the calcaneus, when distracted, can allow for improved visualization of the articular surface and for improved ability to debride osseous and chondral debris (see **Fig. 2**). If a more extensile approach is needed for combination injuries that include the talar neck, an anterolateral approach to the talar neck allows for excellent visualization of the lateral process.

Provisional reduction should be performed with K-wires with final implants placed over the K-wires. Modular plates should be used with screw fixation. Lag screw fixation can be used for simple oblique fractures; however, buttress plating should be used for more comminuted injuries. K-wires can be kept in place to provide stability of smaller articular fragments. These techniques are demonstrated by patient 2 (whose imaging is shown in **Fig. 3**). Locking implants can be used for more complex injuries.

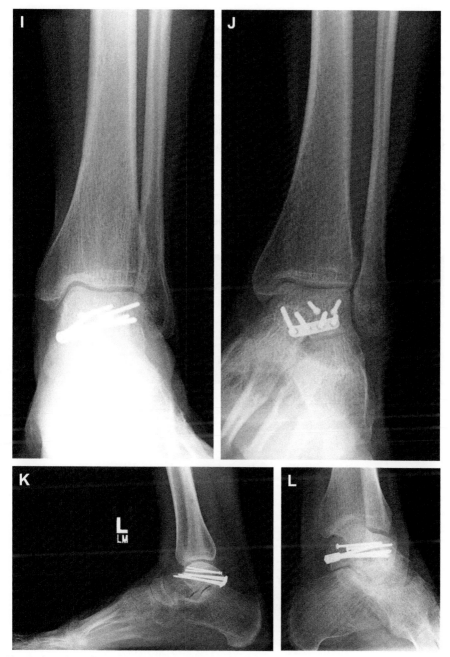

Fig. 5. (*continued*).

Posteromedial

The posteromedial talar body is approached in a prone position (**Fig. 4**A), often with a bump placed beneath the contralateral hip. The knee is flexed to allow for improved fluoroscopic imaging. An intraoperatively placed external fixator or femoral distractor is placed to improve visualization of the ankle and subtalar joints (**Fig. 4**B, C). The posteromedial approach uses the interval between the Achilles tendon and the flexor hallucis longus (FHL). The retinaculum covering the FHL is released to allow improved visualization of the posterior talus (**Fig. 4**D). Retraction of the FHL protects the posterior neurovascular bundle and dissection of the neurovascular bundle should be avoided (**Fig. 4**E).

Provisional reduction should be performed with K-wires with final implants often placed over the K-wires. Modular plates should be used with screws placed through the plate. Separate lag screws can be used if necessary. These techniques are demonstrated by patient 3 (whose imaging is shown in **Fig. 5**). Locking implants can be used for more comminuted injuries.

Talar Head

Talar head injuries can be approached through the distal extension of the anteromedial and anterolateral approach to the talar neck. Direct visualization of the talar head

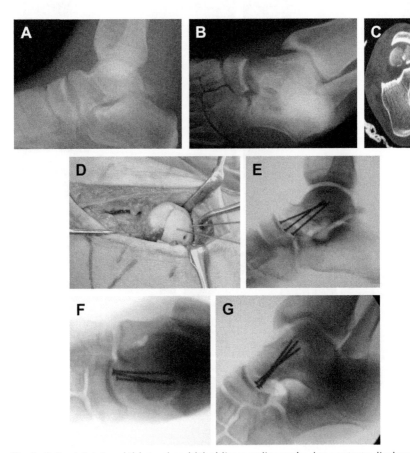

Fig. 6. Patient 4. Injury (*A*) lateral and (*B*) oblique radiographs demonstrate displacement of the talar head. (*C*) Axial CT demonstrates displacement of the articular surface of the talonavicular joint. (*D*) Intraoperative photo with retraction of the navicular to allow access to the talar head. (*E*) Intraoperative fluoroscopic lateral and (*F, G*) oblique imaging demonstrates reduction of the talar head.

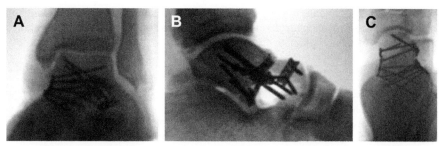

Fig. 7. Patient 5. Postoperative (*A*) mortise, (*B*) lateral, and (*C*) AP foot radiographs on a patient with an injury involving components of the talar neck, lateral process, and talar head.

is easier to achieve through a medial approach. The navicular body is retracted with a bone hook to fully visualize the extent of the articular injury and to allow for open reduction internal fixation of the articular surface. Implants should be buried beneath the articular surface to prevent impingement within the talonavicular joint. These techniques are demonstrated by patient 4 (whose imaging is shown in **Fig. 6**).

COMBINED INJURIES

Injuries that involve multiple components of the talar neck and body and peripheral talus can be treated with dual anteromedial and anterolateral approaches or a combination of anterior and posterior approaches in a staged fashion. These techniques are demonstrated by patient 5 (whose imaging is shown in **Fig. 7**).

POSTOPERATIVE CARE

It is critical to obtain and maintain reduction of the peripheral talus. Early range of motion is critical to long-term outcome. Immediate splint immobilization is performed with conversion to a cast, if needed, to prevent plantarflexion and an eventual equinus deformity. Range of motion should begin as soon as possible, with emphasis on both the ankle and the subtalar joints. Weight bearing is allowed when radiographic union is achieved, generally at 8 to 12 weeks postoperatively, dependent on the degree of comminution and severity of the injury. Long-term follow-up should be performed to assess for arthritic change, avascular necrosis, and collapse of the ankle, subtalar, and talonavicular joints. Complications from these injuries can result in eventual need for ankle, subtalar, or talonavicular arthrodesis.

SUMMARY

Peripheral talus fractures are rare injuries. Careful clinical and radiographic evaluation can lead to prompt diagnosis. An attempt at open reduction internal fixation can potentially improve outcome and delay arthrosis. Conservative treatment or excision should be reserved for smaller avulsion fractures or severely comminuted fractures that are not amenable to open reduction internal fixation. Timely diagnosis and rigid open reduction internal fixation can lead to better results when compared with nonoperative treatment. Obtaining and maintaining a reduction can slow the arthritic process and prevent or delay the need for arthrodesis.

There is a high morbidity with peripheral talus fractures that are treated nonoperatively or that remain undiagnosed. Excision can lead to joint instability and rapid arthrosis. Open reduction internal fixation should be considered for injuries with joint involvement to anatomically restore the articular surfaces of the talus. Open reduction can lead to quicker revascularization of the talus and potentially lead to lower rates of avascular necrosis and collapse.

REFERENCES

1. Langer P, DiGiovanni C. Incidence and pattern types of fractures of the lateral process of the talus. Am J Orthop 2008;37:257–8.
2. Sariali E, Lelievre JF, Catonne Y. Fractures of the lateral process of the talus. Retrospective study of 44 cases. Rev Chir Orthop Reparatrice Appar Mot 2008;94:e1–7.
3. Berkowitz MJ, Kim DH. Process and tubercle fractures of the hindfoot. J Am Acad Orthop Surg 2005;13:492–502.
4. Valderrabano V, Perren T, Ryf C, et al. Snowboarder's talus fracture: treatment outcome of 20 cases after 3.5 years. Am J Sports Med 2005;33:871–80.
5. Sands A, White C, Blankstein M, et al. Assessment of ankle and hindfoot stability and joint pressures using a human cadaveric model of a large lateral talar process excision: a biomechanical study. Medicine (Baltimore) 2015;94(14):e606.
6. Langer P, Nikisch F, Spenciner D, et al. In vitro evaluation of the effect lateral process talar excision on ankle and subtalar stability. Foot Ankle Int 2007;28:78–83.
7. Rammelt S, Goronzy J. Subtalar dislocations. Foot Ankle Clin 2015;20:253–64.
8. Valier HA, Nork SE, Benirschke SK, et al. Surgical treatment of talar body fractures. J Bone Joint Surg Am 2003;32:773–7.
9. Kim DH, Berkowitz MJ, Pressman DN. Avulsion fractures of the medial tubercle of the posterior process of the talus. Foot Ankle Int 2003;24:172–5.

Complex Foot Injury
Early and Definite Management

Tim Schepers, MD, PhD[a],*, Stefan Rammelt, MD, PhD[b]

KEYWORDS

- Complex foot • Reconstruction • Amputation • Outcome

KEY POINTS

- Complex foot occur infrequently, but are life-changing events; treatment is difficult and, if the necessary facilities are not available, referral should be considered.
- The first step in severe trauma should be the trauma screening and resuscitation according to the ABCDE principle following the Advanced Trauma Life Support system.
- The initial treatment of a complex foot injury consists of preventing progression of ischemia/necrosis, prevention of infection, and considering salvage or amputation.
- Definitive treatment (salvage) consists of anatomic reconstruction with stable internal fixation and early soft tissue coverage followed by aggressive rehabilitation and adequate orthopedic shoe modifications.
- Overall, the prognosis is hard to predict and determined by the severity of injury, comorbidities, complications, secondary interventions, and individual demands.

INTRODUCTION

In the fracture epidemiology study by Court-Brown and Caesar,[1] the percentage of fractures involving the foot was approximately 12% out of a total of approximately 6000 patients in 1 year, of which metatarsal and toe fractures accounted for 85%. In an additional analysis on open fractures, the portion of open foot fractures was 10.5% of all open fractures out of almost 2400 open fractures in 15 years.[2] A crude calculation using both studies would show that looking only at the foot injuries (excluding toe fractures) about 1% of all foot injuries is an open fracture, making it a rare injury. In war time, up to 12% to 22% of injuries are foot related.[3,4] A complex trauma to the foot is associated with polytrauma or multiple injury in 22% to 50% of cases, making the management of these injuries an even greater challenge.[5–8]

The authors have nothing to disclose.
[a] Trauma Unit, Academic Medical Center, University of Amsterdam, Meibergdreef 9, PO Box 22660, Amsterdam 1100 DD, The Netherlands; [b] University Center for Orthopaedics and Traumatology, University Hospital Carl-Gustav Carus, Fetscherstrasse 74, Dresden 01307, Germany
* Corresponding author.
E-mail address: t.schepers@amc.nl

An increase in more severe foot ankle trauma has been reported in several studies.[9–11] They occur not only as combat-related injuries, but also in daily life. One theory is that, for example, in car accidents the passenger's upper body is protected well, but the area of the lower leg is less well-protected.[10,12] A second theory relates to the advancing age and a more active elderly population.[13]

Severe injuries of the foot are a life-changing event.[11,14,15] They often lead to some form of disability, and are therefore a real challenge to manage. Injuries of the extremity, and especially of the foot and ankle, are distinct predictors of poor outcome in polytrauma patients.[16–24] Injuries to the foot should, therefore, receive similar attention and treatment as do long bone injuries.[25]

In complex foot trauma, there is a gray area between injuries that are and are not able to be reconstructed. In this article, we present guidance and tools to aid in the treatment and decision making, which, owing to its infrequent occurrence, can be a difficult process at times.

TERMINOLOGY, DEFINITIONS, AND CLASSIFICATION

Complex injuries of the foot are those injuries that occur infrequently, have a major impact on the quality of life, frequently lead to disability, are accompanied by high complication rates, require special expertise, and should therefore be treated in a dedicated level 1 trauma center.[5,26,27] They are often a combination of both bony and soft tissue damage.

Complex injuries of the foot (and ankle) are also called mangled or smashed extremity injuries, or high-energy lower extremity trauma. In an epidemiologic study on open fractures by Court-Brown and colleagues,[2] the most common trauma mechanisms were crush injuries, falls from a height, and motor vehicle accidents. Crush injuries are the result of a body part being forcefully compressed between 2 hard surfaces. Compression of the muscle mass blocks the flow of blood and oxygen to tissues (ischemia), resulting in tissue death (necrosis) within a few hours. A particular entity are combat-related and mine blast injuries ("pied du mine") resulting from explosives.[28–31]

Damage to the soft tissue is often classified by the Tscherne–Oestern classification of closed skin injuries (**Table 1**).[32] It ranges from minimal soft tissue damage to extensive contusion or crush. It is invariably correlated with the energy of the trauma, and therefore also with the severity of the fracture, if present. Closed fractures with skin at risk owing to bone or joint dislocation should be included in this group as well.

Even though Tscherne also proposed a classification for open injuries, the most frequently used classification for open fractures is that by Gustilo and Anderson

Table 1 Tscherne classification of closed fractures	
Grade 0	No or minor soft tissue damage. Indirect injury with simple fracture.
Grade 1	Superficial abrasion or skin contusion. Medium severity fracture pattern.
Grade 2	Deep (contaminated) abrasion with skin or muscle contusion. Severe fracture pattern by direct trauma.
Grade 3	Extensive skin contusion, crush injury with severe damage to underlying muscle. Compartment syndrome, Morel-Lavallee, and/or vascular injury. Complex fracture patterns.

Table 2
Gustilo classification of open fractures

Grade 1	Clean wound (<1 cm). Minimal soft tissue damage. Simple fracture pattern.
Grade 2	Soft tissue damage moderate, no tissue loss, wound >1 cm. Simple fracture pattern.
Grade 3	A. Extensive soft tissue damage, adequate coverage of bone. B. Extensive soft tissue injury, soft tissue loss, bone exposed, periosteal stripping. Wound contamination. C. Open fracture with arterial damage.

(Table 2).[33,34] It classifies open injuries according to the size of the wound and neurovascular involvement. Complication rates are associated strongly with the grade of open injury with complication infectious complication rates of greater than 40% in grade 3 open injuries.[34] Because the interobserver agreement is low for the Gustilo classification, the injury should not be graded in the emergency department, but in the operating room after debridement.[35]

Zwipp and associates[8,27] proposed a scoring system for foot and ankle injuries to define a complex injury **(Fig. 1)**. The foot and ankle are divided into 5 major areas (Lisfranc, Chopart, calcaneus, talus, and ankle/pilon). Each injured area (dislocation or fracture) equals 1 point, to which points are added for the severity of the soft tissue injury according to the Tscherne and Oestern grade in the most affected area. When the sum of the score is 5 points or higher the injury is considered a complex foot trauma. If a hospital is less familiar with a certain injury, it might be deemed a complex injury even at a lower total score and subsequent referral to a trauma center should be considered.

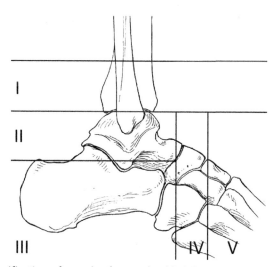

Fig. 1. Zwipp classification of complex foot and ankle injury.

INITIAL TREATMENT

If a patient with a severe injury of the foot presents at the emergency department the following 2 phases can be recognized: (1) initial or early treatment and (2) definite treatment. The initial or immediate treatment of a complex injury of the foot has several goals and can be divided into 3 (overlapping) subphases **(Fig. 2)**: prevention of

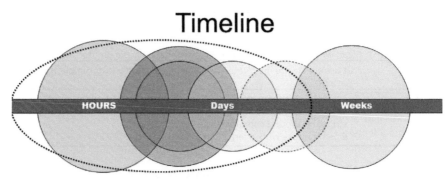

Fig. 2. Timeline of complex foot management. Dotted white field indicates initial treatment.

progression of ischemia and necrosis, prevention of infection, and consideration of salvage or amputation.

Prevent Progression of Ischemia and Necrosis

The first step for every patient with a severe trauma should be the trauma screening and resuscitation according to the ABCDE-principle following the Advanced Trauma Life Support system ("life before limb"; **Fig. 3**). Only gross displacement (at fracture site or dislocation of joints) causing impairment of perfusion can be addressed briefly, ideally at the site of accident. If there are no other life-threatening injuries that need attention first or the patient is stabilized, than the foot injury is assessed and treated.[6]

The second step is diagnostics. Using a physical examination (if possible before intubation), conventional radiographs, and (angio-) computed tomography scans, one should assess vascular injury (palpable pulses, capillary refill, temperature, color, Doppler pulse device), neurologic impairment (sensibility, motoric deficit), soft tissue injury (closed and open), and assess bone and joint injury. Usually at the primary assessment conventional radiographs are sufficient to determine the early treatment (eg, external fixation). During the planning of the definite treatment computed tomography scans are valuable (span–scan–plan principle).

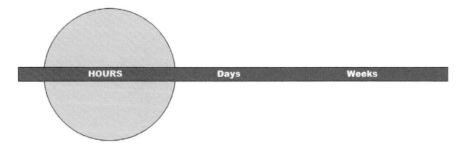

Fig. 3. Phase 1: prevention of progression ischemia/necrosis.

Often in a complex (open) foot injury the strategy chosen is not early total care but damage control orthopedics (limb damage control orthopedics).[36] The individual steps of damage control orthopedics of the foot are as follows:

- Treat the open injury as soon as possible.[37]

- Aggressively debride open wounds using washouts with saline and removal of dead tissue and loose (osseous) fragments.[27,38–42] The use of high-pressure lavage is discouraged.[43]
- Fasciotomy for (impeding) compartment syndrome to prevent ischemia and contractures (**Fig. 4**).[44–49] Early fasciotomy is associated with less morbidity and improved outcomes.[50,51] The sequelae of misdiagnosed or untreated foot compartment syndromes are persistent pain, equinus and cavovarus deformity, clawing of the toes and short foot syndrome.[14,46,48,52–55] The ischemic (dead) tissues can become infected, which has a major impact on future treatment options. The fasciotomy is performed depending on the location of the injury and depending on the subsequent treatment of the injury.[56] A medial approach combined with 2 dorsal approached over the second and forth metatarsals is the workhorse in the release of all 9 compartments of the foot.[49,56] A single incision dorsal (Hannover) approach has been described, as well as an extended single medial approach (Henry approach).[5,57–62] A plantar (Loeffler) approach is not encouraged because it potentially leads to a painful scar. The possibility of a concurrent compartment syndrome of the lower leg and foot through a connection from the deep posterior to the foot with the subsequent need of an extended fasciotomy should be kept in mind.[63]
- Rigid (temporary) fracture fixation using external fixation or Kirschner wires.[64–70] The external frame stabilizes the fracture, allows for frequent inspection and healing of the soft tissues, and prevents the occurrence of equinus deformity.[42] In selected cases with simple fractures and clean wounds, one could decide to perform primary definitive fracture fixation.[71,72] This treatment option should be chosen if both the patient's condition and the local conditions are fit enough to withstand the duration of the procedure and the second hit from surgery. Stabilization of the open fracture is thought to be protective of infection.[37] Many different frame configurations exist (**Fig. 5**), and the type of bone and soft tissue injury are leading in choosing the appropriate frame.[65–67] The tibia is almost always chosen for half-pin placement. Other distal locations are calcaneus (transfixation pin), talus, cuneiform, and the first and fifth metatarsals. The configuration should allow

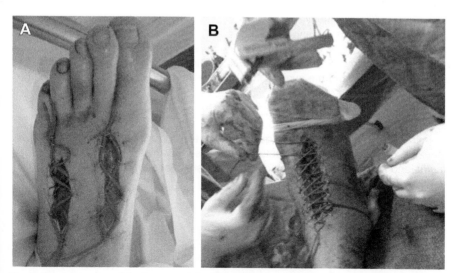

Fig. 4. Two examples of fasciotomy of the foot. (*A*) Classical Manoli approach. (*B*) Hannover approach.

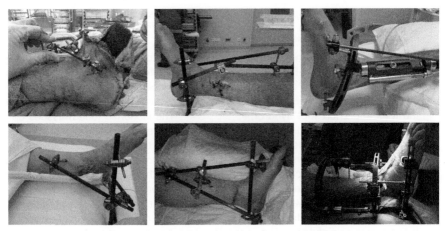

Fig. 5. Various different foot–ankle external fixator configurations.

for wound inspection and dressing (eg, negative pressure wound therapy [NPWT]) changes. Preferably the frame should be on the most injured side, so that the other side is preserved for the definite surgical approach. Attention to pin care should prevent the occurrence of pin track infections.

- Indications for immediate (external) stabilization are as follows[42]:
  - Fracture-(dislocation) with compromised neurovascular structures or skin at risk;
  - Grade 3 open (unstable) fractures;
  - Fracture-(dislocation) with concomitant compartment syndrome; and
  - Gross instability at fracture site or joint.

Although the evidence is not solid, the use of hyperbaric oxygen (HBO) therapy in the treatment of complex foot injuries has been described in several studies.[73,74] Crush injuries are an approved indication for HBO treatment.[74–79] The concept behind the use of HBO in complex trauma is an improved tissue oxygenation (hyperoxygenation), decrease in swelling (vasoconstriction), and preventing the release of toxic oxygen radicals (reperfusion) and its possible aid in the repair of injured tissues (host factors).[74] One randomized trial from 1996 showed improved healing and a reduction in repeat surgery in extensive crush injuries.[73] Therefore, in the presence of ischemia after a crush injury and the availability of a hyperbaric unit, the use of HBO therapy should be considered strongly.

Prevention of Infection

Open fractures should be covered quickly with sterile wound dressings (**Fig. 6**). Fewer than 20% of infections in open fractures are caused by microorganisms present after trauma and more than 90% of infections are hospital-acquired infections.[80–82]

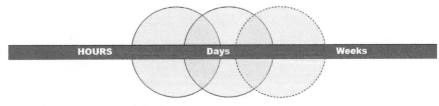

Fig. 6. Phase 2: Prevention of infection.

Digital photographs should be taken to facilitate communication and for patient records.

After the initial washout and debridement, repeated and aggressive debridement and irrigation should be performed as deemed necessary. Depending on the initial contamination and the expectation of ongoing necrosis owing to the force of the trauma (zone of injury),[83] a second (and third if necessary) look should be performed after 24 to 48 hours.[5,27,37,41,52] Traumatized tissue is highly susceptible to infection.[37]

In open fractures, appropriate antibiotics should be started as soon as possible.[41,84,85] A first-generation cephalosporin is usually first choice. Gentamycin might be added in case of gross contamination or grade 3 open fractures.[37] Tetanus prophylaxis should be administered.

When bone defects arise from bone loss or removal owing to infection, necrosis, or gross contamination, gentamycin beads are frequently used.[37,86,87] They release high-dose antibiotics (far higher than serum levels) and maintain therapeutic levels for more than 1 week.[37] However, when used in the treatment of infection, the gentamicin beads act as a biomaterial, which becomes colonized at a high percentage.[88] An alternative solution is the use of polymethylmethacrylate antibiotic-loaded cement spacer (PMMA G/V antibiotic cement).[89–92] The benefit over gentamycin beads is that it fills out the entire cavity, leaving no room for empty voids that can fill with hematoma or debris and might lead to infection. Second, it adds stability to the foot in combination with implants or external fixation (**Fig. 7**). Third, the duration of release is longer than with beads, and can be as long as 8 to 10 weeks.[93,94] Based on the results of cultures from wound swabs, different antibiotics can be added.[93,94] After a chosen period, which depends on the indication of placement, the cement can be removed and

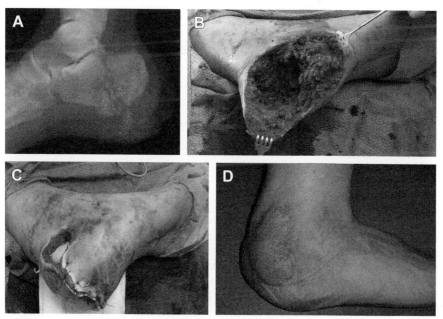

Fig. 7. Use of temporary polymethylmethacrylate antibiotic-loaded (PMMA) cement spacer. (*A*) Radiograph of foot after hail shot to the heel. (*B*) Cavity left after debridement. (*C*) After insertion of vancomycin PMMA spacer. (*D*) Final follow-up with free gracilis flap.

exchanged for tricortical (iliac crest) or cancellous bone graft (eg, from the proximal tibia). Bone grafts may be enhanced with the use of a reamer irrigator aspirator system.[95]

Open wounds in complex foot (and ankle) injuries can be closed temporarily using artificial skin, NPWT (also known as vacuum-assisted closure) or using the antibiotic bead pouch.[96–106] The use of NPWT in open fractures has been investigated more extensively and has shown fewer infectious complications, lesser reoperation rates, and a decrease in hospitalization.[100,103,106,107] In cases in which wounds of open fractures can be closed after the initial debridement, vacuum-assisted closure therapy has been shown to aid in wound healing,[108,109] similar as in high-risk surgical incisions.[110] Combining the concepts of the antibiotic bead pouch and NPWT has been proposed as well, with the fluid-draining effect of the vacuum device on the availability of the antibiotics is still subject to debate.[111,112] For wounds that need soft tissue transfer, early definite flap coverage has been shown to lead to decreased infection rates after complex trauma.[113,114]

Consider Salvage or Amputation

Early in the treatment course, it should be discussed whether the foot is expected to be salvageable or needs to be amputated (**Fig. 8**). The combined rate of primary and secondary amputation is about 15% to 30%, depending on the severity of injury.[5,26,115,116] In case of extreme injury to the limb or when then patient's life is at risk, as in polytraumatized and polymorbid patients, a primary amputation should be performed.[6,27,117,118]

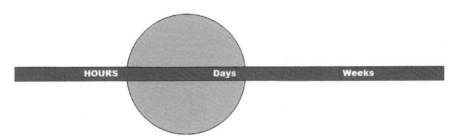

Fig. 8. Phase 3, Consider salvage/amputation.

In cases in which an amputation needs to be performed secondarily, the opinion of the patient should be considered in light of the shared decision making process, if the patients' condition allows for it. It is, however, primarily a decision based on the expertise of the treating physician combined with the results of a multidisciplinary team judgment. This team consists of (but is not limited to) the orthopedic (trauma) surgeon, emergency physician, plastic surgeon, radiologist, pain consultant (anesthesiologist), neurologist, rehabilitation manager, and psychologist.

A recent metaanalysis on severe lower limb trauma showed that reconstruction was psychologically more acceptable to patients compared with an amputation, although outcome scores for both treatment options were comparable.[119] In addition to a primary amputation or a late secondary amputation after failed salvage, regular assessments (early delayed decision) should be performed including the patient's perspective and rehabilitation progress.[120]

Whether or not an amputation is considered is based on patient-related and injury-related factors.[115] In general, an amputation leads to a shorter treatment time, fewer surgical procedures, and a quicker recovery.[121] However, prosthesis costs are greater than reconstruction costs, depending on the patient's age at the time of injury.[122]

Data from the LEAP (Lower Extremity Assessment Project) study showed that severe muscular damage at the lower leg, absence of plantar sensation, venous injury, ischemia, the need for soft tissue coverage, and a high Injury Severity Score are the most important factors leading to amputation.[115] Other factors that should be taken into account are pre-existing peripheral vascular disease and poorly controlled diabetes.[123] Indications for amputation, both primary and secondary, are as follows.[114,124,125]

- Absolute amputation indications
  - Severe polytrauma (previously classified as a score of 3–4 on the polytrauma score by Oestern)[126]
  - Uncontrollable bleeding (Advanced Trauma Life Support system [life before limb])
  - Resources and a lack thereof (war time or less well-equipped hospital)[127]
  - Complete amputation or remaining "skin bridge" only, without the resources for replantation
- Relative amputation indications (**Fig. 9**)
  - Nonreconstructable vascular injury[117]
  - Objectified tibial nerve transection
  - Loss of the talus
  - Loss of the weight-bearing foot sole
  - Crush injury to the forefoot (prolonged ischemia)

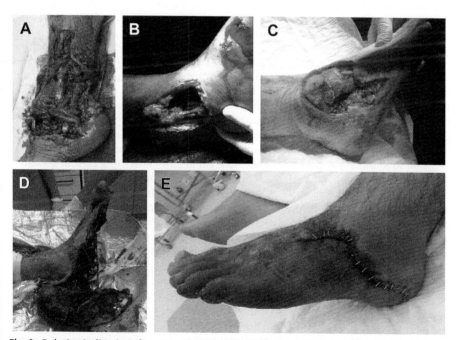

Fig. 9. Relative indications for primary amputation. (*A*) Nonreconstructable (vascular) injury. (*B*) Proven transection of tibial nerve. (*C*) Open talar extrusion with severe cartilage damage. (*D*) Loss of weight-bearing sole of foot. (*E*) Crush injury with ischemia of more than 6 hours.

Box 1
Predictive scores for limb salvage

AIS: Abbreviated Injury Score (A.A.A.M,[154] 1971)

Gustilo classification (Gustilo and Anderson,[33] 1976; Gustilo et al,[34] 1984)

HFS-97: Hannover Fracture Scale-97/98 (Tscherne,[155] 1983)

MESI: Mangled Extremity Syndrome Index (Gregory et al,[156] 1985)

PSI: Predictive Salvage Index (Howe et al,[157] 1987)

MESS: Mangled Extremity Severity Score (Johansen et al,[136] 1990)

LSI: Limb Salvage Index (Russell et al,[158] 1991)

NISSSA: Nerve injury, Ischemia, Soft Tissue Injury, Skeletal Injury, Shock, Age Score (McNamara et al,[159] 1994)

FASS: Foot and Ankle Severity Scale (Manoli et al,[160] 1997)

The Ganga Hospital Injury Severity Score (Rajasekaran,[161] 2005)

List of available limb salvage prediction scores. See text for references.

Over time, many investigators have tried to compute the need for an amputation and successfully predict limb salvage (**Box 1**).[127–137] These limb salvage scores were designed to decrease subjectivity and provide guidance in the difficult process of complex foot injury management. Ideally, a trauma limb salvage system would be 100% specific (all salvaged limbs have scores below the threshold) and 100% sensitive (all amputated limbs have scores at or above the threshold). In daily practice as reflected in the literature on several scoring systems, the specificity is mostly greater than 95%, but sensitivity lies at less than 60% to 70%.[128–137]

Results of the LEAP study showed the inability of scoring systems to predict the need for amputation accurately, although low scores may predict salvage.[130] An initial absence of plantar sensation was a poor predictor, because in one-half of the cases sensation returned.[131] Psychological and social factors proved more important than scoring systems in predicting outcome.[138] Future research should focus on the first postoperative phase, to prevent morbidity from prolonged salvage attempts, late amputations, salvaged limbs without sensation, and functional failures.[123,128]

Scoring systems are of limited use and should not be the sole criterion on which the decision to amputate is based.[139] They may aid in strengthening a clinical decision. One should keep in mind that predicting salvage or amputation is a prediction of neither outcome nor function.[114,132] Although the LEAP study, dealing with all severe lower extremity injuries, revealed no differences in outcome after salvage versus amputation, studies that focused on isolated severe foot injuries ("mangled foot and ankle") showed significantly inferior functional results after foot salvage in both civilian and military cohorts.[29,31,140] All of these studies showed higher rates of complications and revision surgeries as well as prolonged hospitalization and rehabilitation in the salvage groups.[141,142]

DEFINITE TREATMENT

After the initial management and patient counseling, the definite treatment is undertaken. The different strategies are amputation and salvage (**Fig. 10**). Salvage includes anatomic reconstruction of the axial alignment and functional columns of the foot,

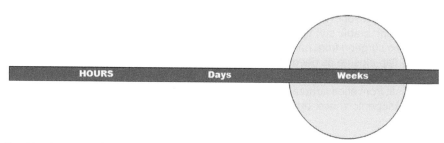

Fig. 10. Phase 4: Definite management.

early stable soft tissue coverage, and primary arthrodesis in cases of severe cartilage injury or gross instability. The timing of definitive treatment depends on the condition of the patient and the soft tissues. A recent prospective study demonstrated that multiply injured patients subjected to secondary definitive surgery between days 2 and 4 had a significantly ($P<.0001$) increased inflammatory response compared with that in patients operated on between days 6 and 8.[143]

Amputation

If primary amputation is warranted, it should be performed at the lowest, most distal level possible.[141,142] In case of high-energy trauma, it is rarely wise to create a definite stump early in the process. Skin and muscle necrosis might develop for several more days, and recurrent debridement is frequently necessary.[118] The type of amputation is largely affected by the level of injury and the availability of viable soft tissues. There is no clear evidence that a certain amputation technique is significantly better. However, in series comparing below the knee, through the knee, and above the knee amputations, the percentage of patients eventually walking with a prosthesis is greater in the below the knee amputation group.[144–146]

After more distal (Chopart, Lisfranc, or transmetatarsal) amputations, muscle balancing is mandatory.[123,147] Flexor and extensor tendons should be reinserted into the most distal remaining bones, if possible. To avoid flexion contracture, primary or secondary fusions may be considered, above all after Chopart amputations.[147] More proximal amputations (Pirogoff and Syme) still allow the patient to load their own heel. After a successful Pirogoff amputation, patients are still able to walk barefoot for short distances without the need for an orthosis. Results with this technique are better for posttraumatic amputation than after amputation for diabetic vasculopathy and the average loss of limb length is less than 3 cm.[147,148]

Stable Internal Fixation

Important surgical principles in posttraumatic foot surgery are precise reconstruction of the foot axes, the functional length of the medial and lateral foot column, and the longitudinal and transverse arches, that is, restitution of the normal foot anatomy.[52] Stable internal fixation has to be accompanied by early and durable soft tissue coverage.[113] Early free tissue transfer has the potential to lower infection rates after third-degree open fractures and allow for functional rehabilitation.[113,149,150]

Reconstruction

- Osseous first (from proximal to distal, but starting with the talus before pilon/ankle).[6,52]
- Primary fusions for severely comminuted intraarticular fractures.[123,151–153]

- Delayed closure using NPWT/vacuum-assisted closure[97-100]
- Early and stable soft tissue coverage (discuss the reconstructive ladder with the plastic surgeon from primary closure or split thickness skin grafts to pedicled or free flap closure as needed).[113,150]
- Frequently, depending on function deficit or deformity, a patient can significantly benefit from shoe adaptations, such as insoles, rocker bottom soles, stabilization in orthopedic shoes, orthesis, or silicone prostheses.

Outcome

There are 6 areas of outcome expectation: (1) the final expected function, (2) cosmesis and chronic swelling, (3) pain and loss of sensation, (4) duration of treatment, (5) cost of treatment, and (6) emotional factors.[123] Few studies report explicitly the results after complex foot trauma. Kinner and colleagues[5] reviewed 50 patients who fulfilled the Zwipp criteria for complex foot trauma[8,52] treated according to the principles as discussed after an average of 4 years follow-up. The mean American Orthopaedic Foot and Ankle Society score was 66.2. The Short Form-12 score showed a physical component of 38.2. And the visual analog scale foot/ankle score was 51.9. Eleven patients underwent primary and 7 patients secondary amputation. Secondary amputation was associated significantly with an Injury Severity Score of greater than 16 and primary soft tissue damage. The overall complication rate was 32%, with 8 patients requiring a free flap for soft tissue coverage. A total of 53% of the patients returned to their preinjury occupation, and 41% were able to perform sports (as compared with 77% before their injury). The complex foot trauma score correlated with the American Orthopaedic Foot and Ankle Society score and the restrictions in the activities of daily living.

When following 19 patients with similar severity of injury over an average of 6 years, Ferreira and colleagues[7] found nearly the same American Orthopaedic Foot and Ankle Society score (average 68.0) but also chronic pain in 15 cases (79%) and a chronic regional pain syndrome in 7 cases (37%). Eleven patients (58%) had a stiff foot, 6 (32%) had chronic ulcerations, and 2 (11%) had chronic osteitis. Still, almost one-half of the patients could return to their previous occupation. Possible reasons for the inferior results as compared with the study of Kinner and colleagues[5] were that most patients were treated with external fixation only and subjected to longer immobilization Most important, Ferreira and colleagues[7] reported 68% as having residual deformities.

Overall, the prognosis after complex injuries to the foot and ankle is hard to predict because of the relatively scarce literature and the high variability of the injury pattern. Results are determined by various confounders, such as overall severity of injury, comorbidities, complications, secondary interventions, and individual demands.[5,7,14] A subgroup analysis of the LEAP population with complex foot injury showed that patients with severe foot and ankle injuries who require free tissue transfer or ankle fusion have Sickness Impact Profile scores that are significantly worse than with below the knee amputations.[140]

SUMMARY

The treatment of complex foot injuries has come a long way in the past decade. One should always keep the end result in mind. Although saving the limb might be psychologically better at first, an insensate, nonfunctional, and/or painful stiff foot with the need for secondary interventions and prolonged hospitalization and rehabilitation might be a far worse outcome. Treatment should be individualized based on patient and injury characteristics. If the necessary facilities are not available, referral should be considered. If the decision to salvage the foot is made, anatomic reconstruction of the foot and ankle with stable internal fixation and early soft tissue coverage followed by an aggressive rehabilitation protocol and adequate orthopedic shoe modifications must be pursued to achieve maximal functional recovery. Complex foot injuries are difficult to treat and may take up to several years to manage.

REFERENCES

1. Court-Brown CM, Caesar B. Epidemiology of adult fractures: a review. Injury 2006;37(8):691–7.
2. Court-Brown CM, Bugler KE, Clement ND, et al. The epidemiology of open fractures in adults. A 15-year review. Injury 2012;43(6):891–7.
3. Bluman EM, Ficke JR, Covey DC. War wounds of the foot and ankle: causes, characteristics, and initial management. Foot Ankle Clin 2010;15(1):1–21.
4. Johnson BA, Carmack D, Neary M, et al. Operation Iraqi Freedom: the Landstuhl Regional Medical Center experience. J Foot Ankle Surg 2005;44(3): 177–83.
5. Kinner B, Tietz S, Muller F, et al. Outcome after complex trauma of the foot. J Trauma 2011;70(1):159–68 [discussion: 168].
6. Rammelt S, Biewener A, Grass R, et al. Foot injuries in the polytraumatized patient. Unfallchirurg 2005;108(10):858–65 [in German].
7. Ferreira RC, Sakata MA, Costa MT, et al. Long-term results of salvage surgery in severely injured feet. Foot Ankle Int 2010;31(2):113–23.
8. Zwipp H. Severe foot trauma in combination with talar injuries. In: Tscherne H, Schatzker J, editors. Major fractures of the pilon, the talus and the calcaneus. Berlin: Springer Verlag; 1993. p. 123–35.
9. De Boer AS, Schepers T, Panneman MJ, et al. Health care consumption and costs due to foot and ankle injuries in the Netherlands, 1986-2010. BMC Musculoskelet Disord 2014;15:128.
10. Richter M, Thermann H, Wippermann B, et al. Foot fractures in restrained front seat car occupants: a long-term study over twenty-three years. J Orthop Trauma 2001;15(4):287–93.
11. Weninger P, Nau T, Aldrian S, et al. Long-term results in the treatment of foot injuries in polytraumatized patients. Zentralbl Chir 2005;130(5):485–91 [in German].
12. Fildes B, Lenard J, Lane J, et al. Lower limb injuries to passenger car occupants. Accid Anal Prev 1997;29(6):785–91.
13. Seeley DG, Kelsey J, Jergas M, et al. Predictors of ankle and foot fractures in older women. The Study of Osteoporotic Fractures Research Group. J Bone Miner Res 1996;11(9):1347–55.
14. Myerson MS, McGarvey WC, Henderson MR, et al. Morbidity after crush injuries to the foot. J Orthop Trauma 1994;8(4):343–9.
15. Westphal T, Piatek S, Schubert S, et al. Quality of life after foot injuries. Zentralbl Chir 2002;127(3):238–42 [in German].
16. Holbrook TL, Anderson JP, Sieber WJ, et al. Outcome after major trauma: discharge and 6-month follow-up results from the Trauma Recovery Project. J Trauma 1998;45(2):315–23 [discussion: 323–4].
17. Holbrook TL, Anderson JP, Sieber WJ, et al. Outcome after major trauma: 12-month and 18-month follow-up results from the Trauma Recovery Project. J Trauma 1999;46(5):765–71 [discussion: 771–3].

18. Probst C, Richter M, Lefering R, et al. Incidence and significance of injuries to the foot and ankle in polytrauma patients–an analysis of the Trauma Registry of DGU. Injury 2010;41(2):210–5.

19. Stalp M, Koch C, Ruchholtz S, et al. Standardized outcome evaluation after blunt multiple injuries by scoring systems: a clinical follow-up investigation 2 years after injury. J Trauma 2002;52(6):1160–8.

20. Tran T, Thordarson D. Functional outcome of multiply injured patients with associated foot injury. Foot Ankle Int 2002;23(4):340–3.

21. Turchin DC, Schemitsch EH, McKee MD, et al. Do foot injuries significantly affect the functional outcome of multiply injured patients? J Orthop Trauma 1999;13(1): 1–4.

22. von Ruden C, Woltmann A, Rose M, et al. Outcome after severe multiple trauma: a retrospective analysis. J Trauma Manag Outcomes 2013;7(1):4.

23. Weninger P, Aldrian S, Koenig F, et al. Functional recovery at a minimum of 2 years after multiple injury-development of an outcome score. J Trauma 2008; 65(4):799–808 [discussion: 808].

24. Zelle BA, Brown SR, Panzica M, et al. The impact of injuries below the knee joint on the long-term functional outcome following polytrauma. Injury 2005;36(1): 169–77.

25. Heckman JD, Champine MJ. New techniques in the management of foot trauma. Clin Orthop Relat Res 1989;(240):105–14.

26. Court-Brown C, Honeyman C, Bugler K, et al. The spectrum of open fractures of the foot in adults. Foot Ankle Int 2013;34(3):323–8.

27. Zwipp H, Dahlen C, Randt T, et al. Complex trauma of the foot. Orthopade 1997; 26(12):1046–56 [in German].

28. Jacobs LG. The landmine foot: its description and management. Injury 1991; 22(6):463–6.

29. Ramasamy A, Hill AM, Phillip R, et al. The modern "deck-slap" injury–calcaneal blast fractures from vehicle explosions. J Trauma 2011;71(6):1694–8.

30. Bevevino AJ, Dickens JF, Potter BK, et al. A model to predict limb salvage in severe combat-related open calcaneus fractures. Clin Orthop Relat Res 2014; 472(10):3002–9.

31. Dickens JF, Kilcoyne KG, Kluk MW, et al. Risk factors for infection and amputation following open, combat-related calcaneal fractures. J Bone Joint Surg Am 2013;95(5):e24.

32. Tscherne H, Oestern HJ. A new classification of soft-tissue damage in open and closed fractures (author's transl). Unfallheilkunde 1982;85(3):111–5 [in German].

33. Gustilo RB, Anderson JT. Prevention of infection in the treatment of one thousand and twenty-five open fractures of long bones: retrospective and prospective analyses. J Bone Joint Surg Am 1976;58(4):453–8.

34. Gustilo RB, Mendoza RM, Williams DN. Problems in the management of type III (severe) open fractures: a new classification of type III open fractures. J Trauma 1984;24(8):742–6.

35. Brumback RJ, Jones AL. Interobserver agreement in the classification of open fractures of the tibia. The results of a survey of two hundred and forty-five orthopaedic surgeons. J Bone Joint Surg Am 1994;76(8):1162–6.

36. Roberts CS, Pape HC, Jones AL, et al. Damage control orthopaedics: evolving concepts in the treatment of patients who have sustained orthopaedic trauma. Instr Course Lect 2005;54:447–62.

37. Acello AN, Wallace GF, Pachuda NM. Treatment of open fractures of the foot and ankle: a preliminary report. J Foot Ankle Surg 1995;34(4):329–46.
38. Investigators F, Bhandari M, Jeray KJ, et al. A trial of wound irrigation in the initial management of open fracture wounds. N Engl J Med 2015;373(27):2629–41.
39. Husain ZS, Schmid S, Lombardo N. Functional outcomes after gunshot wounds to the foot and ankle. J Foot Ankle Surg 2016;55(6):1234–40.
40. Eberl R, Ruttenstock EM, Singer G, et al. Treatment algorithm for complex injuries of the foot in paediatric patients. Injury 2011;42(10):1171–8.
41. Halawi MJ, Morwood MP. Acute management of open fractures: an evidence-based review. Orthopedics 2015;38(11):e1025–1033.
42. Amtsberg G, Seifert J, Ekkernkamp A. Komplexes Fusstrauma. Trauma Berufskrankh 2004;3(6):182–5.
43. Ovaska MT, Madanat R, Makinen TJ. Predictors of postoperative wound necrosis following primary wound closure of open ankle fractures. Foot Ankle Int 2016; 37(4):401–6.
44. Mittlmeier T. Acute compartment syndrome and complex trauma of the foot. Unfallchirurg 2011;114(10):893–900 [in German].
45. Ojike NI, Roberts CS, Giannoudis PV. Foot compartment syndrome: a systematic review of the literature. Acta Orthop Belg 2009;75(5):573–80.
46. Swoboda B, Scola E, Zwipp H. Surgical treatment and late results of foot compartment syndrome. Unfallchirurg 1991;94(5):262–6 [in German].
47. Thakur NA, McDonnell M, Got CJ, et al. Injury patterns causing isolated foot compartment syndrome. J Bone Joint Surg Am 2012;94(11):1030–5.
48. Zwipp H. Reconstructive measures for the foot after compartment syndrome. Unfallchirurg 1991;94(5):274–9 [in German].
49. Sands AK, Rammelt S, Manoli A. Foot compartment syndrome – a clinical review. Fuß Sprunggelenk 2015;13(1):11–21.
50. Farber A, Tan TW, Hamburg NM, et al. Early fasciotomy in patients with extremity vascular injury is associated with decreased risk of adverse limb outcomes: a review of the National Trauma Data Bank. Injury 2012;43(9):1486–91.
51. Han F, Daruwalla ZJ, Shen L, et al. A prospective study of surgical outcomes and quality of life in severe foot trauma and associated compartment syndrome after fasciotomy. J Foot Ankle Surg 2015;54(3):417–23.
52. Zwipp H, Tscherne H, Berger A. Reconstructive foot surgery following complex trauma of the foot. Unfallchirurg 1989;92(3):140–54 [in German].
53. David A, Lewandrowski KU, Josten C, et al. Surgical correction of talipes equinovarus following foot and leg compartment syndrome. Foot Ankle Int 1996; 17(6):334–9.
54. Eisele R. Reconstructive measures for toe deformity after compartment syndrome. Unfallchirurg 2008;111(10):796–803 [in German].
55. Rammelt S, Zwipp H. Reconstructive surgery after compartment syndrome of the lower leg and foot. Eur J Trauma Emerg Surg 2008;34(3):237.
56. Myerson M, Manoli A. Compartment syndromes of the foot after calcaneal fractures. Clin Orthop Relat Res 1993;(290):142–50.
57. Bonutti PM, Bell GR. Compartment syndrome of the foot. A case report. J Bone Joint Surg Am 1986;68(9):1449–51.
58. Fakhouri AJ, Manoli A 2nd. Acute foot compartment syndromes. J Orthop Trauma 1992;6(2):223–8.
59. Frink M, Hildebrand F, Krettek C, et al. Compartment syndrome of the lower leg and foot. Clin Orthop Relat Res 2010;468(4):940–50.

60. Fulkerson E, Razi A, Tejwani N. Review: acute compartment syndrome of the foot. Foot Ankle Int 2003;24(2):180–7.
61. Wright J, Worlock P, Hunter G, et al. The management of injuries of the midfoot and forefoot in the patient with multiple injuries. Tech Orthop 1987;2(3):71–9.
62. Mittlmeier T, Machler G, Lob G, et al. Compartment syndrome of the foot after intraarticular calcaneal fracture. Clin Orthop Relat Res 1991;(269):241–8.
63. Manoli A 2nd, Fakhouri AJ, Weber TG. Concurrent compartment syndromes of the foot and leg. Foot Ankle 1993;14(6):339.
64. Beals TC. Applications of ring fixators in complex foot and ankle trauma. Orthop Clin North Am 2001;32(1):205–14.
65. Chandran P, Puttaswamaiah R, Dhillon MS, et al. Management of complex open fracture injuries of the midfoot with external fixation. J Foot Ankle Surg 2006; 45(5):308–15.
66. Kenzora JE, Edwards CC, Browner BD, et al. Acute management of major trauma involving the foot and ankle with Hoffmann external fixation. Foot Ankle 1981;1(6):348–61.
67. Klaue K. The role of external fixation in acute foot trauma. Foot Ankle Clin 2004; 9(3):583–94, x.
68. Pedrini G, Cardi M, Landini A, et al. Management of severe open ankle-foot trauma by a simple external fixation technique: an alternative during war and in resource-poor and low-technology environments. J Orthop Trauma 2011; 25(3):180–7.
69. Rammelt S, Endres T, Grass R, et al. The role of external fixation in acute ankle trauma. Foot Ankle Clin 2004;9(3):455–74, vii–viii.
70. Seibert FJ, Fankhauser F, Elliott B, et al. External fixation in trauma of the foot and ankle. Clin Podiatr Med Surg 2003;20(1):159–80.
71. Hong-Chuan W, Shi-Lian K, Heng-Sheng S, et al. Immediate internal fixation of open ankle fractures. Foot Ankle Int 2010;31(11):959–64.
72. Johnson EE, Davlin LB. Open ankle fractures. The indications for immediate open reduction and internal fixation. Clin Orthop Relat Res 1993;(292):118–27.
73. Bouachour G, Cronier P, Gouello JP, et al. Hyperbaric oxygen therapy in the management of crush injuries: a randomized double-blind placebo-controlled clinical trial. J Trauma 1996;41(2):333–9.
74. Buettner MF, Wolkenhauer D. Hyperbaric oxygen therapy in the treatment of open fractures and crush injuries. Emerg Med Clin North Am 2007;25(1): 177–88.
75. Strauss MB. The effect of hyperbaric oxygen in crush injuries and skeletal muscle-compartment syndromes. Undersea Hyperb Med 2012;39(4):847–55.
76. Wattel F, Mathieu D, Neviere R, et al. Acute peripheral ischaemia and compartment syndromes: a role for hyperbaric oxygenation. Anaesthesia 1998;53(Suppl 2):63–5.
77. D'Agostino Dias M, Fontes B, Poggetti RS, et al. Hyperbaric oxygen therapy: types of injury and number of sessions–a review of 1506 cases. Undersea Hyperb Med 2008;35(1):53–60.
78. MacFarlane C, Cronje FJ, Benn CA. Hyperbaric oxygen in trauma and surgical emergencies. J R Army Med Corps 2000;146(3):185–90.
79. Mutschler W, Muth CM. Hyperbaric oxygen therapy in trauma surgery. Unfallchirurg 2001;104(2):102–14 [in German].
80. Carsenti-Etesse H, Doyon F, Desplaces N, et al. Epidemiology of bacterial infection during management of open leg fractures. Eur J Clin Microbiol Infect Dis 1999;18(5):315–23.

81. Patzakis MJ, Bains RS, Lee J, et al. Prospective, randomized, double-blind study comparing single-agent antibiotic therapy, ciprofloxacin, to combination antibiotic therapy in open fracture wounds. J Orthop Trauma 2000;14(8):529–33.

82. Patzakis MJ, Wilkins J, Moore TM. Considerations in reducing the infection rate in open tibial fractures. Clin Orthop Relat Res 1983;(178):36–41.

83. Loos MS, Freeman BG, Lorenzetti A. Zone of injury: a critical review of the literature. Ann Plast Surg 2010;65(6):573–7.

84. Hauser CJ, Adams CA Jr, Eachempati SR, Council of the Surgical Infection Society. Surgical Infection Society guideline: prophylactic antibiotic use in open fractures: an evidence-based guideline. Surg Infect (Larchmt) 2006;7(4): 379–405.

85. Rodriguez L, Jung HS, Goulet JA, et al. Evidence-based protocol for prophylactic antibiotics in open fractures: improved antibiotic stewardship with no increase in infection rates. J Trauma Acute Care Surg 2014;77(3):400–7 [discussion: 407–8; quiz: 524].

86. Stabile DE, Jacobs AM. Local antibiotic treatment of soft tissue and bone infections of the foot. J Am Podiatr Med Assoc 1990;80(7):345–53.

87. Agel J, Rockwood T, Barber R, et al. Potential predictive ability of the orthopaedic trauma association open fracture classification. J Orthop Trauma 2014; 28(5):300–6.

88. Neut D, van de Belt H, Stokroos I, et al. Biomaterial-associated infection of gentamicin-loaded PMMA beads in orthopaedic revision surgery. J Antimicrob Chemother 2001;47(6):885–91.

89. Bistolfi A, Massazza G, Verne E, et al. Antibiotic-loaded cement in orthopedic surgery: a review. ISRN Orthop 2011;2011:290851.

90. Ferrao P, Myerson MS, Schuberth JM, et al. Cement spacer as definitive management for postoperative ankle infection. Foot Ankle Int 2012;33(3):173–8.

91. Largey A, Faline A, Hebrard W, et al. Management of massive traumatic compound defects of the foot. Orthop Traumatol Surg Res 2009;95(4):301–4.

92. Schade VL, Roukis TS. The role of polymethylmethacrylate antibiotic-loaded cement in addition to debridement for the treatment of soft tissue and osseous infections of the foot and ankle. J Foot Ankle Surg 2010;49(1):55–62.

93. Anagnostakos K, Kelm J. Enhancement of antibiotic elution from acrylic bone cement. J Biomed Mater Res B Appl Biomater 2009;90(1):467–75.

94. Anagnostakos K, Kelm J, Regitz T, et al. In vitro evaluation of antibiotic release from and bacteria growth inhibition by antibiotic-loaded acrylic bone cement spacers. J Biomed Mater Res B Appl Biomater 2005;72(2):373–8.

95. Karger C, Kishi T, Schneider L, et al. Treatment of posttraumatic bone defects by the induced membrane technique. Orthop Traumatol Surg Res 2012;98(1): 97–102.

96. Joethy J, Sebastin SJ, Chong AK, et al. Effect of negative-pressure wound therapy on open fractures of the lower limb. Singapore Med J 2013;54(11):620–3.

97. Schlatterer DR, Hirschfeld AG, Webb LX. Negative pressure wound therapy in grade IIIB tibial fractures: fewer infections and fewer flap procedures? Clin Orthop Relat Res 2015;473(5):1802–11.

98. Stannard JP, Singanamala N, Volgas DA. Fix and flap in the era of vacuum suction devices: what do we know in terms of evidence based medicine? Injury 2010;41(8):780–6.

99. Liu DS, Sofiadellis F, Ashton M, et al. Early soft tissue coverage and negative pressure wound therapy optimises patient outcomes in lower limb trauma. Injury 2012;43(6):772–8.

100. Stannard JP, Volgas DA, Stewart R, et al. Negative pressure wound therapy after severe open fractures: a prospective randomized study. J Orthop Trauma 2009; 23(8):552–7.
101. Carlson RM, Smith NC, Dux K, et al. Treatment of postoperative lower extremity wounds using human fibroblast-derived dermis: a retrospective analysis. Foot Ankle Spec 2014;7(2):102–7.
102. Baechler MF, Groth AT, Nesti LJ, et al. Soft tissue management of war wounds to the foot and ankle. Foot Ankle Clin 2010;15(1):113–38.
103. Hinck D, Franke A, Gatzka F. Use of vacuum-assisted closure negative pressure wound therapy in combat-related injuries–literature review. Mil Med 2010;175(3): 173–81.
104. Warner M, Henderson C, Kadrmas W, et al. Comparison of vacuum-assisted closure to the antibiotic bead pouch for the treatment of blast injury of the extremity. Orthopedics 2010;33(2):77–82.
105. Seligson D, Henry S, Ostermann PA. Comparison of vacuum-assisted closure to the antibiotic bead pouch for the treatment of blast injury of the extremity. Orthopedics 2010;33(12):868.
106. Kaplan M, Daly D, Stemkowski S. Early intervention of negative pressure wound therapy using Vacuum-Assisted Closure in trauma patients: impact on hospital length of stay and cost. Adv Skin Wound Care 2009;22(3):128–32.
107. Blum ML, Esser M, Richardson M, et al. Negative pressure wound therapy reduces deep infection rate in open tibial fractures. J Orthop Trauma 2012; 26(9):499–505.
108. Suzuki T, Minehara A, Matsuura T, et al. Negative-pressure wound therapy over surgically closed wounds in open fractures. J Orthop Surg (Hong Kong) 2014; 22(1):30–4.
109. Zhang T, Yan Y, Xie X, et al. Minimally invasive sinus tarsi approach with cannulated screw fixation combined with vacuum-assisted closure for treatment of severe open calcaneal fractures with medial wounds. J Foot Ankle Surg 2016; 55(1):112–6.
110. Stannard JP, Volgas DA, McGwin G 3rd, et al. Incisional negative pressure wound therapy after high-risk lower extremity fractures. J Orthop Trauma 2012;26(1):37–42.
111. Large TM, Douglas G, Erickson G, et al. Effect of negative pressure wound therapy on the elution of antibiotics from polymethylmethacrylate beads in a porcine simulated open femur fracture model. J Orthop Trauma 2012;26(9):506–11.
112. Stinner DJ, Hsu JR, Wenke JC. Negative pressure wound therapy reduces the effectiveness of traditional local antibiotic depot in a large complex musculoskeletal wound animal model. J Orthop Trauma 2012;26(9):512–8.
113. Brenner P, Rammelt S, Gavlik JM, et al. Early soft tissue coverage after complex foot trauma. World J Surg 2001;25(5):603–9.
114. Ingram R, Hunter G. Revascularization, limb salvage and/or amputation in severe injuries of the lower limb. Orthopaedics Trauma 1993;7(2):19–25.
115. MacKenzie EJ, Bosse MJ, Kellam JF, et al. Factors influencing the decision to amputate or reconstruct after high-energy lower extremity trauma. J Trauma 2002;52(4):641–9.
116. Omer GE Jr, Pomerantz GM. Initial management of severe open injuries and traumatic amputations of the foot. Arch Surg 1972;105(5):696–8.
117. Moniz MP, Ombrellaro MP, Stevens SL, et al. Concomitant orthopedic and vascular injuries as predictors for limb loss in blunt lower extremity trauma. Am Surg 1997;63(1):24–8.

118. Jacobs C, Siozos P, Raible C, et al. Amputation of a lower extremity after severe trauma. Oper Orthop Traumatol 2011;23(4):306–17.
119. Akula M, Gella S, Shaw CJ, et al. A meta-analysis of amputation versus limb salvage in mangled lower limb injuries–the patient perspective. Injury 2011; 42(11):1194–7.
120. Burdette TE, Long SA, Ho O, et al. Early delayed amputation: a paradigm shift in the limb-salvage time line for patients with major upper-limb injury. J Rehabil Res Dev 2009;46(3):385–94.
121. Hoogendoorn JM, van der Werken C. Grade III open tibial fractures: functional outcome and quality of life in amputees versus patients with successful reconstruction. Injury 2001;32(4):329–34.
122. Chung KC, Saddawi-Konefka D, Haase SC, et al. A cost-utility analysis of amputation versus salvage for Gustilo type IIIB and IIIC open tibial fractures. Plast Reconstr Surg 2009;124(6):1965–73.
123. Hansen ST Jr. Salvage or amputation after complex foot and ankle trauma. Orthop Clin North Am 2001;32(1):181–6.
124. Bakota B, Kopljar M, Jurjevic Z, et al. Mangled extremity–case report, literature review and borderline cases guidelines proposal. Coll Antropol 2012;36(4): 1419–26.
125. Jupiter DC, Shibuya N, Clawson LD, et al. Incidence and risk factors for amputation in foot and ankle trauma. J Foot Ankle Surg 2012;51(3):317–22.
126. Oestern HJ, Tscherne H, Sturm J, et al. Classification of the severity of injury. Unfallchirurg 1985;88(11):465–72 [in German].
127. Ahmed N, Sahito B, Baig N. Evaluation and reliability of Mangled Extremity Severity Scoring in traumatic amputation versus limb salvage. J Pakistan Orthop Assoc 2013;25(2):35–40.
128. Bonanni F, Rhodes M, Lucke JF. The futility of predictive scoring of mangled lower extremities. J Trauma 1993;34(1):99–104.
129. Bosse MJ, MacKenzie EJ, Kellam JF, et al. A prospective evaluation of the clinical utility of the lower-extremity injury-severity scores. J Bone Joint Surg Am 2001;83-A(1):3–14.
130. Bosse MJ, MacKenzie EJ, Kellam JF, et al. An analysis of outcomes of reconstruction or amputation after leg-threatening injuries. N Engl J Med 2002; 347(24):1924–31.
131. Bosse MJ, McCarthy ML, Jones AL, et al. The insensate foot following severe lower extremity trauma: an indication for amputation? J Bone Joint Surg Am 2005;87(12):2601–8.
132. Durham RM, Mistry BM, Mazuski JE, et al. Outcome and utility of scoring systems in the management of the mangled extremity. Am J Surg 1996;172(5): 569–73 [discussion: 573–4].
133. Fodor L, Sobec R, Sita-Alb L, et al. Mangled lower extremity: can we trust the amputation scores? Int J Burns Trauma 2012;2(1):51–8.
134. Helfet DL, Howey T, Sanders R, et al. Limb salvage versus amputation. Preliminary results of the Mangled Extremity Severity Score. Clin Orthop Relat Res 1990;(256):80–6.
135. Hoogendoorn JM, Van der Werken C. The mangled leg, decision-making based on scoring systems and outcome. Eur J Trauma 2002;1:1–10.
136. Johansen K, Daines M, Howey T, et al. Objective criteria accurately predict amputation following lower extremity trauma. J Trauma 1990;30(5):568–72 [discussion: 572–3].

137. Robertson PA. Prediction of amputation after severe lower limb trauma. J Bone Joint Surg Br 1991;73(5):816–8.
138. Busse JW, Jacobs CL, Swiontkowski MF, et al, Evidence-Based Orthopaedic Trauma Working Group. Complex limb salvage or early amputation for severe lower-limb injury: a meta-analysis of observational studies. J Orthop Trauma 2007;21(1):70–6.
139. Brown KV, Ramasamy A, McLeod J, et al. Predicting the need for early amputation in ballistic mangled extremity injuries. J Trauma 2009;66(4 Suppl):S93–7 [discussion: S97–8].
140. Ellington JK, Bosse MJ, Castillo RC, et al. The mangled foot and ankle: results from a 2-year prospective study. J Orthop Trauma 2013;27(1):43–8.
141. Demiralp B, Ege T, Kose O, et al. Amputation versus functional reconstruction in the management of complex hind foot injuries caused by land-mine explosions: a long-term retrospective comparison. Eur J Orthop Surg Traumatol 2014;24(4): 621–6.
142. Shawen SB, Keeling JJ, Branstetter J, et al. The mangled foot and leg: salvage versus amputation. Foot Ankle Clin 2010;15(1):63–75.
143. Pape H, Stalp M, v Griensven M, et al. Optimal timing for secondary surgery in polytrauma patients: an evaluation of 4,314 serious-injury cases. Chirurg 1999; 70(11):1287–93 [in German].
144. Taylor SM, Kalbaugh CA, Blackhurst DW, et al. Preoperative clinical factors predict postoperative functional outcomes after major lower limb amputation: an analysis of 553 consecutive patients. J Vasc Surg 2005;42(2):227–35.
145. Hagberg E, Berlin OK, Renstrom P. Function after through-knee compared with below-knee and above-knee amputation. Prosthet Orthot Int 1992;16(3):168–73.
146. Penn-Barwell JG. Outcomes in lower limb amputation following trauma: a systematic review and meta-analysis. Injury 2011;42(12):1474–9.
147. Rammelt S, Olbrich A, Zwipp H. Hindfoot amputations. Oper Orthop Traumatol 2011;23(4):265–79 [in German].
148. Taniguchi A, Tanaka Y, Kadono K, et al. Pirogoff ankle disarticulation as an option for ankle disarticulation. Clin Orthop Relat Res 2003;(414):322–8.
149. Musharrafieh R, Osmani O, Saghieh S, et al. Microvascular composite tissue transfer for the management of type IIIB and IIIC fractures of the distal leg and compound foot fractures. J Reconstr Microsurg 1999;15(7):501–7.
150. Yazar S, Lin CH, Wei FC. One-stage reconstruction of composite bone and soft-tissue defects in traumatic lower extremities. Plast Reconstr Surg 2004;114(6): 1457–66.
151. MacMahon A, Kim P, Levine DS, et al. Return to sports and physical activities after primary partial arthrodesis for lisfranc injuries in young patients. Foot Ankle Int 2016;37(4):355–62.
152. Schepers T. The primary arthrodesis for severely comminuted intra-articular fractures of the calcaneus: a systematic review. Foot Ankle Surg 2012;18(2): 84–8.
153. Zelle BA, Gruen GS, McMillen RL, et al. Primary arthrodesis of the tibiotalar joint in severely comminuted high-energy pilon fractures. J Bone Joint Surg Am 2014;96(11):e91.
154. Available at: http://www.aaam.org/abbreviated-injury-scale-ais/. Accessed November 10, 2016.
155. Tscherne H. Principles of primary treatment of fractures with soft tissue injury. Orthopade 1983;12(1):9–22.

156. Gregory RT, Gould RJ, Peclet M, et al. The mangled extremity syndrome (M.E.S.): a severity grading system for multisystem injury of the extremity. J Trauma 1985;25(12):1147–50.
157. Howe HR Jr, Poole GV Jr, Hansen KJ, et al. Salvage of lower extremities following combined orthopedic and vascular trauma. A predictive salvage index. Am Surg 1987;53(4):205–8.
158. Russell WL, Sailors DM, Whittle TB, et al. Limb salvage versus traumatic amputation. A decision based on a seven-part predictive index. Ann Surg 1991; 213(5):473–80.
159. McNamara MG, Heckman JD, Corley FG. Severe open fractures of the lower extremity: A retrospective evaluation of the Mangled Extremity Severity Score (MESS). J Orthopaedic Trauma 1994;8:81–7.
160. Manoli A, Prasad P, Levine RS. Foot and ankle severity scale (FASS). Foot Ankle Int 1997;18(9):598–602.
161. Rajasekaran S. Ganga hospital open injury severity score—a score to prognosticate limb salvage and outcome measures in Type III B open tibial fractures. Indian J Orthop 2005;39:4–13.

Index

Note: Page numbers of article titles are in **boldface** type.

A

ABCDE-principle, of trauma resuscitation, 196
Achilles tendon. See also *Gastrocnemius lengthening.*
    calcaneal tuberosity avulsion fractures and, 98
    peripheral talus fractures and, 190
    posterior malleolar fractures and, 136
Advanced Trauma Life Support, for complex foot injury, 196
AITFL. See *Anterior inferior tibiofibular ligament (AITFL).*
Amputation, for complex foot injury, as definite treatment, 203
        indications for, 200–201
        initial consideration of, 200
        predictive scores for, 202
Angle of Gissane, in small incision fixation, of calcaneus fractures, 86–87
Ankle arthrodesis, for tibial pilon fractures, with external fixation, 157–158
    with intramedullary nailing, 152, 154–155, 157, 159
Ankle equinus, with Lisfranc injuries, 17
Ankle joint, posterior, anatomy of, 126–127
    biomechanics of, 126–128
    "rule of threes" ligaments in, 36–37
    syndesmosis zone of, 36, 65, 128
Ankle pain, post-calcaneus fracture treatment, 112
Ankle stability, with Chopart injuries, 167, 172–173
    with peripheral talus fractures, 181, 185
    with posterior malleolar fractures, 134–135
    with syndesmosis injuries, **35–63**. See also *Syndesmosis injuries.*
        biomechanics and, 36–37, 66
        surgical strategies for, 41–58
Anterior inferior tibiofibular ligament (AITFL), in ankle joint, 36–37, 66
    in syndesmosis injuries, 37–40
        anterior inferior tibiofibular ligament and deltoid: stabilization, 50–51
        anterior inferior tibiofibular ligament nonoperative treatment, 49–50
        late treatment and, 73
        posterior malleolus fixation and, 43
Anterior process fractures, of calcaneus, in Chopart injuries, 164
        internal fixation of, 171–172
Anterior-to-posterior fixation, of posterior malleolar fractures, indirect reduction and, 135–136
Anterolateral approach, to peripheral talus fractures, 186, 188, 190
Anteromedial approach, to peripheral talus fractures, 190–191
Antibiotic bead pouch, for complex foot injury, 199–200
Antibiotics, for complex foot injury, 199
    for tibial pilon fractures, 157, 159

Foot Ankle Clin N Am 22 (2017) 215–240
http://dx.doi.org/10.1016/S1083-7515(16)30124-3
1083-7515/17

foot.theclinics.com

AO radiologic classification, of posterior malleolar fractures, 129
    of tibial pilon fractures, 149, 151
Arthritis, post-arthrodesis, for tibial pilon fractures, 159
    posttraumatic, with calcaneus fractures, 109–110
        with Chopart injuries, 177
        with peripheral talus fractures, 185
        with posterior malleolar fractures, 140–141
Arthrodeses, ankle, for tibial pilon fractures, with external fixation, 157–158
        with intramedullary nailing, 152, 154–155, 157, 159
    bone-block subtalar, for calcaneal malunions, 111–112
        as salvage technique, 79–80
    for peripheral talus fractures, 185
    of syndesmosis malunion, as salvage technique, 73–74, 79–80
    primary. See also *Primary arthrodesis (PA).*
        for Chopart injuries, 168, 173–174
        for Lisfranc injuries, **1–14**. See also *Lisfranc injuries.*
        for tibial pilon fractures, **147–161**. See also *Tibial pilon fractures.*
    tibiotalocalcaneal, for tibial pilon fractures, 151, 154–155
Arthrolysis, postoperative, for Chopart injuries, 173, 176
Arthrosis, with peripheral talus fractures, 182–183, 185–186
Articular comminution, with peripheral talus fractures, 184–185, 188
    displacement and, 190–191
    with tibial pilon fractures, 149, 151–156
Articular surfaces, in posterior ankle biomechanics, 126–128
Avascular necrosis (AVN), with Chopart injuries, 173, 176
Avulsion fractures, Chopart injuries as, 164–165, 167
    of calcaneal tuberosity, 94–98
    peripheral talus fractures as, 185
    syndesmosis injuries as, 37

B

Bartonicek and Rammelt classification, 3-D CT, of posterior malleolar fractures, 129–134
        summary of, 129–131
        surgery approaches based on, 135–139
        surgery indications based on, 135
        type 1: extraincisural fragment, 129, 131
        type 2: posterolateral fragment, 129, 132
        type 3: posteromedial, two-part fragment, 129–131, 133
        type 4: large, posterolateral triangular fragment, 131, 133
        type 5: irregular osteoporotic fracture, 131, 134
Beak fractures, of calcaneus, early fixation of, 94, 96
Benirschke and Kramer technique, for gastrocnemius lengthening, 119
Biomechanics, of posterior ankle, 126–128
    of syndesmosis injuries, 36–37, 66
Bohler angle, in calcaneus fracture management, 79–80
Bone defects, with complex foot injury, 199–200
Bone graft, for calcaneal malunions, 111–113
    for Chopart injuries, 169–173
        AVN indication for, 176
    for complex foot injury, 200

for fibula malunions, 72–73
    for tibial pilon fractures, 156–157, 159
Bone scan, radionuclide, of Lisfranc injuries, 20
Bone-block subtalar athrodesis, for calcaneal malunions, 111–112
    as salvage technique, 79–80
Bones, in Lisfranc joint complex, 2–3, 16–17
    open injury management and, 9–12
    in syndesmosis injuries, 37, 65–66
    malreduced, 69

C

Calcaneal malunions, 109–113
    classification of, 110–111
    salvage techniques for, 73–74, 78–80
    treatment of, 111–112
        patient positioning for, 111
        surgical technique for, 111–112
    treatment origins of, 109–110
Calcaneal tuberosity avulsion fractures, closed vs. open reduction of, 95–96
    early fixation of, 94–98
Calcaneocuboid joint, in Chopart joint, 164, 166
    follow-up care for, 173, 176
    primary fusion of, 168, 173–174
    surgical fixation of. See specific anatomical component.
    posttraumatic arthritis of, with calcaneus fractures, 109–110
Calcaneus, anterior process fractures of, in Chopart injuries, 164
        internal fixation of, 171–172
Calcaneus fractures, complications of, **105–116**
        ankle pain as, 112
        cutaneous nerve entrapment as, 114
        cutaneous nerve injury as, 114
        heel exostoses as, 112
        heel pad pain as, 112
        introduction to, 105
        key points of, 105
        malunion as, 109–113
        peroneal dislocation as, 108–109
        peroneal stenosis as, 107–108
        peroneal tenosynovitis as, 107–108
        posttraumatic arthritis as, 109–110
        summary of, 114
        wound, 105–107
    early fixation of, **93–104**
        for calcaneal tuberosity avulsion fractures, 94–98
        for hindfoot fracture-dislocations, 94–95
        for open fractures, 101–103
        in hospitalized patients, 98
        introduction to, 93–94
        key points of, 93
        minimally invasive techniques for, 98–101. See also Sinus tarsi approach.

Calcaneus (*continued*)
    summary of, 103
    management of, **77–91**
        early fixation as, **93–104**
        introduction to, 77–78
        key points of, 77
        nonoperative, vs. operative, 78
        operative, vs. nonoperative, 78
        salvage of malunions in, 73–74, 78–80
        summary of, 89
        surgical, 80–89
    surgical management of, 80–89
        extensile lateral approach to, 80–83. See also *Extensile lateral approach.*
        reconstruction in, 73–74, 78–80
        small incision technique in, 81, 83. See also *Sinus tarsi approach.*
Casts/casting. See *Immobilization.*
Chaput tubercle, syndesmosis injuries and, 37
    late treatment of, 65
Charcot neuroarthropathy, type 3, Chopart injuries vs., 166
Chopart injuries, **163–180**
    assessment of, 164–166
        clinical examination in, 164–165
        radiographic examination in, 165–166
    classification of, 166–167
    complications of, 173, 176–177
    introduction to, . 163–165
    key points of, 163
    mechanisms of, 164–165
    rehabilitation for, 173, 175
    summary of, 177–178
    surgery for, 167–174
        clinical results from literature, 177
        contraindications to, 167
        for combined injuries, 172
        indications to, 167–168
        internal fixation of anterior process fractures of calcaneus, 171–172
        internal fixation of cuboid fractures, 170–171
        internal fixation of navicular fractures, 168–170
        internal fixation of talar head fractures, 168–169
        operative technique for, 168–173
        patient placement and preparation for, 168
        postoperative care of, 173
        primary fusion as, 168, 173–174
        temporary joint transfixation as, 167, 172–173
Chopart joint, anatomy of, 164
    fractures and dislocations at, 163–167. See also *Chopart injuries.*
Closed fractures, in complex foot. See also *Complex foot injury.*
    classification of, 194–195
Closed reduction, of calcaneal tuberosity avulsion fractures, 95–96
    of Chopart injuries, 164, 167, 177
    of Lisfranc injuries, 23–26. See also *Percutaneous reduction and fixation.*

Combat, foot injuries related to, 194

Comminution. See *Crush injuries.*

Comorbidities, evaluation of, with tibial pilon fractures, 149, 152

Compartment syndrome, with Chopart injuries, 167, 173

    with complex foot injury, 197

    with Lisfranc injuries, 17, 20

Complex foot injury, **193–213**

    classification of, 194–195

    definite treatment of, 203–204

        amputation for, 203

        outcomes of, 204

        reconstruction for, 204

        stable internal fixation for, 203

    definitions of, 194

    diagnostic protocol for, 196

    initial treatment of, 195–202

        débridement in, 195, 197, 199

        HBO therapy in, 198

        photographs in, 199

        prevent infection, 197–200

        prevent progression of ischemia and necrosis, 196–198

        step one - trauma screening and resuscitation protocol, 196

        step two - diagnostics in, 196

        step three - damage control in, 196–198

        step four - consider salvage or amputation, 200–202

        timeline for, 195–196

    introduction to, 193–194

    key points of, 193

    summary of, 204–205

    terminology for, 194

    treatment of, 195–204

        definite, 203–204

        initial, 195–202

Compression fractures, Chopart injuries as, 164–165

Computed tomography (CT), of calcaneus fractures, for sinus tarsi approach to fixation, 99–100

        with malunions, 79

    of Chopart injuries, 165, 167

    of Lisfranc injuries, 7–8, 20–21

        3-D, 20

    of peripheral talus fractures, 182, 184, 186–187, 190

    of posterior malleolar fractures, 126, 128

        2-D, 129

        3-D, 129–134

    of posttraumatic arthritis, with calcaneus fractures, 109–110

    of syndesmosis injuries, 43–45

        with malreduction, 66, 68

    of tibial pilon fractures, 148–150, 153, 156

Conservative management. See *Nonoperative management.*

Crush injuries, peripheral talus fractures as, 184–185, 188

        displacement and, 190–191

Crush (*continued*)
 tibial pilon fractures as, 149, 151–156
 to foot and ankle, 164, 177, 194
CT. See *Computed tomography (CT)*.
Cuboidal fractures, in Chopart injuries, 164
  internal fixation of, 170–171
Cuneiforms, in Lisfranc joint complex, 2–3, 16–17
  open injury management and, 9–12
  percutaneous injury management and, 19–20, 26–28
Cutaneous nerve entrapment, with calcaneus fractures, 114
Cutaneous nerve injury, with calcaneus fractures, 114
Cyma line, in Chopart injuries, 165–166

D

Damage control orthopedics, limb, of complex foot injury, 196–198
Débridement, of Chopart injuries, 165, 167–168, 171
 of complex foot injury, 195, 197, 199
 of malreduced syndesmosis injuries, 69–72
 of posterior malleolar fractures, 137
Delayed healing, as wound complication, of calcaneus fractures, 106–107
Deltoid ligament, in ankle joint, 36–37
 injury to, with PER fractures, 55
Diaphyseal comminution, with tibial pilon fractures, 149, 151
Direct injuries, of Lisfranc joint, 16–17
Direct reduction, of posterior malleolar fractures, and posterolateral fixation, 136–138
  and posteromedial fixation, 137–139
Disability, with severe foot ankle trauma, 194
Dislocations, at midtarsal joints, 163–167, 177. See also *Chopart injuries*.
 hindfoot fracture-, early fixation of, 94–95
 peroneal, with calcaneus fractures, 108–109
Distal tibia, high-energy injuries of, 147, 149, 151, 159, 194
 in posterior malleolus biomechanics, 126–128
Distraction devices, for fibula malunions, 71–72
 for salvage of calcaneal malunion, 79
Dorsal ligaments, in Chopart joint, 164
 in Lisfranc joint complex, 3, 17
Dressings. See also *Negative pressure wound therapy (NPWT)*.
 for calcaneus fractures, post-sinus tarsi approach, 88
  with delayed wound healing, 106

E

Ecchymosis, of plantar arch, 5, 165
Entrapment, of cutaneous nerve, with calcaneus fractures, 114
Epidemiology, of complex foot injuries, 193–194
 of Lisfranc injuries, 16
Equinus, ankle, with Lisfranc injuries, 17
 gastrocnemius. See *Gastrocnemius equinus*.
Excision, fracture, for peripheral talus fractures, 181–182
 of fragments, for calcaneal tuberosity avulsion fractures, 96

Exostectomy, lateral wall, for calcaneal malunions, 111–112
Exostoses, heel, with calcaneus fractures, 112
Extensile lateral approach, to calcaneal malunions, 111
    to calcaneus fractures, 80–83
        sinus tarsi approach vs., 97–99
        small incision technique vs., 88–89
        wound complications with, 105–106
External fixation, of tibial pilon fractures, 149, 153–154
    with ankle arthrodesis, 157–158
External frame fixation, of complex foot injury, 197–198
    indications for immediate, 198
    of tibial pilon fractures, 156–158
External rotation fractures, syndesmosis injuries and, degrees of instability with, 39–40, 43
    pronation, 37–38, 40. See also *Pronation external rotation (PER) fractures.*
    supinated foot with posterior malleolus fracture example of, 52–53
    supination, 37–38, 40. See also *Supination external rotation (SER) fractures.*

F

Falls, foot injuries related to, 194
Fasciotomy, for complex foot injury, 197
FHL (flexor hallucis longus) tendon, in peripheral talus fractures, 190
Fibula, in hindfoot fracture-dislocations, 94
    in syndesmosis, 36–37, 65
    in syndesmosis injuries, and medial zone fixation, 42–43
        correction of malunions, 71–72
        fixation of, 42, 45
        fracture pathomechanics of, 37–39. See also *Weber entries.*
            degrees of instability, 39–40
        malreduced, 65–74
            normal appearance vs., 71
        PER fractures and, high fibula, 42, 55–58
            with fibula fracture, and deltoid ligament injury, 55
    in tibial pilon fracture treatment, 155–156
Fibula length, in malreduced syndesmosis injuries, 71–72
Fibular fleck sign, 108
Fixation. See also *specific technique.*
    external. See also *External frame fixation.*
        of tibial pilon fractures, 149, 153–154
            with ankle arthrodesis, 157–158
    internal. See *Internal fixation.*
    of calcaneus fractures, early, **93–104**. See also *Calcaneus fractures.*
    of Chopart injuries, for specific anatomical fractures, 168–172
        temporary, 167, 172–173
    of complex foot injury, rigid (temporary), 197–198
    of Lisfranc injuries, open, **1–14**. See also *Open reduction and internal fixation (ORIF).*
        percutaneous, **15–34**. See also *Percutaneous reduction and fixation.*
        temporary, 5–6
    of posterior malleolar fractures, anterior-to-posterior, indirect reduction and, 135–136
        posterolateral, direct reduction and, 136–138
        posteromedial, direct reduction and, 137–139

Flake fragment sign, of posterior malleolar fractures, 128. See also *Bartonicek and Rammelt classification.*
Flexible stabilization, of syndesmosis injuries, 45–49
    clinical cohort studies of, 47
    complications of, 48
    cost analysis of, 49
    critical analysis of literature, 48–49
    future research on, 48–49
    hybrid technique for, 46–47
    laboratory studies for, 46
    ORIF and, 45
    randomized controlled trials of, 48
    reoperation rates for, 48
    screw fixation vs., 45
    systematic review of, 47–48
    TightRope system for, 46
    vs. no treatment, 45–46
Flexor hallucis longus (FHL) tendon, in peripheral talus fractures, 190
Fluoroscopy, intraoperative, for peripheral talus fractures, 187–189
    for small incision fixation, of calcaneus fractures, 85–88
    for syndesmosis injuries, 44
        malreduced, 68, 71–72
Foot injuries, Chopart, **163–180**. See also *Chopart injuries.*
    complex, **193–213**. See also *Complex foot injury.*
    traumatic. See *Traumatic foot injuries; specific anatomy or injury.*
Force, in Chopart injuries, 164–165
    in Lisfranc injuries, 5–6, 16
    in syndesmosis injuries, 52–53
Fracture excision, for peripheral talus fractures, 181–182
Fractures. See also *specific anatomy or type.*
    at midtarsal joints, 163–167, 177. See also *Chopart injuries.*
    calcaneus. See also *Calcaneus fractures.*
        complications of, **105–116**
        early fixation of, **93–104**
        management of, **77–91**
    complex foot, 194. See also *Complex foot injury.*
        classifications of, 194–195
    pilon, **147–161**. See also *Tibial pilon.*
    posterior malleolar, **125–145**. See also *Posterior malleolus (PM) fractures.*
    syndesmosis injuries and, avulsion, 37
        degrees of instability with, 39–40
        isolated malleolus in, 66
        late treatment of, 65–74
        pronation external rotation, 37–38, 40
        supination external rotation, 37–38, 40
    talus, **181–192**. See also *Peripheral talus fractures.*
Fragment sign, flake, of posterior malleolar fractures, 128. See also *Bartonicek and Rammelt classification.*
Fragments, excisions of, for calcaneal tuberosity avulsion fractures, 96
    posterior tibial rim, 126
    with Chopart injuries, 168, 177

with peripheral talus fractures, 184–185, 188
with tibial pilon fractures, 151, 156
Freer elevator, for peripheral talus fractures, 187
for syndesmosis injury, 69–70
in gastrocnemius lengthening, 122
in small incision fixation, of calcaneus fractures, 86–87
Function assessment, musculoskeletal, following calcaneus fracture fixation, 88–89
Functional anatomy, of Lisfranc joint complex, 3–4
of syndesmosis, 36–37, 65, 74
Functional status, with peripheral talus fractures, 181–183, 185
with severe foot ankle trauma, 194
Fusions. See *Arthrodeses.*
primary. See *Primary arthrodesis (PA).*

G

Gait cycle, midfoot anatomy in, 3–4, 19–20
with tibial pilon fractures, arthrodesis limitations in, 159
Gap sign, of Lisfranc injuries, 17
Gastrocnemius equinus, associated with traumatic foot injuries, 117–118
clinical examination of, 118–119
patient questions for, 118–119
radiographic examination of, 118–119
Gastrocnemius lengthening, at trauma fixation time, **117–124**
injury mechanisms and, 117–118
introduction to, 117–119
key points of, 117
patient evaluation for, 118–119
patient positioning for, 120
postoperative care of, 124
summary of, 124
surgical approach to, 120
surgical procedure for, 120–124
surgical technique for, 119–120
calcaneal tuberosity avulsion fractures and, 94, 98
dissection in, 121–122
Gastrocnemius recession, in gastrocnemius lengthening, 122–123
Gastrocnemius-soleus complex/interval, in gastrocnemius lengthening, 120–121
Gentamycin beads, for complex foot injury, 199
Growth plates, Lisfranc injuries and, 29
Gustilo classification, of open fractures, 194–195

H

Haraguchi classification, 2-D CT, of posterior malleolar fractures, 129
Hardcastle classification, of Lisfranc injuries, 20
Hardware removal, post-late treatment, of syndesmosis injuries, 73
postoperative, for Chopart injuries, 173, 176
post-percutaneous reduction and fixation, for Lisfranc injuries, 28–31
HBO (hyperbaric oxygen) therapy, for complex foot injury, 198
Heel exostoses, with calcaneus fractures, 112

Heel pad pain, post-calcaneus fracture treatment, 112
Heel widening, following nonoperative management of calcaneus fracture, 79
High-energy injuries, of Chopart joint, 164–165
    of distal tibia, 147, 149, 151, 159, 194
    of Lisfranc joint, 5–6, 16–17
    of lower extremity, 194, 203
        classification of, 194–195
Hindfoot fracture-dislocations, early fixation of, 94–95
Hospitalized patients, calcaneus fractures in, early fixation of, 98
Hyperbaric oxygen (HBO) therapy, for complex foot injury, 198

I

Imaging. See also *specific modality.*
    for complex foot injury, 196
    of Chopart injuries, 165–167
    of Lisfranc injuries, 5–8
        advanced, 7–8
        dynamic, 6–7
        initial, 5
    of peripheral talus fractures, 182–187, 189–191
    of posterior malleolar fractures, 126, 128
    of tibial pilon fractures, 148–151, 153, 155–156, 159
Immobilization, for Chopart injuries, 164, 167
        postoperative, 173
    for Lisfranc injuries, 9
    post-gastrocnemius lengthening, 124
    post-late treatment, of syndesmosis injuries, 73
    postoperative, for Chopart injuries, 173
        for peripheral talus fractures, 191
        for posterior malleolar fractures, 138
    post-sinus tarsi approach, to calcaneus fracture fixation, 88
Indirect injuries, of Lisfranc joint, 16–17
Indirect reduction, of posterior malleolar fractures, and anterior-to-posterior fixation, 135–136
Infection, with complex foot injury, 197
        prevention of, 198–200
        treatment decisions related to, 200–204
    with tibial pilon fractures, 151, 153, 158–159
Injuries, complex foot, **193–213**. See also *Complex foot injury.*
    traumatic foot. See also *specific anatomy or injury.*
        gastrocnemius equinus associated with, 117–118
Injury mechanisms, high-energy. See *High-energy injuries.*
    of Chopart injuries, 164–165
    of Lisfranc injuries, 4–5, 16
        high-energy, 5–6, 16–17
    of syndesmosis injuries, 37–39
    of tibial pilon fractures, 149
Instability. See *Ankle stability.*
Intermalleolar ligament, in posterior ankle biomechanics, 126–127
Internal fixation, of Chopart injuries, 167

with anterior process fractures of calcaneus, 171–172
with combined injuries, 172
with cuboid fractures, 170–171
with navicular fractures, 168–170
with talar head fractures, 168–169
of posterior malleolar fractures, anterior-to-posterior, indirect reduction and, 135–136
posterolateral, direct reduction and, 136–138
posteromedial, direct reduction and, 137–139
open reduction and. See *Open reduction and internal fixation (ORIF)*.
Interosseous tibiofibular ligament (IOL), in ankle joint, 36–37, 66
posterior, 126–127
in Lisfranc joint complex, 3, 17
Intramedullary nailing, with ankle arthrodesis, for tibial pilon fractures, 152, 154–155, 157, 159
IOL. See *Interosseous tibiofibular ligament (IOL)*.
Ischemia, with complex foot injury, 194, 196
classification of, 194–195
prevention of progression, 196–198

J

Joint transfixation. See *Temporary joint transfixation*.
Jowett and Main classification, of Chopart injuries, 166

K

Kirschner wire (K-wire) fixation, of calcaneus fractures, in sinus tarsi approach, 87, 99–100
of Chopart injuries, 167–171
removal of, 173, 176
of complex foot injury, 197
of fibula malunions, 72
of Lisfranc injuries, Puna and Tomlinson technique for, 26–29
of peripheral talus fractures, 184, 187–188, 190
of posterior malleolar fractures, 136–137
of tibial pilon fractures, 156
Kramer and Benirschke technique, for gastrocnemius lengthening, 119
Kuss and Quenu classification, of Lisfranc injuries, 20

L

Lamina spreader, for calcaneal malunions, 112
for fibula malunions, 72
Lateral approach, direct, to hindfoot fracture-dislocations, 94
extensile. See *Extensile lateral approach*.
Lateral ligaments, in ankle joint, 36–37
Lateral wall exostectomy, for calcaneal malunions, 111–112
Lauge-Hansen fractures, of syndesmosis, pronation external rotation, 37–38
supination external rotation, 37–38
Ligaments. See also *specific ligament*.
in ankle joint, injury mechanisms of, 37–39, 66
with fractures, 37–38

Ligaments (*continued*)
    "rule of threes," 36–37
    in Chopart joint, 164
        rupture of, 164–165
    in Lisfranc joint complex, 3, 17
        open injury management and, 9–12
    in peripheral talus fracture surgery, 187–188
    in posterior ankle biomechanics, 126–127
    in syndesmosis injuries, 36–37, 65–66
        late treatment and, 73
Limb damage control orthopedics, of complex foot injury, 196–198
Limb salvage, with complex foot injury. See *Salvage procedures.*
Lisfranc injuries, **1–14**
    classification of, 8, 20, 22
    diagnosis of, 5–8
    imaging of, 5–8
        advanced, 7–8, 20–21
        dynamic, 6–7, 18–20
        initial, 5, 17–18
    introduction to, 1–2
    key points of, 1
    mechanisms of, 4–5, 16
    nonoperative management of, 9
    open reduction and internal fixation for, 9
        anatomy in, 2–4
        discussion on, 10–12
        percutaneous technique vs., 23
        primary arthrodesis vs., 10
    operative management of, 23
        open reduction and fixation for, 9–12, 23
        percutaneous reduction and fixation for, **15–34**
        primary arthrodesis for, 9–10, 23
    percutaneous reduction and fixation for, **15–34**
        anatomy in, 16–17
        clinical findings in, 17
        incidence of, 16
        introduction to, 15–16
        key points of, 15
        other operative options vs., 23
        prevalence of, 16
        Puna and Tomlinson technique for, 23–31
        radiologic findings in, 17–21
        summary of, 31
    physical examination of, 5–6, 17
    primary arthrodesis for, 9–10
        anatomy in, 2–4
        discussion on, 10–12
        ORIF vs., 10
        percutaneous technique vs., 23
    summary of, 12–13
Lisfranc joint complex, anatomy of, functional, 3–4

ligamentous, 3, 17
  osseous, 2–3, 16–17
Lisfranc ligament, in Lisfranc joint complex, 3, 17
  open injury management and, 9–12
Load, in Chopart injuries, 164–165
  in Lisfranc injuries, 6
Locking implants, for peripheral talus fractures, 188, 190–191

M

Magnetic resonance imaging (MRI), of Lisfranc injuries, 7–8, 20
  of peripheral talus fractures, 182–183
  of syndesmosis injuries, 39
Main and Jowett classification, of Chopart injuries, 166
Maisonneuve fractures, posterior malleolar fractures and, 135
  syndesmosis injuries and, 37
    missed, 40–41
Malalignment, with posterior malleolar fractures, 139–141
Malleolus, syndesmosis injuries and, isolated fractures of, 66
    medial. See *Medial malleolus (MM)*.
    posterior. See *Posterior malleolus (PM)*.
Malreduction, of syndesmosis injuries, 66–67
    surgical treatment of, 66, 68–74
Malunion, with calcaneus fractures, 109–113. See also *Calcaneal malunions*.
  with Chopart injuries, 176
  with posterior malleolar fractures, 140
Medial malleolus (MM), in posterior ankle biomechanics, 126–127
  syndesmosis injuries and, 41–43
    with PER fractures, and Tillaux fracture, 53–54
Medial zone fixation, of syndesmosis injuries, 42–43
Metaphyseal comminution, with tibial pilon fractures, 149, 151–154, 156
Metatarsals, in Lisfranc joint complex, 2–4, 16
    open injury management and, 9–12
    percutaneous injury management and, 18–19
MFA (musculoskeletal function assessment) scores, following calcaneus fracture fixation,
    88–89
Midfoot, functional anatomy of, 3–4
  injuries of, in Lisfranc injuries. See *Lisfranc injuries*.
  sprains of, 167. See also *Chopart injuries*.
Midtarsal joints, fractures and dislocations at, 163–167. See also *Chopart injuries*.
Minimally invasive techniques, for fixation, of calcaneus fractures, 98–101. See also *Sinus tarsi approach*.
Mining, foot injuries related to, 194
MM. See *Medial malleolus (MM)*.
Motor vehicle accidents, foot injuries related to, 194
MRI. See *Magnetic resonance imaging (MRI)*.
Muscles, in Chopart joint, 164
  in complex foot injuries, 194
    classification of, 194–195
    treatment decisions related to, 200–204
    posterior malleolar fractures and, 136–137

Musculoskeletal function assessment (MFA) scores, following calcaneus fracture fixation, 88–89
Myerson classification, of Lisfranc injuries, 8, 20, 22

N

Nailing, intramedullary, with ankle arthrodesis, for tibial pilon fractures, 152, 154–155, 157, 159
Navicular fractures, in Chopart injuries, 164
    AVN of, 173, 176
    internal fixation of, 168–170
Naviculocuneiforms, in Lisfranc joint complex, 2–4, 16
    open injury management and, 9–12
Necrosis, avascular, with Chopart injuries, 173, 176
  soft tissue, with calcaneal fractures, 80–82, 94–97
    with Chopart injuries, 173
    with complex foot injury, 194, 196
      classification of, 194
      prevention of progression, 196–198
      treatment decisions related to, 200–204
Negative pressure wound therapy (NPWT), for complex foot injury, 198, 200, 204
    post-ORIF, of calcaneus fractures, 101–102, 107
Nerve entrapment, cutaneous, with calcaneus fractures, 114
Nerve injury, cutaneous, with calcaneus fractures, 114
Neuroarthropathy, Charcot type 3, Chopart injuries vs., 166
Neuropathy, peripheral, tibial pilon fractures and, 149, 154–155
Neurovascular bundles. See also *Sural nerve.*
    fractures and, 114, 136, 190
Nonoperative management, of calcaneal malunions, 111
  of calcaneus fractures, 78
    complications with, 78–80
  of Lisfranc injuries, 9
  of peripheral talus fractures, 181, 183–185
Nonunion, with Chopart injuries, 176–177
  with posterior malleolar fractures, 140
  with tibial pilon fractures, 157–159
NPWT. See *Negative pressure wound therapy (NPWT).*

O

Open fractures, in Chopart injuries, 165, 170
  in complex foot. See also *Complex foot injury.*
    classification of, 194–195
  of calcaneus, early fixation of, 101–103
  of tibial pilon, 151, 157–158
Open reduction, of calcaneal tuberosity avulsion fractures, 96
  of Chopart injuries, 167
  of peripheral talus fractures, 185
  of syndesmosis injuries, 44–45
Open reduction and internal fixation (ORIF), of calcaneal fractures, 101–103
    indications for, 101–102

        operative technique for, 102–103
    of calcaneal malunions, 111
    of Lisfranc injuries, **1–14**
        anatomy of, 2–4
            functional, 3–4
            ligamentous, 3
            osseous, 2–3
        classification of, 8
        diagnosis of, 5–8
        discussion on, 10–12
        imaging of, 5–8
            advanced, 7–8
            dynamic, 6–7
            initial, 5
        introduction to, 1–2
        key points of, 1
        mechanism of, 4–5
        nonoperative management vs., 9
        operative procedure for, 9
            vs. primary arthrodesis, 10
        physical examination of, 5–6
        summary of, 12–13
    of peripheral talus fractures, 181, 185, 191
    of syndesmosis injuries, with fibular fracture, 45
        with PER fractures, 54–55
    of tibial pilon fractures, with ankle arthrodesis, 157–158
        with primary arthrodesis, 149, 151, 154, 156–157
Osteomyelitis, with calcaneus fractures, 107
Osteophytes, in malreduced syndesmosis injuries, 69, 71
Osteotomies, for calcaneal malunions, 112
    for fibula malunions, 71

P

PA. See *Primary arthrodesis (PA)*.
Pain, post-calcaneus fracture treatment, ankle, 112
        heel pad, 112
    postoperative, with Chopart injuries, 173, 175
    post-traumatic foot injury, 118–119
    with peripheral talus fractures, 182
    with syndesmotic injuries, 66, 73
Passive pronation-abduction test, for Lisfranc injuries, 17
Patient positioning, for and after gastrocnemius lengthening, 120, 124
    for calcaneal malunions, 111
    for Chopart injuries surgery, 168
    for percutaneous reduction and fixation, of Lisfranc injuries, 24–25
    for peripheral talus fracture surgery, 186
    for sinus tarsi approach, to calcaneus fractures, 83–84
    for syndesmosis injury treatment, 68
    for tibial pilon fracture treatment, 154
PER. See *Pronation external rotation (PER) fractures*.

Percutaneous reduction and fixation, as temporary, of complex foot injury, 197–198
    of Lisfranc injuries, 5–6
  of calcaneal tuberosity avulsion fractures, 96
  of Lisfranc injuries, **15–34**
    anatomy in, 16–17
    as temporary, 5–6
    clinical findings in, 17
    incidence of, 16
    introduction to, 15–16
    key points of, 15
    other operative options vs., 23
    prevalence of, 16
    Puna and Tomlinson technique for, 23–31
      closed reduction, 24–26
      hardware removal, 28–31
      indications for, 23–24
      K-wire fixation, 26–29
      palpation and marking, 25–26
      patient positioning, 24–25
      screw fixation, 26–30
      stab incision, 26–27
      wound closure, 27–28
    radiologic findings in, 17–21
    summary of, 31
Peripheral neuropathy, tibial pilon fractures and, 149, 154–155
Peripheral talus fractures, **181–192**
  conservative treatment of, 181, 183–185
  introduction to, 181
  key points of, 181
  precise identification of, 184–185
  summary of, 191–192
  surgical treatment of, 185–191
    anterolateral approach to, 186, 188, 190
    anteromedial approach to, 190–191
    approaches to, 187–191
    equipment for, 186–187
    for combined injuries, 191
    literature review for, 181
    posteromedial approach to, 186–190
    postoperative care of, 191
    preoperative planning for, 186
    primary arthrodesis as, 186
    pros and cons of, 185–186
    sinus tarsi approach to, 183–185, 187–188
    talar head in, 190–191
  treatment of, conservative, 183–185
    indications for, 185–186
    optimal, as controversial, 181–183, 185–186
    surgical, 181, 184–191
Peroneal dislocation, with calcaneus fractures, 108–109
Peroneal retinaculum, superior, in hindfoot fracture-dislocations, 94

Peroneal stenosis, with calcaneus fractures, 107–108
Peroneal tenolysis, for calcaneal malunions, 111–112
Peroneal tenosynovectomy, for calcaneal malunions, 111
Peroneal tenosynovitis, with calcaneus fractures, 107–108
Photographs, of complex foot injury, 199
Physical examination, of Chopart injuries, 164–165
   of complex foot injury, 196
   of Lisfranc injuries, 5–6, 17
   of tibial pilon fractures, 149
Physical therapy, for Lisfranc injuries, 9
   postoperative, for Chopart injuries, 173, 175
      for peripheral talus fractures, 191
      for posterior malleolar fractures, 139
Pilon, tibial, fractures of, **147–161**. See also *Tibial pilon fractures.*
   in posterior malleolus biomechanics, 126–127
Pin fixation, of calcaneus fractures, 99–100
      with hindfoot fracture-dislocations, 94–95, 97
      with small incision technique, 85–86
   of Chopart injuries, 168
   of posterior malleolar fractures, 137
   of tibial pilon fractures, 156
Pin placement, with external frame fixation, for complex foot injury, 197–198
PITFL. See *Posterior inferior tibiofibular ligament (PITFL).*
Pituitary rongeur, 72
Plantar arch, ecchymosis of, 5, 165
Plantar ligaments, in Chopart joint, 164
      rupture of, 164–165
   in Lisfranc joint complex, 3, 17
Plantaris resection, in gastrocnemius lengthening, 121
Plantaris tendon recession, in gastrocnemius lengthening, 122–123
Plate fixation, of calcaneal fractures, 96–97
      with sinus tarsi approach, 99–100
   of Chopart injuries, 168, 171–172, 177
   of peripheral talus fractures, 184, 188, 190
   of posterior malleolar fractures, 137–138
   of tibial pilon fractures, 154, 156–157
Plating systems, for fibula malunions, 71–72
PMMA G/V antibiotic cement, for complex foot injury, 199–200
Posterior inferior tibiofibular ligament (PITFL), in ankle joint, 36–37, 66
   in syndesmosis injuries, posterior malleolus fixation and, 43
Posterior malleolus (PM), fixation of, syndesmosis zone and, 43–45
      tibial pilon fractures and, 149, 154, 156
Posterior malleolus (PM) fractures, **125–145**
   anatomy of, 126
   Bartonicek and Rammelt 3-D CT classification of, 129–134
      summary of, 129–131
      type 1: extraincisural fragment, 129, 131
      type 2: posterolateral fragment, 129, 132
      type 3: posteromedial, two-part fragment, 129–131, 133
      type 4: large, posterolateral triangular fragment, 131, 133
      type 5: irregular osteoporotic fracture, 131, 134

Posterior (*continued*)
    biomechanics of, 126–128
    classifications of, 128–134
        AO radiologic, 129
        Bartonicek and Rammelt 3-D CT, 129–134
        Haraguchi 2-D CT, 129
    complications of, 139–141
    evaluation of, 128
    introduction to, 125–126
    key points of, 125
    malalignment with, 139–141
    summary of, 141
    surgery for, 134–139
        approaches to, 135–139
        direct reduction and posterolateral fixation, 136–138
        direct reduction and posteromedial fixation, 137–139
        indications to, 134–135
        indirect reduction and anterior-to-posterior fixation, 135–136
        postoperative care of, 138–139
        results of, 141
        transfibular reduction according to Weber, 136
    vs. posterior pilon fractures, 134
Posterior tibial rim fragment, 126
Posterior tubercle, of distal tibia, in ankle biomechanics, 126–127
Posterolateral fixation, of posterior malleolar fractures, direct reduction and, 136–138
Posteromedial fixation, of peripheral talus fractures, 186–190
    of posterior malleolar fractures, direct reduction and, 137–139
Primary arthrodesis (PA), for Chopart injuries, 168, 173–174
        clinical results from literature, 177
    for Lisfranc injuries, **1–14**
        anatomy of, 2–4
            functional, 3–4
            ligamentous, 3
            osseous, 2–3
        classification of, 8
        diagnosis of, 5–8
        discussion on, 10–12
        imaging of, 5–8
            advanced, 7–8
            dynamic, 6–7
            initial, 5
        introduction to, 1–2
        key points of, 1
        mechanism of, 4–5
        nonoperative management vs., 9
        operative procedure for, 9–10
            vs. ORIF, 10
        physical examination of, 5–6
        summary of, 12–13
    for peripheral talus fractures, 186
    for tibial pilon fractures, **147–161**

ankle procedures in, 155, 157–158
    complications of, 148–149
    indications for, 151–155
        delayed definitive treatment as, 151, 153
        multiple medical comorbidities as, 149, 152
        nonreconstructibility as, 151–152
        patient factors as, 152, 154–155
        peripheral neuropathy as, 149, 154–155
    limitations of, 159
    postoperative care for, 148, 157
    proposal of, 148–149
    results of, 148, 157–159
    staged, 154, 159
    surgical technique for, 154–157
        initial treatment, 154–156
        with ORIF, 149, 151, 154, 156–157
Pronation external rotation (PER) fractures, syndesmosis injuries and, 37–38, 40
    high fibula, 42, 55–58
    ORIF for, 54–55
    with fibula fracture, and deltoid ligament injury, 55
    with medial malleolus, 43
    with medial malleolus and Tillaux fracture, 53–54
Puna and Tomlinson technique, for Lisfranc injury management, 23–31. See also
    Percutaneous reduction and fixation.

Q

Quality of life, with severe foot ankle trauma, 194
Quenu and Kuss classification, of Lisfranc injuries, 20

R

Radiography, dynamic. See *Stress radiography.*
    of Chopart injuries, 165–166
    of complex foot injury, 196
    of Lisfranc injuries, for open managment, 5
        for percutaneous management, 17–20
    of malreduced syndesmosis injuries, 66, 68–70
    of midfoot, 3-column classification for, 3–4
    of peripheral talus fractures, 182, 184–185, 187, 189–191
    of posterior malleolar fractures, 128
        AO classification based on, 129
    of posttraumatic arthritis, with calcaneus fractures, 109–110
    of tibial pilon fractures, 148–151, 153, 155, 159
    of traumatic foot injuries, 118–119
    post-sinus tarsi approach, to calcaneus fracture fixation, 88
Rammelt classification. See *Bartonicek and Rammelt classification.*
Range of motion, with Chopart injuries, 168, 173
    with malreduced syndesmosis injuries, 68
    with peripheral talus fractures, 185, 191
Reconstructive surgery, for calcaneal malunion, 79–80

Reconstructive (*continued*)
    for complex foot injury, 194
        as definite treatment, 204
        indications for, 200–201
        initial consideration of, 200
        predictive scores for, 202
    for peripheral talus fractures, 185
    for syndesmosis malunion, 73–74
    for tibial pilon fractures, 151, 157, 159
Reduction, of calcaneal tuberosity avulsion fractures, closed vs. open, 95–96
    of calcaneus fracture, with sinus tarsi approach to fixation, 86–88, 99–100
    of Chopart injuries, closed, 164, 177
        open, 167
    of fibula, with tibial pilon fractures, 155–156
    of Lisfranc injuries, closed, 23–26
        open, **1–14**. See also *Open reduction and internal fixation (ORIF)*.
        percutaneous, **15–34**. See also *Percutaneous reduction and fixation*.
    of peripheral talus fractures, open, 185
        provisional, 188, 190
    of posterior malleolar fractures, direct, and posterolateral fixation, 136–138
        and posteromedial fixation, 137–139
        indirect, and anterior-to-posterior fixation, 135–136
        transfibular, according to Weber, 136
    of syndesmosis injuries, open, 44–45
    of tibial pilon fractures, 149, 151
Rehabilitation, postoperative, for Chopart injuries, 173, 175
        for Lisfranc injuries, 9
        for peripheral talus fractures, 191
        for posterior malleolar fractures, 139
Resuscitation protocol, for complex foot injury, 196
Roman arch, in Lisfranc joint complex, 2, 16
Rotation deformities, with fibula malunions, 71
Rotation fractures. See *External rotation fractures*.
Rotational force, in Chopart injuries, 164–165

    S

Salvage procedures, for Chopart injuries, 177
    for complex foot injury, as definite treatment, 204
        indications for, 200–201
        initial consideration of, 200
        predictive scores for, 202
    for syndesmosis malunion, 73–74, 79–80
Sanders and Stephens classification, of calcaneal malunions, 79, 110–111
Sanders IIC fractures, hindfoot fracture-dislocations and, 94
Schanz pin, for calcaneus fracture fixation, in sinus tarsi approach, 99–100
        with hindfoot fracture-dislocations, 94–95, 97
        with small incision technique, 85–86
Screw fixation, of calcaneal fractures, with extensile lateral approach, 81
        with sinus tarsi approach, 88, 99–100
    of calcaneal malunions, 112

of calcaneal tuberosity avulsion fractures, 96–97
of Chopart injuries, 168–169, 172
of Lisfranc injuries, discussion on, 10–12
   techniques for, with open reduction, 9–10
      with percutaneous reduction, 26–31
of peripheral talus fractures, 184, 187–188, 190
of posterior malleolar fractures, 136–138
of syndesmosis injuries, 42–44
   problems with, 45
   vs. no fixation, 45–46
   with fibula malunions, 71–73
of tibial pilon fractures, 154, 156–157
SER. See *Supination external rotation (SER) fractures.*
Sinus tarsi approach, to calcaneus fractures, advantages of, 81, 83, 89, 94
   as minimally invasive, 98–99
   extensile lateral approach vs., 88–89
   for open fractures, 101
   surgical fixation technique with, 83–88
      fluoroscopy for, 85–88
      patient positioning for, 83–84
      skin markings for, 84–85
   with hindfoot fracture-dislocations, 94–95
   wound complications with, 106
  to peripheral talus fractures, 183–185, 187–188
Skin grafts, for complex foot injury, 200, 204
Skin markings, for gastrocnemius lengthening, 120
  for percutaneous reduction and fixation, of Lisfranc injuries, 25–26
  for sinus tarsi approach, to calcaneus fracture fixation, 84–85
Small incision technique, for calcaneus fractures, 81, 83, 94. See also *Sinus tarsi approach.*
Sofield retractors, for gastrocnemius lengthening, 120
Soft tissue, calcaneal fractures impact on, 81, 94, 101–102, 105
  calcaneal tuberosity avulsion fractures impact on, 95–98
  in Chopart injuries, 164, 167, 173, 177
  in complex foot injuries, 194
    classification of, 194–195
    treatment decisions related to, 200–204
  in Lisfranc injuries, 4–5, 16, 24
  necrosis of. See *Necrosis.*
  tibial pilon fractures impact on, 149, 151–153
Soft tissue flap, in extensile lateral approach, to calcaneus fractures, 80
  in tibial pilon fracture treatment, 156–157
Soleus, in gastrocnemius lengthening, 120–121
Splints/splinting. See *Immobilization.*
Splitting, for calcaneal tuberosity avulsion fractures, 95
SPR. See *Superior peroneal retinaculum (SPR) injury.*
Sprains, of midfoot, 167. See also *Chopart injuries.*
Spur sign, of posterior malleolar fractures, 128. See also *Bartonicek and Rammelt classification.*
Stability. See *Ankle stability.*
Stabilization, of syndesmosis injuries, **35–63**. See also *Syndesmosis injuries.*
  flexible, 45–49. See also *Flexible stabilization.*

Stenosis, peroneal, with calcaneus fractures, 107–108
Stephens and Sanders classification, of calcaneal malunions, 79, 110–111
Stress mechanism, of Chopart injuries, 164–165
Stress radiography, of Lisfranc injuries, for open management, 6–7
    for percutaneous management, 18–20
  of malreduced syndesmosis injuries, 66, 69–70
Subtalar arthrodesis, bone-block, for calcaneal malunions, 111–112
    as salvage technique, 79–80
Subtalar joint, in Chopart injuries, 164, 168
  in peripheral talus fractures, 182, 184–187, 190
Superior peroneal retinaculum (SPR) injury, with calcaneus fractures, 108–109
  with hindfoot fracture-dislocations, 94
Supination external rotation (SER) fractures, syndesmosis injuries and, 37–38, 40
    force type 4 with posterior malleolus fracture: ORIF, 52–53
    medial side fixation, 42–43
    type 2: stable, non-operative, 51–52
Sural nerve, Chopart injuries and, 171, 173
  in extensile lateral approach, to calcaneus fractures, 80–81
  in gastrocnemius lengthening, 122
  posterior malleolar fractures and, 136
  tibial pilon fractures and, 154
Suture anchors, for calcaneal tuberosity avulsion fractures, 96
Suture fixation, of calcaneal tuberosity avulsion fractures, 96, 98
Syndesmosis, tibiofibular, in posterior ankle biomechanics, 126–128
    instability with posterior malleolar fractures, 134–135
Syndesmosis injuries, **35–63**
  anatomy of, 36–37, 65, 74
  instability and, degrees of, 39–40
    missed injuries and, 40–41
    pathomechanics of, 37–39
      pronation external rotation fractures and, 37–38, 40
      purely ligamentous injuries and, 38–39
      supination external rotation fractures and, 37–38, 40
    surgical strategy for, 41–58
  introduction to, 35–36
  key points of, 35
  late treatment of, **65–75**
    ankle joint in, 71
    arthrodesis in, 73–74
    débridement in, 69–72
    dissection in, 69–70
    fibula malunions and, 71–72
    imaging evaluation of, 66, 68–70
    key points of, 65
    patient positioning for, 68
    reconstruction in, 73
  malreduction of, 66–67
    surgical treatment of, 66, 68–74
  mechanisms of, 37–39
    fracture patterns and, 40
    ligaments only, 40

zones and, 39–40
stability of, biomechanics and, 36–37, 66
   surgical strategies for, 41–58
stabilization case studies of, 49–58
   anterior inferior tibiofibular ligament and deltoid: stabilization, 50–51
   anterior inferior tibiofibular ligament nonoperative treatment, 49–50
   pronation external rotation, fibula fracture, and deltoid ligament injury, 55
   pronation external rotation, high fibula, 42, 55–58
   pronation external rotation injury: ORIF, 54–55
   pronation external rotation injury with medial malleolus and Tillaux fracture, 53–54
   supinated foot subjected to external rotation force type 4 with posterior malleolus
      fracture: ORIF, 52–53
   supination-external rotation type 2: stable, non-operative, 51–52
stabilization surgery for, 41–58
   examples of, 49–58
   fibula and medial zone fixation, 42–43
   judicious use of hardware, 41–42
   late, **65–75**
   primary goal of, 41
   syndesmosis flexible stabilization, 45–49. See also *Flexible stabilization.*
   syndesmosis zone fixation, 43–45
summary of, 58

T

Talar body fractures, peripheral talus fractures and, 186–187, 189, 191
Talar head fractures, in Chopart injuries, 164
   internal fixation of, 168–169
  peripheral talus fractures and, 190–191
Talar neck fractures, peripheral talus fractures and, 186, 188, 191
Talometatarsal angle, in Lisfranc injuries, 19
Talonavicular joint, in Chopart joint, 164, 166
   follow-up care for, 173, 176
   primary fusion of, 168, 173–174
   surgical fixation of. See *specific anatomical component.*
Talus fractures, **181–192**. See also *Peripheral talus fractures.*
Tarsals, in Lisfranc joint complex, 2, 16
Tarsometatarsal joint complex. See also *Lisfranc joint complex.*
  injuries of. See also *Lisfranc injuries.*
   classification of, 8, 21–22
Tarsometatarsals (TMTs), in Lisfranc joint complex, 2–4, 16
   open injury management and, 9–12
   percutaneous injury management and, 19–20, 24–29
  reproducible pain in, 5–6
Temporary joint transfixation, of Chopart injuries, 167, 173–174, 177
  of complex foot injury, 197–198
  of Lisfranc injuries, 5–6
Tenolysis, peroneal, for calcaneal malunions, 111–112
Tenosynovectomy, peroneal, for calcaneal malunions, 111
Tenosynovitis, peroneal, with calcaneus fractures, 107–108
3-Column classification, in Chopart joint, 164

3-Column (*continued*)
  of midfoot, 3–4
3-D computed tomography, intraoperative, of Lisfranc injuries, 20
  of posterior malleolar fractures, classification based on, 129–134. See also *Bartonicek and Rammelt classification.*
Tibia, distal, high-energy injuries of, 147, 149, 151, 159, 194
    in posterior malleolus biomechanics, 126–128
  in syndesmosis, 36–37, 65
    fracture pathomechanics of, 37–39
      degrees of instability, 39–40
Tibial pilon, in posterior malleolus biomechanics, 126–127
Tibial pilon fractures, **147–161**
  ankle arthrodesis for, with external fixation, 157–158
    with intramedullary nailing, 152, 154–155, 157, 159
  complications of, 148–149
  evaluation and workup of, 149–151
  external fixation for, 149, 153
    with ankle arthrodesis, 154, 157–158
  introduction to, 147–149
  key points of, 147
  mechanism of injury, 149
  posterior, posterior malleolar fractures vs., 134
  primary arthrodesis for, ankle procedures in, 155, 157–158
    indications for, 151–155
      delayed definitive treatment as, 151, 153
      multiple medical comorbidities as, 149, 152
      nonreconstructibility as, 151–152
      patient factors as, 152, 154–155
      peripheral neuropathy as, 149, 154–155
    limitations of, 159
    postoperative care of, 148, 157
    proposal of, 148–149
    results of, 148, 157–159
    staged, 154, 159
    surgical technique for, 154–157
      initial treatment, 154–156
      with ORIF, 149, 151, 154, 156–157
  summary of, 159
Tibial plafond, posterior malleolar fractures and, 137
Tibial rim fragment, posterior, 126
Tibiofibular ligaments, in posterior ankle biomechanics, 126–128
  interosseous. See *Interosseous tibiofibular ligament (IOL).*
Tibiofibular syndesmosis, in posterior ankle, 126–128
  instability with posterior malleolar fractures, 134–135
Tibiotalocalcaneal (TTC) arthrodesis, for tibial pilon fractures, 151, 154–155
TightRope device, for syndesmosis stabilization, 45–49
    as flexible system, 46
    clinical cohort studies of, 47
    complications of, 48
    cost analysis of, 49
    critical analysis of literature, 48–49

description of, 46

future research on, 48–49

hybrid technique for, 46–47

laboratory studies for, 46

ORIF and, 45

randomized controlled trials of, 48

reoperation rates for, 48

screw fixation vs., 45

systematic review of, 47–48

vs. no treatment, 45–46

Tillaux fractures, syndesmosis injuries and, 37

open reduction of, 44

PER fractures with, medial malleolus and, 53–54

syndesmosis zone fixation and, 43–45

TMTs. See *Tarsometatarsals (TMTs)*.

Tomlinson technique. See *Puna and Tomlinson technique*.

Tongue-type calcaneus fractures, small incision technique for, 81, 83, 94

extensile lateral approach vs., 88

Transfibular reduction, of posterior malleolar fractures, according to Weber, 136

Transfixation, joint. See *Temporary joint transfixation*.

Transverse intermetatarsal ligaments, in Lisfranc joint complex, 3, 17

Trauma screening, for complex foot injury, 196

Traumatic foot injuries. See also *specific anatomy or injury*.

Chopart injuries and, **163–180**. See also *Chopart injuries*.

complex, **193–213**. See also *Complex foot injury*.

gastrocnemius equinus associated with, 117–118

gastrocnemius lengthening, at trauma fixation time, **117–124**. See also *Gastrocnemius lengthening*.

long-term sequelae of, 118–119, 194. See also *Arthritis*.

resuscitation protocol for, 196

Triple joint complex, in Chopart injuries, 164, 168, 177

Tscherne–Oestern classification, of closed fractures, 194

TTC (tibiotalocalcaneal) arthrodesis, for tibial pilon fractures, 151, 154–155

Tuberosity avulsion fractures, calcaneal, early fixation of, 94–98

2-D computed tomography, of posterior malleolar fractures, classification based on, 129

V

V identification, in gastrocnemius lengthening, 120–121

Vacuum-assisted closure (VAC), of complex foot injury, 198, 200, 204

post-ORIF, of calcaneus fractures, 101–102, 107

Varus alignment, following nonoperative management of calcaneus fracture, 79

Vascular perspectives, in gastrocnemius lengthening, 120–121

W

Wagstaff fractures, syndesmosis injuries and, 37

late treatment of, 65

syndesmosis zone fixation and, 43–45

Weber B fractures, of fibula, syndesmosis injuries and, 37, 40

posterior malleolar fractures and, 128, 135

Weber (*continued*)
    surgery approaches based on, 136
Weber C fractures, of fibula, syndesmosis injuries and, 37–38, 40, 42
    posterior malleolar fractures and, 128, 135
    surgery approaches based on, 136
Weight-bearing radiography. See *Stress radiography.*
West Point Grading system, for purely ligamentous injuries, of syndesmosis, 39
Wire fixation, K-wire. See *Kirschner wire (K-wire) fixation.*
    percutaneous, as temporary, of complex foot injury, 197–198
        of Lisfranc injuries, 5–6
        of Lisfranc injuries, as permanent. See *Percutaneous reduction and fixation.*
        as temporary, 5–6
Wound closure, in calcaneal malunions, 112
    in complex foot injury, 200, 204
    in gastrocnemius lengthening, 122–124
    in percutaneous reduction and fixation, of Lisfranc injuries, 27–28
    in sinus tarsi approach, to calcaneus fracture fixation, 88
    in tibial pilon fracture treatment, 157
Wound complications, of calcaneus fractures, 105–107
        delayed healing as, 106–107
        extensile lateral approach and, 80–81, 105–106
        osteomyelitis as, 107
        sinus tarsi approach and, 81, 106
Wrinkle sign, of tibial pilon fractures, 151, 156

Z

Zone fixation, of syndesmosis injuries, 43–45
        medial, 42–43
Zwipp classification, of Chopart injuries, 166–167
    of complex foot and ankle injuries, 195

Moving?

Make sure your subscription moves with you!

To notify us of your new address, find your **Clinics Account Number** (located on your mailing label above your name), and contact customer service at:

Email: journalscustomerservice-usa@elsevier.com

800-654-2452 (subscribers in the U.S. & Canada)
314-447-8871 (subscribers outside of the U.S. & Canada)

Fax number: 314-447-8029

Elsevier Health Sciences Division
Subscription Customer Service
3251 Riverport Lane
Maryland Heights, MO 63043

*To ensure uninterrupted delivery of your subscription, please notify us at least 4 weeks in advance of move.

Printed and bound by CPI Group (UK) Ltd, Croydon, CR0 4YY

08/05/2025

01864699-0003